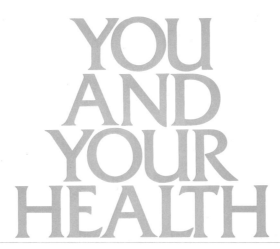

YOU AND YOUR HEALTH

WILLIAM FASSBENDER
TRENTON STATE COLLEGE

JOHN WILEY & SONS

NEW YORK   SANTA BARBARA   LONDON   SYDNEY   TORONTO

PREPARED IN COOPERATION WITH EDUCATIONAL BOOKCRAFTERS, INC.

THIS BOOK WAS SET IN OPTIMA BY GRAPHIC ARTS
COMPOSITION, INC.

IT WAS PRINTED BY MURRAY PRINTING
COMPANY AND BOUND BY BOOK PRESS.

COVER AND TEXT DESIGN BY SUZANNE G. BENNETT

PICTURE EDITING BY MAJORIE GRAHAM

PRODUCTION SUPERVISED BY THERESA A. HARMSEN.

Library of Congress Cataloging in Publication Data:

FASSBENDER, WILLIAM V
YOU AND YOUR HEALTH.

INCLUDES BIBLIOGRAPHIES, FILMOGRAPHIES, DISCOGRAPHIES,
AND INDEX.
1. HYGIENE. I. TITLE.
RA776.F24   613   76-28402
ISBN 0-471-60503-4

PRINTED IN THE UNITED STATES OF AMERICA

10 9 8 7 6 5 4 3 2 1

TO MY ENTIRE FAMILY FOR THEIR MANY YEARS OF LOVE AND ENCOURAGEMENT,
BUT ESPECIALLY TO JACKIE.

PREFACE

You and Your Health was written from the beginning with today's student in mind. The author and publisher agreed, in the planning stages, that a unique health textbook was needed to meet the requirements of a more informed student population. Most students have studied some form of health science since elementary school. In addition, many schools teach courses in sex and drug education. Therefore, it was our conclusion that a health science textbook must be relevant to today's more informed student.

You can get an idea of what this book is about by skimming through the table of contents. In addition, you can get a preview of each chapter by reading the chapter introduction and the list of major concepts that follows. You will find the introductions and concepts lists to be useful aids to the teaching-learning process.

When skimming the contents, you will find chapter titles that are familiar to you. How then, you might ask, is this book different? *You and Your Health* emphasizes what is happening now in health and how it relates to you and to society. Current topics have been discussed and information has been taken from contemporary research and literature. Many of the books referred to in this textbook are recent best-sellers or are classics in their field. In addition, you will find anecdotes throughout the book that relate to contemporary life.

This book has a "real world" approach which takes major social issues into consideration throughout the topic discussions. Controversial issues are neither glossed over nor avoided. When a controversial issue is presented, the author has attempted to give all meaningful viewpoints. You are encouraged to reach a conclusion based on what is read and discussed both in and out of class. A second emphasis of *You and Your Health,* therefore, is that the informed individual will make informed decisions, based on facts not feelings.

This brings us to the third emphasis of this textbook: *valuing.* This is a term that has appeared in recent educational jargon. It simply means the ability to recognize the positive and negative aspects of a situation and to "value" or place these points in their proper perspective so that you can best cope with the situation. *You and Your Health* has stressed valuing through a questioning technique used frequently throughout the text.

Many paragraphs contain open-ended questions based on the topic discussed. You are encouraged to "value" or use your own judgment in answering these questions. These questions are thought exercises and do not require a written response. Of course, there is no right or wrong answer. The "right" answer will be your own thoughts on a particular subject based on the factual information presented and any additional information that you may have.

To help you assimilate the terms presented, each chapter contains a glossary of key words that is readily accessible at the end of the chapter. Each chapter also includes sections entitled Thinking It Over and Getting Involved. The Thinking It Over section poses thought-provoking questions that will guide you in your review of the chapter and also assist in the "valuing" process. In the Getting Involved section, books and movies, both contemporary and classic, are listed and annotated.

This section provides opportunities for further involvement in the teaching-learning process.

It is important to remember that health information is constantly changing. It is impossible for any book to keep up with daily changes in the field. We hope that you will supplement text information with relevant articles and books. This information will expose you to current trends involving health issues.

We strongly feel that you will find *You and Your Health* a unique book that provides both stimulating and entertaining reading. We hope that you will get involved in the learning process and carry over your new knowledge of health matters into your daily life.

William Fassbender

ACKNOWLEDGMENTS

The last two years have been both professionally rewarding and intellectually stimulating for me. I have learned that the writing of a health textbook is not a task to be taken lightly. The variety and depth of the body of knowledge known as health science sometimes seems overwhelming. The planning and research that was conducted in order to make *You and Your Health* an up-to-date and relevant textbook reflects the collective wisdom and cooperation of many dedicated professionals.

I was fortunate to work with Mr. Harold Miller, President of Educational Book Crafters, throughout the entire project. I deeply appreciate his faith in me, as well as his unique administrative and technical skills. His cheerful and thoughtful personality was always appreciated. To the staff that Harold assembled for this project I am deeply indebted. Many thanks go to Ms. Fran Kaplan for her research efforts, and to the genius of Ms. Myra Madnick, I am forever grateful.

As the manuscript developed and was reviewed, the opinions of those who continually teach health science were both humbling and challenging. I'm grateful to Thomas Storer (El Camino College), Harold Hauben (Southern Connecticut State College), Charles Kegley (Kent State University), Murray Vincent (University of South Carolina), and Wayne Oberparleiter (Kingsborough Community College) who separately and collectively helped shape the final form and content of this text.

I have received a great deal of assistance and advice from professional associates and friends. My thanks go to Dr. Jonathan Levine and Dr. Franklyn Greenberg from Hunter College. I am deeply indebted to Mr. Joseph Herzstein from Trenton State College, my colleague and friend, for his advice and critical reviews. A great deal of thanks to my aunt, Dr. J. C. Vanlooy, recently retired from Glassboro State College, not only for her help and assistance in preparing this book, but, more importantly, for her many years of encouragement and support. Thanks also are extended to Mrs. Judy Simon and Mrs. Marie Hendricks for their assistance.

Many other people lent their support, and there are numerous friends and teachers to whom I am deeply indebted. There is one person to whom I am especially grateful for he introduced me to the profession, had faith in me, and has always been a source of encouragement. To my friend, Dr. Gere Fulton, I say thanks.

Of course, I must also acknowledge Jackie, Barbara, and Elizabeth for their many years of patience, perseverance, and love.

W.V.F.

INTRODUCTION

Why should you study health science? One very important reason is that it can increase levels of "wellness" or health. This occurs when health education helps you to better understand yourself emotionally and physically. Health information helps you to recognize symptoms and to be aware of methods of coping with apparent symptoms. In this way, health science is a form of preventive medicine. Many conditions can be prevented if you have a good understanding of basic health concepts.

A recent newspaper article reported that a thirteen-year-old girl had saved her father's life through cardiac resuscitation. She had learned the method that same day in her health class. This story suggests another reason why health is studied. Health knowledge has many practical applications in our everyday life. Health is an *applied science*. You may apply health knowledge in many different ways each day.

Another reason for studying health science is to present the most accurate and up-to-date information that will enable you to make decisions regarding health that are best for you and your environment.

You are faced with health decisions each day. Whether to smoke, go on a diet, buy a health-related product, or visit a doctor are all health decisions. In order to make the best decision, you must have *accurate* information. Can you think of any other reasons why you should study health science?

"health": what does it mean?

Although the word *health* is certainly not new to you, have you ever thought about its meaning? If you were to ask five different people what health means to them, you would most likely get five different answers.

Health is much more than the "absence of disease." Being "sick," as we know it, is only one aspect of health. A state of health or "wellness" is a forceful quality of life.

No sharp lines can be drawn between being healthy and unhealthy.

Your health can be viewed as a straight line. No separate parts can be recognized. How you feel, look, and behave are all part of this line. Your total health is equally dependent on how you feel emotionally and physically. This can best be indicated by the following straight-line diagram.

Your state of health is complex. People cannot look at you and determine that you are healthy simply because there are no obvious signs of disease or distress. There are many factors to consider that not only include the physical, but the mental, emotional, and social as well.

All three aspects are interrelated and each aspect affects all of the others. If you are physically ill,

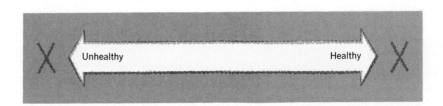

then, in many cases, your mood and behavior are also affected. The opposite is also true. A depressed mood can cause physical symptoms. This interrelationship is expressed in the diagram at the right.

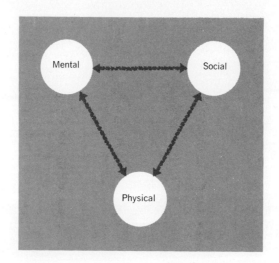

Health behavior is complex. It is based on attitudes and knowledge. For example, you may know that cigarette smoking is hazardous to your health, but you may continue to smoke in spite of this knowledge. The same people who smoke may not want their children to smoke and yet they cannot control their own smoking habit. The following is a diagram of the relationship between attitude, knowledge, and behavior.

Health education provides you with an understanding of this relationship. It is not enough to warn people of the hazards of smoking. They must also be made aware of why they smoke and that they probably share a common attitude of "nothing can happen to me." Many people think that they are the only ones who may feel a certain way. Health education helps us to appreciate behavior that is shared by many people.

Very often, behavior patterns can be changed. Your knowledge and attitudes may serve to deter or reinforce the existing behavior. Health education provides the knowledge that will, we hope, affect attitudes and lead to positive changes in behavior.

As you can see from this introduction, health science exerts an important influence on many aspects of your life. I sincerely hope that you will not only learn from this book but will also find it enjoyable, exciting, and entertaining.

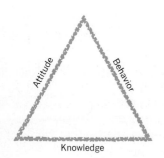

CONTENTS

PART I
CONFLICT, JOY, AND THE GOOD LIFE

1
YOUR UNIQUE PERSONALITY

In order to better understand "why you are like you are," the influences of heredity and environment on your personality are explored in this chapter. The impact that learning processes, your family and friends, and various psychological theories has on your unique personality is discussed. Once you have an understanding of "why you are like you are," then the question "do you like yourself" is explored. In this part of the chapter you learn about who you are and how you can feel better about yourself. The "now I can like you," section of the chapter expresses a few popular views on how you can learn to relate better to other people.

While reading this chapter think about the following concepts:

■ No two people react in the same way in a given situation.

■ Your physical environment, as well as your family and friends, have a unique influence on your personality.

■ People can be conditioned to think and act in a particular way.

■ The way you feel about yourself can affect your behavior.

■ Friends of your own age contribute to your personality development.

■ Honesty is essential to healthy interpersonal relationships.

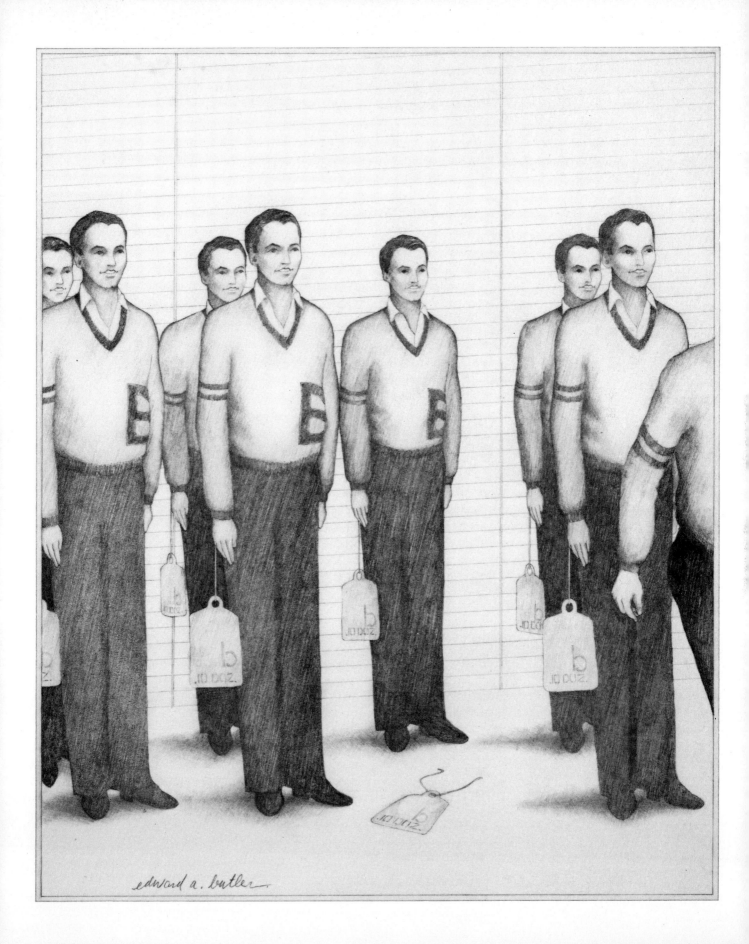

edward a. butler

4

why are you like you are?

Three girls were watching a television program when it was suddenly interrupted by a news bulletin. The bulletin spoke of tornado warnings for that section of the country. One of the girls became frightened and tears came to her eyes. Another girl began to speak rapidly and appeared to be nervous, while the third girl calmly turned off the television and guided her friends to the safety of the basement.

Why did these girls react so differently? Perhaps the frightened girl had been injured in a tornado when she was a small child. The girl who seemed to be at loose ends probably reacts in a similar manner to any crisis or "would-be" crisis situation. The girl who took charge of the others and remained calm probably has a mature attitude and leadership qualities.

The way you react in a given situation is directly related to your personality. What makes you act one way and your friend, sister, or brother act in an entirely different way is your unique personality. You may wonder how your personality came to be so unique. There are many factors involved in the development of personality. These factors and the role they play in making you the person you are today are considered in this chapter.

personality and heredity

You are different from other people the moment you are born. Newborn babies in a hospital nursery show different personality traits while only a few hours old. Some may cry continuously while others seem to be very placid most of the time. Any mother of a young baby will tell you that her new baby is very different from her other children and other babies she knows.

The inherited traits that make you both look and act differently from other individuals are passed on to you from your parents. This "passing on" of traits is your heredity and certain traits help to form your basic personality

and physical characteristics. However, both personality and physical characteristics may be affected positively or negatively by your environment. For example, although your physical structure may be small and slender, overeating may soon change your appearance. The influence of environment on your personality is discussed later in this chapter.

YOUR BODY TYPE

Body type is an inherited characteristic that can be determined by measuring the body's muscle bulk and testing for fatty tissue deposits beneath the skin. Body types are usually classified according to the system that Dr. William H. Sheldon, a noted physician, introduced many years ago. Sheldon referred to his method of classifying body builds as somatotyping. His classification system included three body types or builds: ectomorph, endomorph, and mesomorph.

The ectomorph, according to Sheldon and other researchers, has a long, lean, fragile-looking body and a greater sensory development than the other body types. The endomorph is described as short and stocky, having a round, soft appearance. This type usually has short, tapered arms and legs and a prominent abdomen. Endomorphs tend to gain weight easily and are not very muscular. The mesomorph is very muscular and is frequently described as having a strong, athletic body. Mesomorphs tend to have great strength and massive muscular development. They usually have broad shoulders, narrow hips, and prominent muscles. When they gain weight, they tend to develop muscular size rather than an increase in fatty tissue deposits. Do you have the traits of any of these body types? Do you think you might like to have a different body type? If so, which body type would you choose?

Body build is something you inherit and it cannot be changed. However, you can learn to accept your build and change your outward appearance if that is what you

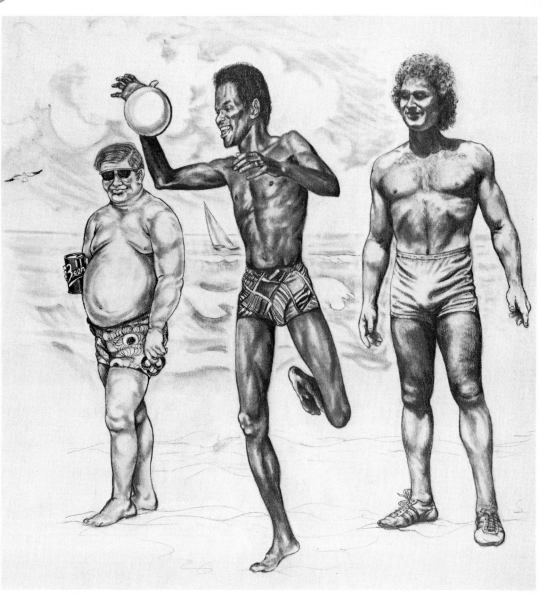

Three body types: Endomorph, ectomorph, and mesomorph.

would like to do. For example, if you have the build of an endomorph and are unhappy with the way you look, strict dieting and proper exercise can help to alter your physical appearance. In addition, style and color of dress, hair style, and even your attitude can alter the way you look.

You may be wondering what body build has to do with personality. Research has found that certain personality types are associated with particular body builds. In addition, the way you feel about your body build has a

very important effect on personality development. This is discussed later in this chapter.

A study (conducted in 1971 at Case Western Reserve Medical School, Cleveland, Ohio) explored the relationship between body build and heart attacks. This study provided some interesting information regarding body type and personality. Several hundred patients who had suffered heart attacks were studied from the time they entered a rehabilitation center until their death. Each patient was psychologically tested, evaluated, and classified according to Sheldon's body types.

It was found that generally the short-term survivors were more uncertain about their illness and were less able to accept the fact that a limitation had been placed upon their physical freedom. The body type of these individuals was predominantly mesomorph, the more muscular body type. Endomorphs proved to be more relaxed, even-tempered, and easygoing. They lived many more years following heart attacks than did those individuals who had been classified as mesomorphs. Endomorphs tended to accept their condition more easily and did not complain of the long periods of bed rest and lack of physical exercise. The ectomorph was also found to tolerate the effects of a heart attack better than the mesomorph.

This study and others like it seem to indicate that endomorphs have a more easygoing personality while mesomorphs tend to have an aggressive and restless personality. Ectomorphs seem to be somewhere in the middle of the other two. It is important to stress here that very few people will fit perfectly into a body type category and have the exact personality traits of the body type. A person's body type may be generally designated but he may have characteristics of other body types in both his physical and personality makeup.

personality and the environment

Your environment and all of your life experiences have had an important effect on your personality. Parents, brothers and sisters, friends, teachers, and all of the people you come into contact with affect your personality.

Personality development starts from the moment you are born; even the way you were cared for as an infant has helped to form your present personality. For example, many studies have shown that infants who are deprived of loving care over long periods of time will withdraw from their environment and show few of the normal human responses that are typical of a baby of that age.

Personality development is very closely related to the way we learn. Learning in this sense is not only the formal learning associated with school and books, but also the learning of behavior. A four-year-old might have a temper tantrum if his balloon breaks, but a 14-year-old is not apt to scream, kick, and cry if he doesn't make the basketball team. What accounts for this difference in behavior? By learning what behavior is appropriate and acceptable at different stages, behavior patterns change and so does the personality. In the next section, learning theory (the way people learn) is explored in some detail.

HOW BEHAVIOR IS LEARNED

Learning in the psychological sense may be defined as a change in behavior that results from doing something over and over again or because of an enviromental influence. Learning in this sense does not include learning that results only from physical growth or body maturation. For example, a child does not have to be taught how to chew; this ability comes about naturally at a certain stage of physical development.

Learning is made possible by three major functions of the brain: perception, association, and memory. Perception allows us to receive sensory stimuli (agents that promote responses) such as odors and visual images and to form impressions about these and other stimuli. Association allows us to draw from our past experiences and relate these experiences to present happenings. Our memory helps us to remember what has already happened and what we have learned in the past. Can you think of an example of association and memory that has recently helped you to learn something?

CONDITIONING

Conditioning is one way that people learn to behave in a certain manner. It can best be explained by reviewing Ivan Pavlov's classic experiment in this area. Pavlov, a well-known Russian physiologist (one who

7

Ivan Petrovich Pavlov (1849–1936), a Russian physiologist, is noted for his conditioning experiments with dogs. While studying the digestive glands of dogs he noticed that the dogs he was experimenting on started salivating before they actually began to eat. The dogs were responding to a signal, or stimulus, that they had learned to associate with food. Pavlov concluded that human beings as well as animals could be taught, or conditioned, to give a response to an artificial stimulus. His studies into the nature of conditioning form the basis of *behavioral psychology and modern learning theory.*

studies body function) conducted a series of experiments that involved dogs and their release of saliva when a weak acid was placed in their mouths. Pavlov's dogs were enclosed in a cage-like apparatus. Weak acid was placed in the dog's mouth causing the dog to salivate. At the same time, a turning fork was struck giving off a very loud noise. The acid served as the *stimulus* that caused the dog to salivate. At first, the loud noise was incidental to the salivation. However, as the experiment was repeated numerous times, the noise came to have an important effect on the dogs. The dogs began to associate the loud noise with the weak acid and after a while the loud noise *alone* was sufficient to make the dogs salivate. In other words, the dogs had learned a type of behavior through conditioning (a response to an artificial stimulus that has replaced the original or natural stimulus). In Pavlov's experiments, the artificial stimulus (the loud noise) had replaced the natural stimulus (the acid).

This type of conditioning, or conditioned response as it is sometimes called, has probably happened to you. Think of a food that you really enjoy eating (a delicious pizza pie)! Close your eyes and picture it in your mind. Are you beginning to salivate? Sometimes, by thinking of a food you can recall the pleasant associations of eating that food and salivation will begin.

OPERANT CONDITIONING

Operant learning or conditioning (response to a given situation in order to receive a reward) is a more advanced form of learning than conditioning. In operant learning, an animal has to solve a problem in order to receive food or another type of reward. Rats are often used in these types of experiments. If a rat is able to find his way through a maze, he will be rewarded with food or water. This type of learned behavior is called operant conditioning because the rat has worked with the environment (the maze) in order to receive the reward (food or water).

People, especially young children, often exhibit operant conditioning. The child who is rewarded following a certain action will repeat the action to receive the reward. Children learn very early in life that certain actions are positively rewarded while others are negatively received. Rewards do not always have to be in the form of food or a tangible item. Clapping hands, hugging, and happy noises are often reward enough for a young child to modify his behavior through operant learning.

PROGRAMMED LEARNING

Many of you may be very familiar with programmed learning or learning through the use of a teaching machine or similar apparatus. The teaching machine works on the same principle as operant conditioning. The subject manipulates his or her environment (in this case the teaching machine) in order to receive a reward (the correct answer). Teaching machines are programmed or written in small units. The student reads each item (called a frame) and writes down his answer. The correct answer is shown immediately so the student does not have to wait for the reward. The reward in this case is called reinforcement because it reinforces the satisfaction of having arrived at the correct answer. Programs are written for workbooks as well as machines and they provide an excellent method of allowing students to learn at their own speed. In addition, the student can immediately see his errors and correct them as he goes. Programmed learning is just one method of learning that must be accompanied by teacher–student interaction and other learning techniques.

SOCIAL LEARNING

Social learning, learning from individuals and society in general, is another way by which learning takes place. Children learn certain behavior patterns by following the example set by their parents. Children will imitate the actions of their parents and older

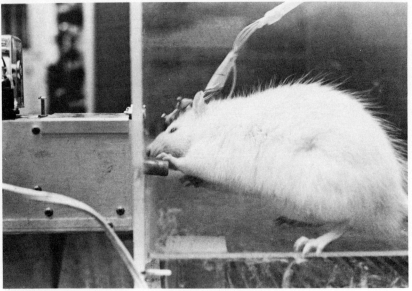

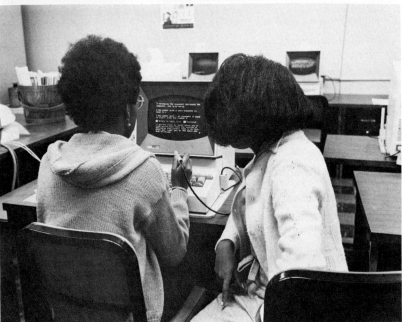

This laboratory rat has been conditioned to press a lever to receive "pleasure" impulses. Teaching machines operate on the same principle by providing immediate positive reinforcement.

brothers and sisters and begin to take on certain behavior patterns. A young child will learn correct table manners by eating with his family and doing what they do. Soon, using correct table manners becomes a part of his own behavior pattern and he comes to internalize, accept the value system of society as his own, a certain way of behaving.

Children will also internalize their parents' attitudes concerning right and wrong, acceptable forms of behavior, and what is generally expected of them. Social behavior will differ from culture to culture depending on what behavior is considered acceptable in that society. Many studies have shown the important influence social learning has on behavior patterns. One such study conducted by Dr. C.H. Kluckhohn, a noted anthropologist (one who studies man), classified newborn white American babies and Zuñi Indian babies according to energy levels. The babies were observed to be "unusually active," "average," or "quiet." It was found that although more white babies were placed in the "unusually active" group, many Indian babies also showed this behavior pattern. However, the Zuñi culture is restrained and quiet, and when the study was followed up two years later, the white babies who had been classified as "unusually active" were much more active than their Zuñi counterparts. You may conclude from this study and other similar studies that inherited personality patterns may change as a result of social experience. This conclusion may become quite clear if you visit a nursery school session at the beginning of the year. It is interesting to observe how many "anti-social" three-year-olds become quite socialized after only a few weeks of the school experience. Can you think of a social experience that has altered your personality? If so, how did it change you?

social behavior is developmental

Social behavior develops gradually and children go through distinct stages in their ability to get along with other people. The infant's first and closest social contact is his mother or the person who is tending to his immediate needs. Soon the father, other relatives, and brothers and sisters become a part of the baby's social world. Although the two- or three-year-old child may play in a group with other children, he tends to play by himself and has difficulty in sharing toys or playing games that require cooperation.

From four years of age until the pre-teen years (10 to 12), children begin to play cooperatively and the sexes usually play well together. However, during the pre-teen years or a little before, children seek out the friendship of others of the same sex. Most of you can probably remember attending a dance or party when you were ten or eleven. Most likely the boys and girls sat separately and if they danced there was little conversation.

By the time one enters the teen years, friendships and interests begin to include the opposite sex and dating begins. In the late teens, serious dating occurs and persons are able to form lasting friendships with many members of both sexes. In order to be able to relate to people of both sexes in a mature manner, the individual had to go through a slow learning process. Do you find that some people of your age have difficulty in relating to others of both sexes? If so, think about some of the possible reasons for their social behavior.

CONSCIENCE

What do you mean when you use the word conscience? Conscience may be defined as that part of our personality that tells us what is considered an acceptable form of behavior. The conscience gradually develops as the child learns what is acceptable in his family and in the larger society. The conscience develops as the child experiences different social interactions with parents, friends, and

Early adolescent sexual behavior is likely to be playful.

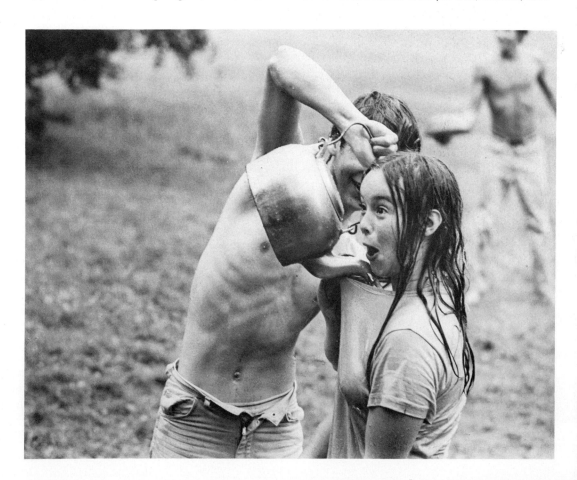

others with whom he comes into frequent contact. Conscience develops to differing degrees depending on a child's social experiences. As learning progresses, one's conscience may become more liberated (letting go). Cognitive or intellectual learning will affect the conscience as it does all behavior. This aspect of learning is discussed in the next section of this chapter.

COGNITIVE LEARNING

Cognitive learning is often defined as learning that utilizes the processes of reasoning, judgment, and perception (our own impressions of an experience). Jean Piaget (pee-ah-jhay), a Swiss psychologist, has done much of the classic research concerned with cognitive learning in children.

Piaget has observed that cognitive learning takes place in four stages. The first or sensori-motor stage begins at birth and lasts until the child is around 18 months old. During this stage the child is primarily concerned with his senses and body movement. The second or preoperational stage continues from 18 months until around seven years of age. In the first half of this stage (until around four years of age), the child learns to talk, see mental images, and solve simple problems. The latter half of this stage or the intuitive phase continues from four to seven years of age. During this stage, the child is able to see relationships between differing experiences and is able to solve more complex problems. The third major stage is that of concrete operations which includes children from about seven to eleven years of age. The term "concrete" is used in the title because it is during this stage that children develop the ability to understand such concrete problems as size, age, weight, and classification of items according to dimension or weight. The ability to solve abstract problems is not developed until the final or abstract operations stage, which takes place between the ages of eleven and fifteen. At this stage, children are able to look at a problem from many points of view and solve complex problems that are not of a concrete nature.

Piaget has written numerous books and conducted many studies concerning cognitive development. If you decide to become a teacher, psychologist, sociologist, or physician, you will no doubt read many of his works. On the basis of his research, Piaget concludes that cognitive development is closely linked to the maturation levels of children, and certain tasks or skills cannot be taught before the child is ready to learn them. Many of you have probably heard this theory expressed in relation to walking, toilet-training, and reading. A child cannot be taught to do any of the previousty mentioned tasks if he is not physically and emotionally ready. Many a parent is surprised to find that his 15-month-old child who he thought was toilet-trained really was not trained at all. The explanation may simply be that the child may have been habitually placed on a toilet seat at a certain time of day and would go to the bathroom at that time. His parents were trained to put him there, but he was not trained to do this by himself. The child may not be able to consider what he is doing at this age and he is often physically unable to control his body functions.

HOW LEARNING TAKES PLACE

Conditioning, social learning, and cognitive learning are the three basic ways by which we learn. Although they may occur by themselves, most frequently two or three different learning processes are required to alter behavior patterns. A young child being taught to drink from a cup may learn partially through conditioning, partially through social learning, and to some extent through cognitive means. If he is rewarded by attention or given something he likes to eat after drinking correctly from the cup, his behavior is reinforced and conditioning has taken place. By watching parents and other family members he is learning how to imitate them in order to hold the cup and drink from it without spilling. In addition, cognitive learning takes place by the child's ability to control the body movements and sensations necessary

Jean Piaget (b. 1896) is a Swiss psychologist whose studies of children have influenced child psychology (Developmental psychology). Piaget is chiefly interested in the development of intelligence. He believes that all behavior, including thought, represents an adaptation to the environment. Thus he believes that in children, intelligence develops in age-related stages, each stage representing another step away from thought about physically present objects and toward abstract thought.

to manipulate the cup and drink from it. Can you think of an example of learned behavior that involves conditioning, social learning, and cognitive skills?

your unique home and community

No two families or communities are exactly alike. The number of people in your family, the ages of your parents and brothers and sisters, and whether or not other relatives share your home all contribute to making your immediate environment very different from that of other people. The size of the community in which you live, whether you reside in an urban (city), suburban (area close to a city), or rural (country) area, and the population of the area all contribute to making your community very different in character from other communities. Though you may never have thought about it, your personality has been affected by your family and by the community where you have been raised. You might be a very different person had you been brought up on a farm and had eleven sisters or brothers as opposed to being raised in a large city and being a part of a small family.

In this section of the chapter the effect of parents, siblings (brothers or sisters), and birth order on personality development are explored.

YOUR PARENTS

Parents have a significant effect on the personalities of their children. In some cultures children show very similar personality traits because of a certain type of parental influence. For example, Balinese infants are shown great love and outward affection during their first two years of life. Then the mother begins to tease the child, ignore its demands, and foster jealousy in the child by showering her attention on a neighbor's younger child. Because of this treatment, the Balinese child will begin to withdraw and look for satisfaction within himself rather than from others.

Different cultures as well as different people tend to affect the personality of their children. In some cultures the parents are very outgoing, loving, and affectionate. Other parents tend to be cold and unable to show affection easily. The child will come to understand that the type of attention he receives from his parents is a result of *their* desires rather than his own. Very few children are able to change the personality and cultural patterns of their parents.

Some homes are matriarchal or mother-dominated, while other homes are patriarchal or father-dominated. If there is such domination in the family, the child's personality will reflect this domination. Through imitation, his own family may be dominated in the same manner. Do you feel that your family is dominated by one parent or the other? If so, has this affected your personality in any specific way?

Many books habe been written about the effect of divorce on the personality of children. This is a very valid topic to consider because of the increased incidence of divorce in the United States. Statistics indicate that one out of every three marriages ends in divorce. Young children may be greatly affected by divorce. They frequently feel that they are the reason why a parent has left the home. They sometimes feel that they must have done something very wrong in order for a parent to have left them. If the child is spoken to and is made to understand that he or she is not responsible for what has happened, the child will be better able to cope with the situation. However, the child's personality will in some way be affected by the divorce.

Older children may not react in the same way as younger ones, but they are often hurt, embarrassed, or tend to take sides in the dispute. Mature parents can handle these situations tactfully by speaking openly with their children, avoiding placing blame on the other person, and keeping the channels of communication open between the parents and the children.

12

YOUR
BROTHERS AND SISTERS

Your relationship with your brothers and sisters has had a very important effect on your personality. At a very young age sibling rivalry, rivalry between brothers and sisters, takes place. A two-year-old child may react in a physically harmful manner toward a new baby that is taking his mother's attention from him. Parents are frequently told by pediatricians (doctors who treat babies and children) that the older child needs more emotional attention than the new baby. Rivalry often diminishes with age and the awakening of separate interests, ideals, and goals. However, in some families, adult children still feel very competitive toward their brothers and sisters. Can you think of some of the reasons why this behavior pattern has not changed over the years?

The personalities of children who are members of large families are frequently quite different from those of children in smaller families. Children (especially older ones) in large families frequently have responsibility for caring for the younger children and for taking on a greater number of household chores. The children in a large family often feel great attachment to each other and are very protective of their younger sisters and brothers. From your own experience, can you think of any families where the size of the family bears no direct relationship to an increase in responsibility among the children. What are some of the reasons for this occurrence?

BIRTH ORDER
AND PERSONALITY

There is strong research that supports the assumption that the order of birth (first, second, or third child) has a very important influence upon your personality. Generally speaking, firstborn children tend to be more achievement-oriented (seeking accomplishment) than their siblings. This may occur because they try to imitate their parents to a greater degree than do their brothers and sisters. First children often have responsibility for younger brothers and sisters and this experience affects their personality development.

Many research studies have been conducted that indicate personality traits of firstborn children. According to such studies, firstborn children tend to: (1) show a great desire for achievement; (2) attend colleges and

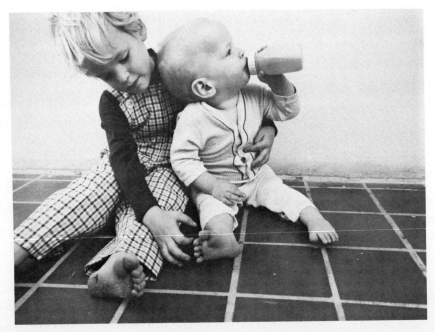

The first-born has a monopoly on parental love and attention until the second child is born. The older child learns to take responsibility for his sibling.

universities in greater numbers; (3) score very well on tests of mental ability; (4) hold more memberships in social groups; and (5) be listed more often in *Who's Who in America.*

The middle and youngest child also have distinct personality traits. Much of a child's personality forms as a reaction to what his or her parents expect from that child. Parental expectations often vary with the child's birth order. The oldest or firstborn may be expected to have greater responsibility and achievement levels than his younger siblings and often conforms in his behavior to these expectations. A middle child may find himself in a difficult position in that he does not have the responsibility of the older child and he is not protected as much as the younger child. Middle children may tend to show greater independence because of their unique postion in the family.

The "baby" or youngest child is usually treated protectively by his parents and siblings. Youngest children may have difficulty asserting themselves and some tend to act "spoiled" or "bratty" because so much is done for them. A parent tends to see the youngest child as immature, even when he or she is in the teen years. You may have heard parents talking about a mature adult and saying, "he is still my baby!"

What about the only child? Only children have a very distinct place in the family. They are frequently showered with attention by parents and close relatives. They often show very mature personality traits at a young age because they are frequently in the company of adults and have adult models to imitate. Only children may have difficulty in adjusting to children their own age unless they are exposed to play situations in their neighborhoods or in nursery groups.

Although much research has been conducted concerning birth order, it is important to remember that birth order alone will not affect your personality to any great extent. There are some very general personality traits attributed to a person's birth order; however, there are many other influences that are simultaneously at work. Children of

the same birth order in different families will have unique personalities because of differing parental treatment and expectations, financial and social factors, and a multitude of other influences.

According to birth order, what is your place in the family unit? Think about the personality traits you exhibit and how they may or may not be related to your birth-order position.

PEER GROUP

Your peer group is made up of those people usually around your own age and generally in a similar socioeconomic group. Peer groups become increasingly important as one enters the teenage years. As teenagers become more and more independent, they feel a great need to be with others of their age who will support them in their new roles. Parental interest, love, and attention are still very much required, but teenagers need to be given the freedom to make their own decisions and choose their own friends. A peer group provides a feeling of security to a teenager because they are persons he can relate to on his own level. Many teenagers are unsure of how to handle their new roles and the security of a peer group makes the transition from teenager to adult an easier one.

Peer groups often take the form of single sex or mixed social groups that limit their membership. These groups are sometimes called clubs, sororities, fraternities, or gangs. This type of group provides social status as well as security and friendship to its members. In the 1950s gangs were very popular and violence was an essential part of the nature of the group. The well-known play and movie, *West Side Story,* depicted the racial hatred between two gangs during the 50s. Violent gangs seemed to diminish in number during the 1960s; however, a resurgence of these groups has been reported in recent years.

Sometimes teenagers live with a peer group because there is no one else to take an interest in them. One such group was recently

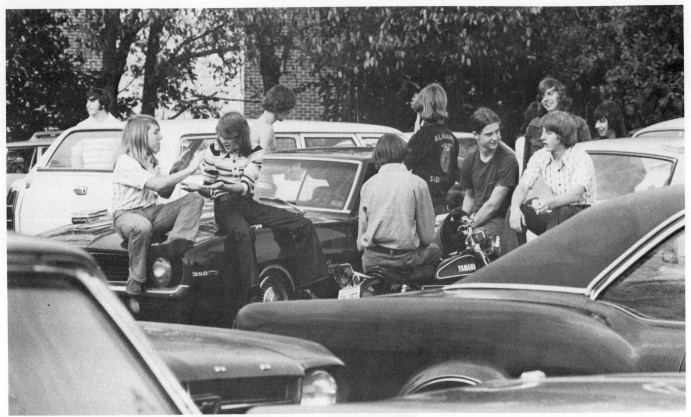

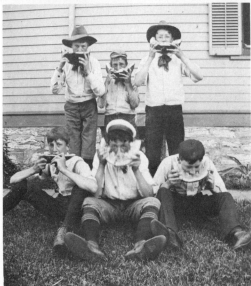

Peer groups have always played an important role in the lives of teenagers.

discussed in a December 1973 article by Claude Brown in *The New York Times Magazine*. The 21 teenagers (15 boys and six girls) in this group range in age from 14 to 17. The group lives in an abandoned, deteriorating building in Harlem in New York City. Only nine members of the group live in the building on a permanent basis, but others will stay there if home life becomes too unbearable of if they have nowhere else to go. Members of the group have a genuine concern for each other and are united by feelings of friendship and belonging. The group disapproves of cutting classes, and nine out of ten members hope to go to college. Fights between group members are rare and fights in general are frowned upon. The taking of hard drugs is also disapproved of as many group members were brought up in homes where one or both parents were addicts. This type of peer group provides many advantages to its members. There is the usual security through identification with persons of the same age and the additional security of living with people who care about what happens to you. What purposes, other than social interaction, are served by peer groups with which you are familiar?

SEX ROLE IDENTIFICATION

This term refers to the way in which boys and girls learn patterns of behavior associated with their sex and then identify themselves as members of that sex. Sex roles are learned by imitation of parents and other members of the family and through a process referred to as socialization (adopting the values of a particular society). Socialization begins to occur very early in life and the learning of sex roles usually takes place without the child being completely aware of what is happening. For example, a mother may dress her small daughter in pastel dresses and warn her not to get dirty. By doing this the mother is telling the child that girls wear dresses and should not get dirty. The message is implied in the action and the child will begin to identify with the role.

In recent years, much has been written about how sex roles are assigned and how these roles affect the personalities of boys and girls. Much of this information has come to light as a result of the woman's movement and more people today are aware of sex-role stereotyping (behavior associated with one sex or the other) than ever before. Sex-role stereotyping can perhaps best be explained by the following example: Julie and Michael were sister and brother. She was four and he was two. Julie's toys consisted mainly of dolls, carriages, some books, and a nurse kit which was her favorite toy. Michael had many trucks, balls, riding toys, and a small baseball glove which he always carried with him. Michael's father would refer to his son as a future baseball player or doctor and would always ask Julie about how many boyfriends she had in nursery school.

Obviously this example has been oversimplified to point out sex-role stereotyping and what it can do to a child's personality.

Parents unknowingly teach their girls to assume "mother" roles by providing girls' toys. Career goals for girls are often limited to those of teacher, mother, or nurse. On the other hand, boys are given toys that require more aggressive actions and they are primed for professional careers. This type of stereotyping can be most harmful to children of both sexes. Girls need as much freedom of expression as boys and likewise boys should experience the fun of playing with dolls, doing crafts, and appreciating non-aggressive play.

Because of a great amount of publicity stressing the avoidance of sex-stereotyping, today's generation of children are generally less role-stereotyped than ever before. Young mothers exposed to the media have, in many cases, gone out of their way to avoid sex-stereotyping. The author is familiar with one mother who took a children's book about a boy becoming a pilot and inserted a girl's name throughout so that her daughter would be able to visualize women as pilots.

Some psychologists disapprove of the trend away from sex-role stereotyping. They strongly feel that a child in grade school will have greater difficulty in understanding what it means to be a boy or girl if he or she is not exposed to the traditional roles of men and women. These psychologists urged that same-sex orgainzations such as Little League (which recently changed its policy to admit girls), Boy Scouts, and Girl Scouts provide a necessary social experience that helps children to achieve healthy sex role identification. How do you think you will handle this problem if you have your own children?

It is also thought that boys and girls need exposure to traditional sex roles so that they will be able to be good parents and not be confused about their roles. Those who do not wish to become parents should be able to reach this conclusion after considering all the available information. Some psychiatrists have come across cases of teenage girls who are deeply disturbed because they are looking forward to marriage and raising a family but think that it is embarrassing

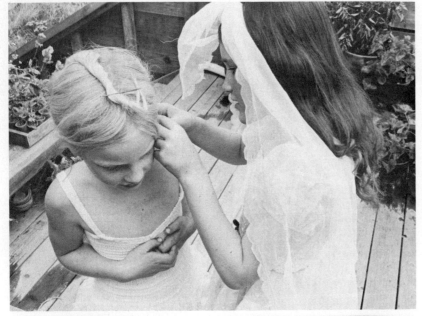

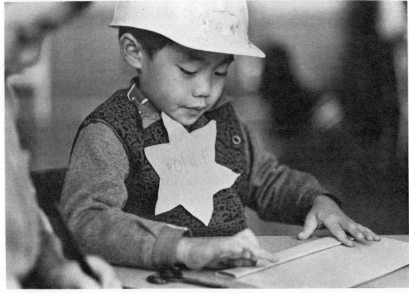

Children learn their sex roles by using their parents and other adults as models, and, beginning early in life, they practice the roles in their play.

for a girl in today's society to have such desires.

There is an obvious controversy concerning sex-roles and "pat" answers cannot be given. As in most other learning experiences, extremes should be avoided and children should be encouraged to be themselves and discover their own potentialities.

Sigmund Freud, a renowned psychiatrist, has provided us with the psychoanalytic theory of personality. His classic studies and interpretations of personality development including sex-roles are discussed in the next section of this chapter.

FREUDIAN THEORY

No chapter concerned with personality would be complete without studying the Freudian or psychoanalytic theories of per-

Sigmund Freud (1856–1939) began his career as a physician in Vienna. He became interested in treating neuroses and soon developed the theory that behavior is based upon unconscious emotions and motivations. His method of treatment, psychoanalysis, attempts to release unconscious feelings.

An easily angered man, Freud quarreled with many of his associates, including Jung and Adler, who subsequently formed their own theories. Today it is acknowledged that Freud's theories have greatly influenced psychological thought and that Freud is largely responsible for the "psychological" way in which we think of ourselves today.

sonality. Freud concluded from his studies that most adult personality problems were the result of a confused or inadequate child-parent relationship. Freud's "Oedipus complex" (derived from Oedipus the tragic legendary Greek hero who unwittingly killed his father and married his mother) theorizes that small boys initially develop strong attachments to their mothers. At the same time they may show obvious dislike for their fathers. This dislike is based on the father's relationship to the mother. As a boy matures, he comes to realize that his feelings are unreasonable and a more positive attitude toward the father develops. Identification with father occurs at this time. Girls, on the other hand, show the opposite pattern, known as the Electra complex. The Electra complex is like the Oedipus complex except that it denotes that young girls develop strong feelings about their fathers and hostility toward their mothers. This is resolved as a girl matures and begins to identify with her mother. According to Freudian theory, if these patterns are not resolved, adult mental and emotional disturbance might result.

Freud's concept of personality involves three basic elements: "id," "ego," and

"superego." The "id" is that part of the personality that represents the primitive, instinctual, and childlike feelings. The "ego" represents the conscious, intellectual, reality feelings. The "superego" is the conscience, internalized values, and the source of guilt feelings. Freud's view of human personality is basically that of a dominant "id" held back by the "ego" and "superego." He also theorized that the unconscious area of personality "contained" many experiences that were repressed (held back) because of their painful, frustrating, or embarrassing nature. Freudian theory also concludes that the sex drive is an important component of the personality and underlies many human actions.

Freud's theories did not meet with immediate acceptance. The very nature of the "id" acting as a dominant force in human personality was unacceptable to most people of his era. (in the late 1800s to early 1900s). In addition, the importance that Freud placed on the sex drive and his theory of infant sexuality were shocking to most people.

His methods of dealing with mental and emotional disturbances were also unique

Freud's concept of personality: The id, the ego, and the superego.

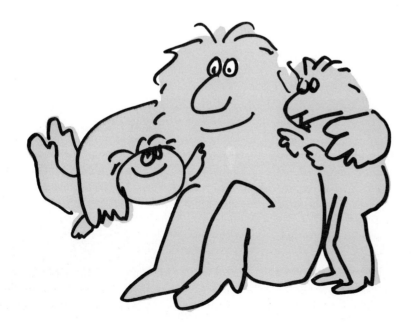

to his period. Freud encouraged his patients to talk freely about their problems and feelings. He sometimes employed hypnosis to free people to delve into their past experiences that had remained repressed for many years. He also used the technique of free association. Patients would express their thoughts and feelings as they came to mind. Dreams and their meanings would also be discussed. Much of Freud's writing deals with dreams and their interpretations. This type of treatment often referred to as psychoanalysis (a treatment for mental and emotional problems where the patient is encouraged to recall early life experiences) is very much a part of today's treatment for mental and emotional illness. During psychoanalysis, the patient and psychoanalyst (one who has had specialized training in this field) try to get to the root of mental problems through discussions of thoughts and attitudes and to eventually attain breakthroughs that will help the patient to cope with his particular situation.

The process of psychoanalysis may be better understood by studying the following simplified example. Paul was a middle-aged man who graduated from college and became a librarian. After many years, his responsibilities increased until he had become the chief librarian of a county library system. Paul's family and friends considered him to be well-adjusted and successful in both his job and family life. However, over the years he had developed a habit of washing his hands many times during the day. After seeking psychiatric help, psychotherapy was advised. In psychotherapy, Paul became aware of the guilt feelings he felt at not living up to his father's expectations. He felt that his father thought library work was for women and disapproved of his son entering this career. Paul's hand washing was a symptom of the subconscious desire to wash away the guilt that he felt.

Psychiatrists and psychologists with psychoanalytic training most frequently use psychotherapy in helping their patients to overcome mental or emotional problems.

Psychoanalysis is not a "surecure" but rather a method of helping people to understand and cope with their problems and to adjust to the demands of society. Other methods of treatment for the mentally and emotionally ill are discussed in Chapters 3 and 4.

do you
like yourself?

Your answer to this question should immediately tell you a great deal about how you feel about yourself and about your personality. Your self-concept (the way you see yourself both physically and emotionally) is an integral part of your unique personality.

If you think back to an earlier section of this chapter, you will recall a discussion of body type. Closely related to body type is a person's feeling about his physical self and how these feelings affect personality development. Some people use their feelings about their physical appearance to adversely affect relationships with others. You probably have heard someone say, "I'm so fat and ugly—no one could ever like me." What is this person really saying? If he or she *really* is fat and ugly, will it affect friendships with other people? It is not the physical characteristics of people that make other people like or dislike them. What is important is a person's friendliness or genuine interest in other people. If the person who stated he was "fat and ugly" was very unhappy with his looks then he might make an attempt to alter his looks through dieting and paying more attention to his appearance. Many persons who speak this way are hiding behind their supposed unattractive appearance because they may be afraid to make new friends and are unsure about the way others will receive them. Do you know any people who fit into this type of personality pattern? Can you think of any ways that they could be helped to gain a more positive self-concept?

In the preceding paragraph, a part of one sentence read as follows, "if he or she really is fat . . . ." The word *really* was placed

19

in that sentence to stress a specific thought concerning a person's self-concept. Read the following illustrative example and think about its relationship to the word "really." Marilyn was in the neighborhood "jeans only" shop trying on a pair of jeans in the dressing room. Disgusted with how fat she thought she looked she was ready to leave without buying anything. As she changed, she thought she heard some familiar voices outside the dressing room. One of the girls said to the other, "those white jeans would look great on Marilyn—she has the perfect figure for them." Marilyn soon recognized the voices as belonging to two of her closest friends.

The point made in this example is quite obvious. People frequently have a different body image of themselves than others have of them. Certain people are very "hard" on themselves and never feel that they are the people they really would like to be physically or emotionally. Can you think of some reasons why one would have a negative body-image when others do not share that opinion?

It is impossible to separate one's self-concept into physical and emotional parts. Each part is completely dependent on the other. The way a person feels about his body is reflected in the way he behaves and the way others perceive his personality.

Important psychological interpretations of self-concept are explored in the following sections of this chapter.

ON BECOMING A PERSON

This heading is also the title of a well-known book by a respected psychotherapist, Carl Rogers. The following paragraph from *On Becoming a Person* explains Rogers' theory of self-concept and how this theory of behavior helps people to better all of their human relationships:

"If I can create a relationship characterized on my part:
by a genuineness and transparency, in which I am my real feelings;
by a warm acceptance of and prizing of the other person as a separate individual,
by a sensitive ability to see his world and himself as he sees them;

Then the other individual in the relationship:
will experience and understand aspects of himself which previously he has repressed;
will find himself becoming better integrated, more able to function effectively;
will become more similar to the person he would like to be;
will be more self-directing and self-confident;
will become more of a person, more unique and more self-expressive;
will be more understanding, more acceptant of others;
will be able to cope with the problems of life more adequately and more comfortably." [1]

In this excerpt, Rogers is expressing the theory that a person who is able to truly be himself without creating a false image will encourage others he encounters to act in a similar manner. Rogers believes that underlying all personal and interpersonal problems is a person's need to find out who he or she is and get in touch with this self. People should ask themselves the question, "how can I become myself?" How would you answer this question?

So often the "self" we present to others and even the "self" we may think is the "real" self is a personality that has become masked or protected by life experiences. For example, a young girl who tends to be a quiet person may be called shy by a parent or teacher. She may soon begin to feel that she is shy and her quiet nature takes on a new dimension of withdrawal. As the years go by, shyness becomes an accepted part of her self-concept and she acts the part of a shy individual.

Carl Rogers (1902–), an American psychologist, originated "client-center-ed" therapy, a way of treating people by en-couraging them to express how they feel about themselves and their world. Rogers is known as a *humanistic psy-chologist*, because he believes that, given the chance, people will express distinctly human values and behave in distinctly human ways— even if this behavior goes against their animal instincts of survival.

[1] From Carl P. Rogers, *On Becoming a Person*. (Boston: Houghton Mifflin Company, 1961.)

In order for her to "become herself" she would have to explore the reasons for her shyness and try to find the hidden "real self." Psychotherapy or counseling can help the individual with mental or emotional problems to "uncover" the real self and live up to that self's potential.

Abraham Harold Maslow (1908–1970), an American humanistic psychologist, is best known for his theory of a "hierarchy of needs." In Maslow's opinion, people have different levels of needs. On the first level are the bodily needs: hunger, thirst, sex. Once these needs are satisfied, a person concentrates on the next levels—security, affection, and success, in that order. The highest need of all is for *self-actualization*—or the development of all one's potential. But this need cannot be fulfilled until all the lower needs are.

SELF-ACTUALIZATION

Self-actualization may be defined as the expression of the highest potentialities of which a person is capable. According to the late Abraham Maslow, the concept of self-actualization is the most advanced of the five basic needs of the human personality. These needs develop in sequence and progress to the need for self-actualization. Maslow's hierarchy (order) of needs includes the primary need for physical necessities. Neither the body nor the personality can grow if hunger or thirst persist. In order for a person to be interested in education or religion, for example, these basic needs must first be satisfied. People also have safety needs and one's physical security is essential to personality development.

A third and most important need is that of affection and friendship. People need to feel they are loved and needed; that they belong somewhere, whether it be to a family, social group or club, or friendship group at work. People also have a need for affection often satisfied by an involved relationship with one or more individuals.

Esteem needs according to Maslow are important when physical, safety, and affection needs have been satisfied to an acceptable degree. Often called "self-esteem," these needs include status, prestige, power, and respect. The need for self-esteem varies but most people express a basic need to be accepted and respected as an individual having one's own feelings and ideas. The need for recognition and status varies greatly among different personality types. Some persons have a need to achieve which is so important to them that little else matters. Others are satisfied with a feeling of self-

respect and acceptance by other persons whose opinions they value.

The ultimate need according to Maslow is the need for self-fulfillment beyond purely selfish motives. This need is satisfied by a total involvement or commitment to an ideal or goal. An example of self-actualization would be a nurse who is so completely committed to her patients that salary and working hours become secondary to the people she is helping. Her concern is totally the welfare of the people she is caring for and through this commitment she becomes free of selfish concerns. As with the other needs described, one cannot fully satisfy the need for self-actualization unless the basic needs are satisfied to an acceptable degree. However, Maslow feels that those who are able to satisfy the need for self-actualization enjoy a freedom of self and a feeling of "wholeness" that they could not otherwise achieve.

On a sheet of paper jot down Maslow's five basic needs, leaving space between them. Briefly write down to what extent you feel that each of these needs is being satisfied in your life. Do you feel that you have to some degree satisfied the need for self-actualization? Do you agree with Maslow that this need represents the highest form of human needs? Think carefully about your answer to this question.

TRANSACTIONAL ANALYSIS

Transactional analysis is the study of interpersonal relationships and the social defenses, "games," and masking that people use when relating to other people. It is not a form of psychoanalysis, as it usually deals with observable behavior and how this behavior can be modified in order to help people to be more honest with themselves and with each other. Transactional analysis does not attempt to deal with past experiences and tends to remain on a superficial level. The founder of transactional analysis, Eric Berne, wrote about his theories in the book *Games People Play*. In the next section of this chapter you will explore some of the "games" that people play and see how these games affect your unique personality.

GAMES, GAMES, GAMES

According to Berne, all people exhibit certain behavior patterns that may differ depending on their social encounters. He refers to these behavior patterns as those of the Parent, Adult, and Child. All of us sometimes act the role of each of these patterns. For example, have you ever had the experience of going shopping with your parents and seeing something that you wanted, although it was very expensive. How did you react? Did you play the child role and in a sense "beg" for the item as a youngster might have done? This was your Child behavior pattern. In a setting that required a different response you may have been an Adult or a Parent. The Parent pattern refers to having that state of mind that you identify with your parents or parent substitutes. The Adult is that objective, thoughtful state of mind that comes from independent thoughts in a particular area. The Child is the behavior pattern you exhibited as a small boy or girl. These three patterns are referred to by Berne as ego states. It may be said that everyone has a Child, Parent, and Adult within him.

Each of these ego states has its own very important value to the individual. The Child provides intuition, creativity, and joy. The Adult provides objectivity, reasoning, and the pleasure received from more complicated tasks such as appreciating sports or problem solving. The Parent has two primary functions. One function is the ability to act as an effective parent of actual children. The second function is to make automatic decisions that conserve time and energy.

A game has two chief characteristics: (1) a motive that is other than the one seemingly expressed, and (2) a payoff. The payoff is ultimately derived from a social encounter or transaction (social interaction). For example, in the game referred to as SWYMD (see what you made me do), a woman may be busy sewing a dress when her child asks her for a glass of water. Annoyed at being interrupted, she hurts her finger on the needle and screams, "see what you made me do!" Of course, the child really had nothing to do with the mother injuring her finger but the payoff that results is that the child may leave the room. This is what the mother had really desired though she was not able to express it. How many times have you used the SWYMD game? Which of the ego states do you think is acting in this game?

Another popular game is termed IWFY (if it weren't for you). IWFY can be used in many different situations, but a common example may involve a man who would like to better his career by taking a job that requires a great deal of traveling. His response to his wife about why he hasn't taken the job is "if it weren't for you." He is implying that she is preventing him from taking the job for any number of possible reasons: too much time away from home, family responsibilities, or social obligations. However, the payoff for him may be that he is not taking the job because he really doesn't want to be away from home and cannot express his feelings to his wife or family. The IWFY game accomplishes the desired payoff and the individual doesn't have to face the responsibility of having made the desired decision. Suggest another set of circumstances where one would employ the IWFY game.

As in all of these games, some type of deception is implied. If people were totally honest about their feelings, such games wouldn't be necessary and the character of their interpersonal relationship would probably improve. If one person relies on a game to gain a certain payoff, then the other people involved in the game will probably employ other games to counter the effects of the first game.

Game play can be much more involved than the examples indicate. There are different levels of game-playing with differing involvements and payoffs. If you are interested in learning more about Berne's theories, you should read his interesting and informative book, *Games People Play*.

22

Thomas Anthony Harris
(1910–   ), a Texas-born
psychiatrist, uses Trans-
actional Analysis as a
method of treatment.
Transactional Analysis
(TA) focuses on how
people interact and how
they communicate with
each other. What it's all
about is well illustrated
in Harris's book *I'm OK–
You're OK* (New York:
Harper and Row, 1969),
as well as in *Games
People Play* (New York:
Grove, 1964) by Eric
Berne, the movement's
founder.

I'M OK—YOU'RE OK

This is the title of another very popular book dealing with transactional analysis. Written by Thomas Harris, *I'm OK—You're OK* also stresses the "parent, adult, child," concept of personality. One's *life position* or the way a person views himself and his relationship to others is another major theme of this book. There are four possible life positions with respect to yourself and others:

1. I'm Not OK—You're OK
2. I'm Not OK—You're not OK
3. I'm OK—You're Not OK
4. I'm OK—You're OK

Harris believes that by the end of the second year of life or sometime during the third year, the child has decided on one of the first three life positions. These positions are discussed in some detail in the following paragraphs.

The first position of I'm Not OK—You're OK is the general position of infancy. The child sees others who care for him as OK, but he is not OK because of his helplessness and passiveness. This of course is not a conscious thought on the part of the infant but becomes a part of his unconscious self.

I'm Not OK—You're Not OK is a second position. This often occurs by the end of the first year of life when the mother's physical and emotional attention have diminished to some degree. The adult who remains in this life position may give up, have little hope, and may ultimately suffer from severe withdrawal (inability to cope with society).

I'm OK—You're Not OK is the third position. A child who comes to accept this life position has probably been able to provide himself with the affection that was lacking from his parents. Adults who remain in this position are often criminal types who see everyone else as being at fault but not themselves. They often are persons "without a conscience" who feel little or no guilt as a result of their actions.

I'm OK—You're OK is the fourth and most hopeful life position. It differs from the others because it is a conscious position that a person has thought about and accepted. The other three positions are subconscious and occur early in life. Most people tend to remain in the first or I'm Not OK—You're OK position. The second and third positions are less frequently held by adults. One must make an active decision to accept the I'm OK—You're OK position and see himself and others as being acceptable and worthy of affection and respect.

To better understand what is meant by a life position, study the following example: A small boy in the I'm Not OK—You're OK position is frequently told how bad he is and how dirty he gets. He cannot see any worth in himself and feels that he is helpless and defenseless. However, he sees the parent as powerful, all-knowing, and having all the answers.

Many children are placed in a position where they are not able to feel OK about themselves. As they get older, they have to consciously seek out and accept OK'ness in order to enter the I'm OK—You're OK position.

As mentioned earlier, Harris also stresses the PAC (Parent, Adult, Child) concept of personality. In any social situation, these parts of the personality express themselves. Any interaction between two people may involve the Parent, Child, or Adult of an individual involved in the transaction. There are Parent–Parent, Child–Child, and Adult–Adult responses and any combination of these. An example of a Parent–Child trans-action might be:

Parent: "Boy, Wall Street is really going to the dogs this year. I just know it's not the time to invest—the whole country is in for a bad time!"

Child: "So what!"

This transaction wasn't between a real parent and child but between a husband and wife. The *Parent* (husband) was talking in a man-ner similar to his own parents. The Parent usually speaks easily about subjects that are not that familiar to him. The *Child* (wife) is acting as she might have when she was a child—showing no interest in what the parent was saying.

Choose a PAC transaction and write it down. One from your own experience would probably be most meaningful. Have you ever thought about people interacting in this way?

The book *I'm OK—You're OK* is a fascinating study of life position and its relationship to PAC transactions. It discusses PAC in relationship to common problem areas of most people (use of time, marriage, children, etc.) and gives some startling insights into our everyday behavior and how we see ourselves and others.

now I can like you

Once an individual understands who he is in relation to his heredity and environment, he can better understand how he feels about himself (self-concept) and if he likes himself. If a person can understand some of the reasons for his behavior, he is then able to have better, more joyful relationships with other people. There are many books written on the subject of people interacting with and appreciating each other. No one book could possibly cover the multitude of theories and approaches concerned with getting along better with others. In this section of the chapter, three very interesting and innovative methods of improving one's relationship with others are discussed.

GESTALT THERAPY

Gestalt therapy is related to the Gestalt school of psychology that believes in looking at behavior as a whole rather than as separate parts. Gestalt therapy is based on the way in which a person perceives his environment. In Gestalt therapy, seeing, hearing, touching, and moving are important aspects of helping a person to overcome his problems and relate better to other individuals. Gestalt therapists often deliberately touch their patients and are very aware of a patient's bodily movements. The therapist feels that by using bodily contact the patient will become more aware of himself. Shy in-

dividuals often find Gestalt therapy helps them to come into immediate physical contact with others. This is often the first experience of this type for some persons. Gestalt therapy is helpful in aiding people to "let go" and express their true feelings. However, the Gestalt therapist must be very careful not to push certain people too fast. This type of therapy concentrates mainly on what is happening right now and what can be done to modify behavior patterns so that people can be happier with themselves and their relationships with other people.

THE ART OF LOVING

This is the title of a very famous book by an equally well-known psychoanalyst, Erich Fromm. Fromm believes that love is the answer to man's problem of living. He feels that love is an active state and that it is primarily *giving,* not receiving. By *giving,* Fromm implies a sacrifice on the part of an individual. Fromm believes that love must include the four basic elements of care, responsibility, respect, and knowledge. *Care* is implied, for example, in the nurturing that a mother gives a child. Caring takes into consideration one's feeling of protectiveness for those he loves. *Responsibility* is a voluntary act and concerns the ability to respond to those we love. Too often responsibility is looked at in an economic rather than an emotional sense. According to Fromm, *respect* is that abiltiy to see a person for what he is and to understand his unique personality. Respect should not be confused with domination of another individual. If you truly respect a person, you want very much for him to be himself in every way and live up to his own potential. *Knowledge* in this sense is the desire for people to know about "who they are" as human beings. Fromm theorizes that only through love can you *know* yourself, those you love, and all of mankind.

This discussion can only begin to express Erich Fromm's, *The Art of Loving.* It is a small but powerful book that you will enjoy reading over and over again.

24

ON CARING

On Caring is the title of a book that expresses the importance of being cared for and caring. Written by Dr. Milton Mayeroff, *On Caring* is concerned with the significance of caring for another individual. Mayeroff feels that one can grow and best realize his potential by truly caring for another. Mayeroff's definition of caring is helping another person to grow and be himself. Caring for someone in this sense can involve a variety of different relationships. The way a parent *cares* for a child, a teacher *cares* for a student, or a doctor *cares* for a patient. Caring can simply be stated as a way of helping people to grow by putting a special effort into all interpersonal relationships.

THINKING IT OVER

1. Do you think that your environment or your heredity has had a greater influence on your unique personality? Explain your answer.
2. Create your own example of conditioning and explain how it works.
3. Do you think that one's home or community environment can really affect heredity?
4. Do you feel that sibling rivalry may be consciously or unconsciously fostered by parents? What circumstances may lead to this?
5. Explain why you accept or reject the concept of birth order and personality.
6. Have peer groups had an important influence on your personality? Explain and give relevant examples.
7. How were you raised in respect to sex-role stereotyping? Do you approve or disapprove of stereotyping? Explain your answer.
8. Do you agree with Freud that sex drive is a crucial part of the personality? Explain your answer.
9. Discuss Rogers' theory of self-concept and whether you are open to such a theory.
10. Do you think that most people are truly "self-actualized" according to Maslow's definition?
11. After thinking about your relationship with others, can you come up with a "game" that people play?
12. Devise your own PAC transaction and explain the personality roles of the individuals involved.

KEY WORDS

Abstract operation. Ability of people to deal with abstract thought.

Association. Ability to draw from our past experiences and relate these experiences to the present.

Body type. An inherited characteristic that classifies people according to body build.

Cognitive learning. Learning that utilizes the processes of reasoning, judgment, and perception.

Concrete operations. Ability of persons to deal with concrete aspects of thought.

Conditioning. A response to an artificial stimulus that has replaced the orginal or natural stimulus.

Conscience. That aspect of one's personality that tells us what is an acceptable or unacceptable form of behavior.

Ectomorph. A long, lean, fragile appearance or body type.

Endomorph. A short, stocky, round appearance or body type.

Gestalt therapy. A type of therapy based upon how a person perceives his or her environment.

Heredity. Those physical, emotional, and mental traits that are passed on from one's parents.

Internalize. Accepting the value system of society as one's own.

Intuitive phase. A phase of cognitive learning.

Learning theory. The way people learn social behavior and acquire knowledge.

Memory. Recall of past events.

Mesomorph. A muscular, strong, athletic appearance or body type.

Operant conditioning. A response to a given situation in order to receive a reward.

Pediatrician. A doctor who specializes in the care of babies and children.

Peer group. Those persons of the same age and socioeconomic position that have an influence on one's personality development.

Perception. Receiving of sensory stimuli and

ability to form impressions about the stimuli.

Physiologist. One who specializes in the study of body function.

Preoperational stage. A stage of cognitive learning.

Programmed learning. A form of conditioning where responses are recorded in small units with immediate feedback to the questions.

Psychiatrist. A doctor who specializes in the treatment of mentally and emotionally ill persons.

Psychoanalysis. A treatment for mental and emotional problems that includes recall of early experiences.

Self-actualization. The highest expression of human potential that involves unselfish commitment to an ideal.

Self-concept. How you feel about yourself.

Sensorimotor stage. Stage of cognitive learning.

Sex-role stereotyping. Behavior associated with one sex or the other.

Sibling rivalry. Rivalry between brothers and sisters.

Social learning. Learning from individuals and society in general.

Socialization. Adopting the values of society as your own.

Somatotyping. A general term that describes body-type classification.

Stimulus. A factor that promotes a response.

Transactional analysis. The study of interpersonal relationships through the analysis of present behavior.

GETTING INVOLVED

Books and Periodicals

Berne, Eric. *Games People Play*. New York: Grove, 1964. The basic premises of Transactional Analysis, written by the movement's founder.

Brown, Claude. "The Group," *The New York Times Magazine,* New York: December 16, 1973. A group of teenagers living together in New York's Harlem.

Freud, Sigmund. *The Basic Writings of Sigmund Freud*. New York: Modern Library, n.d. The founder of psychoanalysis tells what it's all about.

Fromm, Erich. *The Art of Loving*. New York: Harper & Row, 1956. Explores "love" in various kinds of relationships.

Harris, Thomas A. *I'm OK—You're OK*. New York: Harper & Row, 1969. More about TA.

Maslow, Abraham H. *Towards a Psychology of Being*. New York: Van Nostrand Reinhold, 1968. Man's needs expounded.

Mayeroff, Milton. *On Caring*. New York: Harper & Row, 1971. Relates "caring" to all kinds of interpersonal relationships.

Piaget, Jean. *The Origins of Intelligence in Children*. New York: Norton, 1963. Theories of child development.

Rogers, Carl. *On Becoming a Person*. Boston: Houghton Mifflin, 1970. How human beings can achieve their potential.

Movies

Freud, with Montgomery Clift, 1962. Freud's life, in the original settings. Distributed by Cine-Craft, Clem Williams, The Movie Center, Universal 16.

Record

"Older Sister," Carly Simon, *Hotcakes* album, Elektra label

2
EMOTIONAL GROWTH AND HEALTH

What does it mean to "grow up" emotionally? Are we not "emotionally" grown when we are "physically" grown? This question and others concerned with emotional growth and health are answered and discussed in this chapter.

You will also read about psychological theories concerning personality development and their relationship to emotional growth. You will find out about the four basic "wants" in life — and you can discover whether they apply to you.

The second part of this chapter discusses how to go about achieving good emotional health. It is one thing to understand what it means to be emotionally healthy and quite another to be able to <u>become</u> emotionally healthy. You will learn about the factors involved in achieving emotional health.

An important aspect of emotional health is the need to develop a personal value system. You will learn about the term "valuing" and what it means to the individual.

After you have completed this chapter you will better be able to evaluate your own emotional health and to also achieve a higher degree of emotional health.

While reading this chapter, think about the following concepts:

■ Emotional development is closely interwoven with personality development.

■ Emotional growth is an on-going process.

■ Emotional growth is linked to human "wants."

■ There are certain essential factors involved in achieving good emotional health.

■ People need to establish personal value systems.

■ Emotional health is a crucial part of good total health.

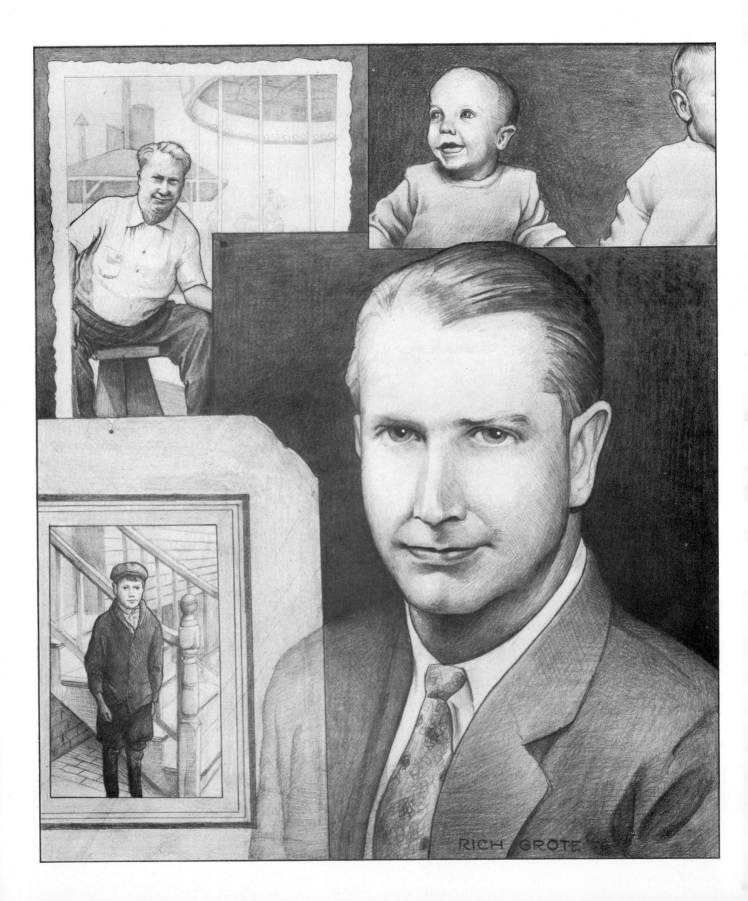

RICH GROTE '46

The title of this chapter, "Emotional Growth and Health," is really what this chapter is all about. The key words are *emotional* and *growth*. Do we all of a sudden reach a point where we are "emotionally grown" or "completely mature"? The answer, of course, is "no." Emotional growth is an on-going process. Most people continue to grow emotionally throughout their lives. Most people do become more responsible and exhibit greater emotional control, but they continue to "grow" in their attitudes and methods of coping emotionally.

The person who continues to grow emotionally is far healthier mentally than the person who has stopped growing or who has "turned off" emotionally. These are some of the topics that are explored in this chapter.

growing up emotionally

Emotional development is closely interwoven with the development of the personality. Both are closely related to physical development and well-being. You may recall that Chapter 1 stressed the idea of *total health*. You cannot be totally healthy unless you are emotionally and physically healthy. If you feel terrible *physically*, most likely you also feel terrible emotionally. This, of course, works both ways. When would this not be the case?

AN ON-GOING PROCESS

A person does not go to sleep one night and awake the next morning to find himself emotionally mature. This, as previously mentioned, is an on-going process. One's behavior does change from childhood to adulthood, but it is a progressive change that occurs slowly. For example, a young child may have temper tantrums two or three times a day over "silly" things. Of course, these "things" are only "silly" to the adult not to the child. Do people stop having temper tantrums when they reach adulthood? Your first answer may be "yes"; but think about it for a minute. You certainly

may have fewer tantrums, but you probably still have them. When was the last time you were locked out of your house and tried to kick the door down? What would be another example of this type of behavior?

Emotional growth is *not* necessarily linked to one's chronological age. We all know people who are well into adulthood who react to situations as if they were four or five instead of 45. Some people have great difficulty in growing up and tend to face responsibility in an immature manner.

There are particular times in one's life when one can be called mature because he has reached a certain age or stage in life. One does not suddenly become mature, for example, when one gets married. In fact, some people become "less" mature after marriage because they depend more heavily on someone else to make decisions for them or to "protect" them.

Like the "3 R's" in education, there are "2 R's" in emotional maturity: *responsibility* and *reality*. Responsibility is one aspect of the emotionally mature person. That person is able to cope with the responsibility for his own actions and those of others. Reality is the ability to know who you are and what your capabilities are. If an individual can cope with the "2 R's," he or she has a head start on emotional growth. These factors will be discussed again later in this chapter.

STAGES OF PERSONALITY DEVELOPMENT

Many psychiatrists and psychologists have put forth their theories on the developing personality and how it matures emotionally over the years. One of the most well-known theories was proposed by Erik Erikson in his book, *Childhood and Society,* 1960. Erikson's eight stages of personality development or "eight stages of man" are as follows:

1. *Oral sensory stage.* Trust versus distrust.
2. *Muscular anal.* Anatomy versus shame and doubt.

29

Erik Homburger Erikson (1902—) is an American psychoanalyst. He believes that each stage of life is characterized by specific problems, and the way in which an individual solves these problems influences his personality. In the teen years, the problem is to discover one's individual identity; Erikson called this problem the "identity crisis," and the term made him famous.

3. *Locomotor genital.* Initiative versus guilt.
4. *Latency.* Industry versus inferiority.
5. *Puberty and adolescence.* Identity versus role diffusion.
6. *Young adulthood.* Intimacy versus isolation.
7. *Adulthood.* Generativity versus stagnation.
8. *Maturity.* Ego integrity versus disgust and despair.

As you can gather from reading these eight stages, each has its positive goals as well as its negative risks. Let us take a closer look at each of Erikson's stages and see what the alternatives are. The first stage *(oral sensory stage)* requires the personality to trust someone else; however, by trusting, he is opening himself to distrust. In the second or *muscular anal stage,* the person becomes interested in his body but risks shame and doubt because of it. In the third *(locomotor genital)* stage, the personality learns to take the initiative, but may be risking guilt at the same time. The *latency stage* is a period of wanting to do things (industry); but along with industry one faces the risk of being inferior at what he wants to do. These developmental stages occur prior to puberty.

In the fifth stage or *adolescent stage* the individual experiences identity and the risk of role diffusion. Identity involves the formation of one's own values, where role diffusion is the identification with various leaders or with other adolescents (gang or group). While the individual is trying to define his own values, he is also being influenced by others. During this stage, the adolescent's frequent crushes and love interests are seen as another way of finding himself and at the same time preparing for the development of a love relationship.

Erikson's sixth stage is that of *young adulthood.* This is the stage of intimacy versus isolation. The young adult desires intimate relationships with others but risks isolation from others if he "cuts" himself off too much. In the seventh or *adulthood stage,* the individual is faced with the goal of wanting to produce versus the risk of not being able to produce or stagnating.

The *maturity stage* is one where the ego is integrated but the individual risks disgust or despair. The mature individual knows who he is but may not like what he finds out about himself. This, too, is tied up with reality and being able to face up to it.

BASIC WANTS IN LIFE

Erikson's eight stages of personality development explore the growth of the individual. Here we are going to explore the "wants" that differ from the physical needs of food, air, clothing, and shelter. Everyone "needs" these physical necessities or they would not be able to go on living. However, once these factors are satisfied to some degree then people look to the psychological needs.

The four basic "wants" are simple desires that everyone of you probably agree are important to happiness. These "wants" include the following:

1. Want to live.
2. Want a feeling of importance.
3. Want someone to love me.
4. Want variety.[1]

Let us explore each of these "wants" and find out a little more about them. The first "want" is the "want" to live. Everyone wants to live a long life. You may have heard someone say, "I don't care if I live or die." And yet the next day he will be at the doctor's office to find out what is wrong with him. People generally *do* want to live. Those who attempt to commit suicide may be communicating a "I want to live" message so that someone will hear them and respond to their needs. Those who do commit suicide may not have gotten their message across in sufficient time or are adjusting in their own way to life's problems. This topic is discussed in more detail in Chapter 3.

The second "want" is expressed as the desire to feel important. You may not think

[1] From a record by Dr. Murray Banks, *How to Live With Yourself...or What to do Until the Psychiatrist Comes.* (New York: Murmil Associates, Inc., 1965.)

you have this "want" but it does exist in all of us to a certain degree. Importance is expressed by different people in different ways. Importance may be job success or position to some; money to others; praise to still others. Some people need to feel important by having status, money, and praise. Where people live, what they do, the car they drive, and the clothes they wear are all ways of conveying their feeling of self-importance.

You may be thinking, "What about the person who is unconcerned with money and success?" What about him? He also wants to feel important. His importance may be involved with the fact that he is "different" from others and somewhat intellectually better off because he is not caught up in the traditional "rat-race." Still, he has a need to be important or recognized in his own way. How do you express your need to feel important?

A third basic want is for someone to love you. A small child may ask his mother or father many times a day "do you love me?" All he wants to hear is a reassuring "yes." Love is his new "security blanket." As long as he knows he is "loved" he can go on to face the problems of that day. It isn't much different with adults. Love provides for the need of being wanted and cared for on a one-to-one basis. A person can love "mankind" much more easily if he is first loved for himself.

The fourth "want" is for variety. What does this mean? Variety is change; the desire to occasionally do something that is different. People who follow the same routine every day at work and at home are more likely to be less emotionally happy than those who have some variety in their lives. The need for variety can be achieved by having many different interests. Some people tend to live their lives with one consuming interest, whether it be their families or jobs. When this interest is gone, the person "falls apart."

Dr. Banks, the psychiatrist who discusses these "wants in life," tells about the need for variety on his record. He says that one

would never purchase a house that had one column for support. However, many people tie their emotional lives to only one column of support. This column might be a husband, a wife, a child, or a job. When that one support collapses, so does the person's life. Have you known people who built their entire lives around one interest? How did they react when the interest was taken away from them? Many women face this problem when their children are grown and many men face the same problem when they retire from their jobs.

You may have read this section and concluded that one must have all of these "wants" fulfilled all of the time in order to live a satisfactory life. No one can have *complete* satisfaction in all these "wants." Everyone will experience some degree of frustration in his life at some time. This is normal. Life is unpredictable and unfortunate things happen that ruin the best made plans. However, if these four needs are satisfied to some degree and one has developed the ability to adjust and adapt to problems, then that person will have a better chance at a happy, fulfilled life.

This brings us to the next part of this chapter, which is concerned with how one can achieve a healthy adjustment to life. This is where a lot of people have problems; they are not able to "roll with the punches" and adjust to the constant changes in their lives.

achieving good emotional health

Throughout this chapter so far, we have been discussing emotional growth. What about the other half of the chapter title—*emotional health*? How does one go about achieving emotional health? It does not just happen to some people and not to others. Those who are emotionally healthy work at it. Some of the factors involved in emotional health are discussed in this section.

One of the most crucial aspects of emotional health is the ability to adjust and adapt. Life and its situations are constantly changing and an inability to adjust may lead to fear, anxiety, and other problems. An emotionally

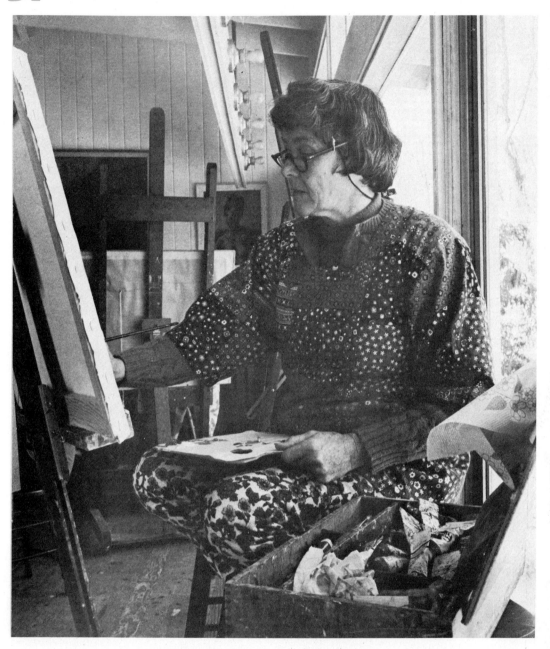

With children grown and
gone, midlife can become
the time for developing
artistic talents.

healthy individual has the ability to adapt easily to a wide variety of situations and people. This does not mean that one has to agree with everyone; but one should be able to be flexible and hear people out.

Adaptability is based on a number of personality factors including self-confidence, feeling comfortable with one's values, and a generally positive self-concept. Adaptive individuals are people who are able to observe themselves in a constructive, objective manner. They are able to see themselves as they really are. Adaptive individuals do not approach each problem in the same way; they can alter their behavior to fit the particular situation at hand. Adaptive people are flexible and understand that each situation presents a different type of problem. Would you consider yourself adaptive?

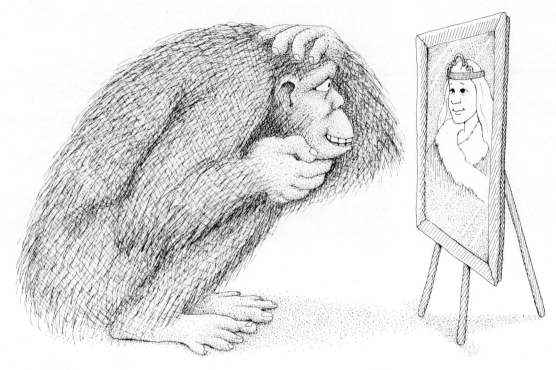

Facing reality?

Earlier in this chapter, the term *reality* was introduced. Reality may be simply defined as knowing one's strengths as well as one's limitations. Reality is the world that we live in and not the world we wished that we lived in. You have probably known some people who are forever living in a "daydream." The "real world" does not exist for them. Daydreams are fine as long as you recognize them for what they are—brief escapes from reality. If people escape too often from reality, then they may become unable to live in the "real" world. Many patients in mental institutions suffer from an inability to live with reality. Facing reality is another important factor in being able to achieve good emotional health.

The ability to love other people is also essential to good emotional health. Love for other people involves a caring, responsible feeling, not a selfish, all-consuming love. It is a desire to be involved with others without any thought of exploitation. Emotionally healthy individuals are able to respond to both the expressed and unexpressed needs of the people they love. To be emotionally healthy, one must also be highly sensitive to the needs of others.

Another factor involved in achieving good emotional health is enjoyment of one's work. *Work,* in this sense, is whatever you are devoting most of your time to at the moment. For some people it is school, for others home and children, and for others a job. Whatever it is, if you are enjoying it then your emotional health is positively affected.

All of you have probably had days when the last thing you wanted to do was to get up for work or class. You are probably shaking your head in agreement right now. Occasional feelings like this are normal. It would be difficult to find someone who is exhilarated about work or school each day. However, if a person consistently dreads his "work," then something is very wrong. It may be the job; the people with whom he has to associate; a feeling of not getting any place; or doing something that he really does not want to do. Each of these possibilities should be explored by the individual and perhaps discussed with a mental health professional.

Since so much of one's time is spent at "work," it should be a generally satisfying experience. Of course there are people who, because of their education or background, might not be able to find a job that they consider enjoyable. For these people, family, friends, recreation, and other outside interests should help to fill the void left by an unenjoyable job.

Emotionally healthy individuals have a capacity to give of themselves in all situations. The immature individual may always be looking for an angle, "What can I get from this?" The mature person, on the other hand, looks to what he can give, not what he can get. Many people are afraid to give of themselves for fear of being taken advantage of at times. However, this is another aspect of facing reality. Yes, you may be taken advantage of and you may sometimes feel frustrated, but you will know that you have given the most you could in a given situation.

Do you have empathy for others? Empathy may be defined as the ability to understand how other people feel in a certain situation. Empathy is another aspect of the emotionally healthy individual. It can only be developed once you are able to look beyond yourself and to others. If you have a disagreement with someone, think about how the other person feels about the situation. You know how *you* feel, but what about the other person? This is what empathy is all about.

Are you able to challenge and control your anger? If so, you have a head start on emotional health. The ability to understand the emotion of anger and what is behind it is a valuable asset to the individual. Most anger is a cover-up of another feeling such as hurt or loneliness. Anger can usually be challenged along more positive lines than "blowing up." Try to use your anger to change the situation that is making you angry.

This is not to say that the "blow up" anger never occurs in an emotionally mature person. Of course it does, but less frequently than in the emotionally immature person. People who are secure in themselves have a much healthier and easier time of handling anger. They respond to its causes and not to its being a threat to them.

The last factor to be mentioned here concerning emotional health is *attitude*. How do you look at things? Are you an optimist, a pessimist, or a middle-of-the-roader? Optimists generally have a better chance of developing and keeping their emotional health. There are many "tests" given to deter-

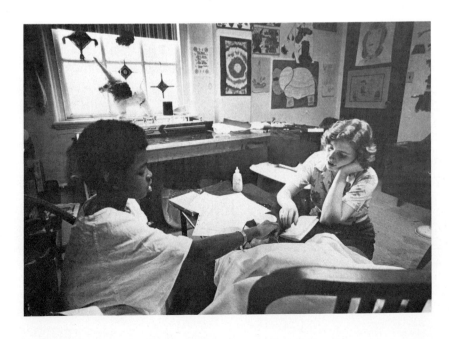

A college volunteer working with a patient at a children's hospital.

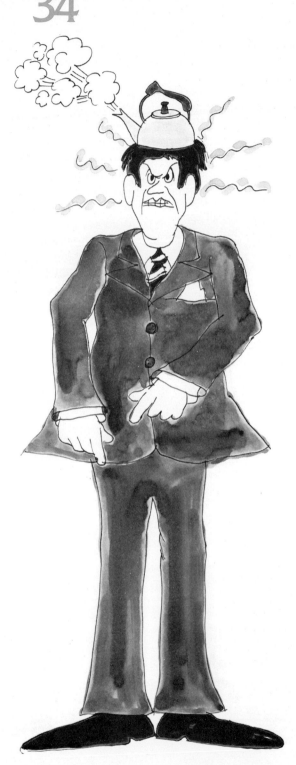

Try to make your anger work for you.

mine if one is an optimist or pessimist. The classic one is to hold up a glass that is half full of water and ask someone to describe what they see. The optimist will say "the glass is half-full;" the pessimist will say "the glass is half-empty." Try it on a few friends and see if you have them pegged correctly.

The story the author likes best in relation to optimism and pessimism is the one about the mother of twin boys. She goes to the psychiatrist and explains that one boy is an optimist and the other is a pessimist and asks what can she do to "balance" them. The doctor responds that she should give the pessimist a room full of toys and the optimist a box of horse manure. She follows his advice and the next day looks into their rooms to see how they are reacting. The pessimist is scowling and calling the toys "a bunch of junk." The optimist is happily digging through the manure. When his mother asks him what he's doing, he responds "where there is ma- nure—there must be a pony!"

Attitude colors the way one looks at every aspect of life. If you enter into something hopefully, there is a much better chance that you will derive greater enjoyment from the experience. This is not to say that at times we might be pessimistic. If, for example, your house burns down and your car is demol- ished in an accident and on top of that you forgot to mail the insurance premium for both the house and car, then you are entitled to be pessimistic. In fact, you might cer- tainly have a "reality" problem if you *were* optimistic. This, of course, is a very extreme example. Optimism is a generally healthy attitude but there are times in everyone's life when they have the right and the need to feel pessimistic about a situation.

In general, optimism is just a way of looking at a situation until one has reason for not being optimistic. At least this allows you to give a person or situation a chance and avoids prejudgment. Do you tend to come to a con- clusion about people and situations without really knowing about them?

All the factors discussed in this section are important to emotional health. You may be wondering, can a person be emotionally healthy without having all of these capacities? Yes, one can be as long as most of the elements are either represented or at least understood. Very few people exhibit all of these qualities. Some people have the ability to exhibit them but not the desire to consciously work at them. Others are unable to exhibit these qualities without some professional help. Still others fall into the category of "emotional cripples" and because of their damaged self-concept and inability to relate, they may never be able to be emotionally healthy.

As a brief review of this section, consider the following checklist of factors involved in good emotional health. How many of these qualities do you possess? Which are your strong points and which are your weak points? Do you consider yourself emotionally healthy based on these eight factors?

1. Ability to adjust and adapt.
2. Ability to face reality.
3. Ability to love others.
4. Satisfaction in one's work.
5. Ability to give of oneself.
6. Ability to empathize with others.
7. Ability to challenge and control anger.
8. Generally optimistic attitude toward life.

Take a piece of paper and write down the numbers that correspond to these factors in the order that you think is most important to emotional health. If you think that some are equally important put those numbers on the same line. Are there any that you think are unimportant? Are there any other factors that you would add?

the need to develop a personal value system

Your personal values are formed by the influences placed on you throughout life. These influences are both conscious and unconscious; overt and subtle. Personal values are not a "set" thing. They grow and change as you do depending on your experiences and the people who have a role in influencing your life. The value system you have today may be quite different from the one you will have in ten years. For example, think about some of the values you had ten years ago. How are they different from those values you have today?

You may be asking yourself, "Why does one need a value system?" Values give one a head start on making decisions. The way you feel about something, or "value" it, will to a great degree affect the course of your actions. For example, if you value education, then you would be more likely to make those decisions that will advance your educational desires. Values help one to decide about the choice of friends, work, and numerous other decisions.

How does one develop a value system? There are a few basic guidelines that one could follow. First, be flexible and willing to change; nothing; including values, is not subject to some change. Secondly, set goals for yourself. These goals are important to keep you from aimless drifting. This is often called goal orientation. However, set goals that are reasonable for you. This takes us back to the important principle of *reality*. Do not set your goals too high or too low. Remember, it is always easier to set higher goals than to step backward and set lower goals. Lastly, make decisions that are your own and that are meaningful to you. You are the one that has to live with those decisions.

The word "valuing" is heard more frequently these days. Valuing is a process by which one learns *how* to value; not *what* to value. This is an important aspect of emotional health. Many individuals have never learned how to value and how to place values in their proper perspective. Do you think that you have the ability "to value?"

Let us conclude this chapter with this ob-

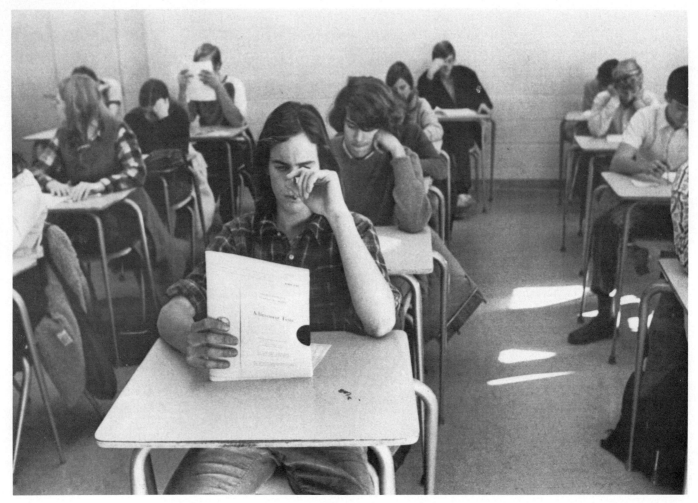

If your goal is a college education then a
necessary first step is preparing for and
taking college boards.

servation: good emotional health is an essential part of good total health. An "unhealthy"
physical self would find it difficult to have
a "healthy" emotional self and vice versa.

THINKING IT OVER

1. Discuss the following statement: Emotional development is closely interwoven
   with personality development.
2. Why is emotional growth considered
   to be an on-going process?
3. Discuss Erikson's eight stages of personality development.
4. What are the four basic "wants" in
   life? Do you feel that there are any
   other "wants" that are essential to an
   emotionally healthy life?
5. Discuss some of the factors that are
   important to achieving good emotional
   health.
6. Why is it so important to be able to
   adjust and adapt?
7. Discuss the term *reality*. What does it
   mean to you?
8. Do you think a person could be emotionally healthy without the ability to
   love? Explain your answer.
9. Do you think it is important to be able
   to enjoy one's work? Discuss your
   answer.

10. Discuss the need for a personal value system. Do you have a value system that you have given serious thought to over the years? Explain your answer.
11. What is meant by "valuing?" Do you think that people can be taught to "value?" Explain your answer.
12. Discuss the following statement: Good emotional health is an essential part of good total health.

KEY WORDS

Emotional growth. An on-going process by which one develops emotional maturity.

Emotional health. An ability to cope with life's situations with a degree of ease.

Goal orientation. Having realistic long-range goals.

Reality. Knowing one's strengths and one's limitations.

Role diffusion. Identification with leaders or other adolescents.

Value system. Personal guidelines and goals that help a person to make decisions that will affect his life.

Valuing. The ability of *how* to value; not *what* to value.

GETTING INVOLVED

Books and Periodicals

Erikson, Erik H. *Identity, Youth and Crisis.* New York: Norton, 1968. The "identity crisis" explained.

Newman, Mildred, Berkowitz, Bernard, and Jean Owen. *How To Be Your Own Best Friend.* New York: Ballantine Books, 1971. Helps you to discover who you are and how to like yourself.

Pirsig, Robert M. *Zen and the Art of Motorcycle Maintenance: An Inquiry into Values.* New York: Morrow, 1974. A father tries to help his son grow up.

Terkel, Studs. *Working: People Talk about What They Do All Day and How They Feel about What They Do.* New York: Pantheon, 1974. Interviews with all kinds of working people.

Movies

David and Lisa, with Keir Dullea, Janet Margolin, 1963. Two disturbed young people find new hope when they fall in love. Distributed by Clem Williams, Twyman, Walter Reade 16.

Making It, with Kristoffer Tabori, 1971. A teenager's growing-up problems. Distributed by Films Incorporated.

Records

How to Live with Yourself . . . or What to Do until the Psychiatrist Comes, Dr. Murray Banks, Murmil Associates, Inc., 8 East 63 Street, New York, New York 10021.

"Friends," Bette Midler, *The Divine Miss M,* Atlantic.

"You've Got a Friend," Carole King, *Carole King Tapestry,* Ode.

3
MENTAL HEALTH

If someone asked you to define <u>mental health</u> and <u>mental illness</u>, could you do it? It is not easy, as you will learn in this chapter. The fine line that divides these classifications is explored in this chapter. You will learn what makes some actions "normal," while others are considered "abnormal." You will also examine some of the misunderstandings concerning mental illness.

The nature of mental disorders is discussed and symptoms of each classification are explored. You will learn about

psychoses, neuroses, personality disorders, and suicide. You will also learn about current methods of treatment, including drug therapy and community mental health centers. Controversies concerning these and other areas are also explored.

Prevention of mental illness is also examined and you are cautioned to be attuned to your own symptoms and those of your family and friends. A good friend can be most helpful in recognizing symptoms of mental illness and helping a person to seek treatment.

While reading this chapter, think about the following concepts:

■ Mental health and mental illness are not absolute, but rather a matter of degree.

■ Mental illness is perhaps better described as emotional illness.

■ Mental illness does not strike without warning — there are a number of early, easily recognizable symptoms.

■ Mental illness can be prevented.

■ Mental illness can be treated by many forms of therapy.

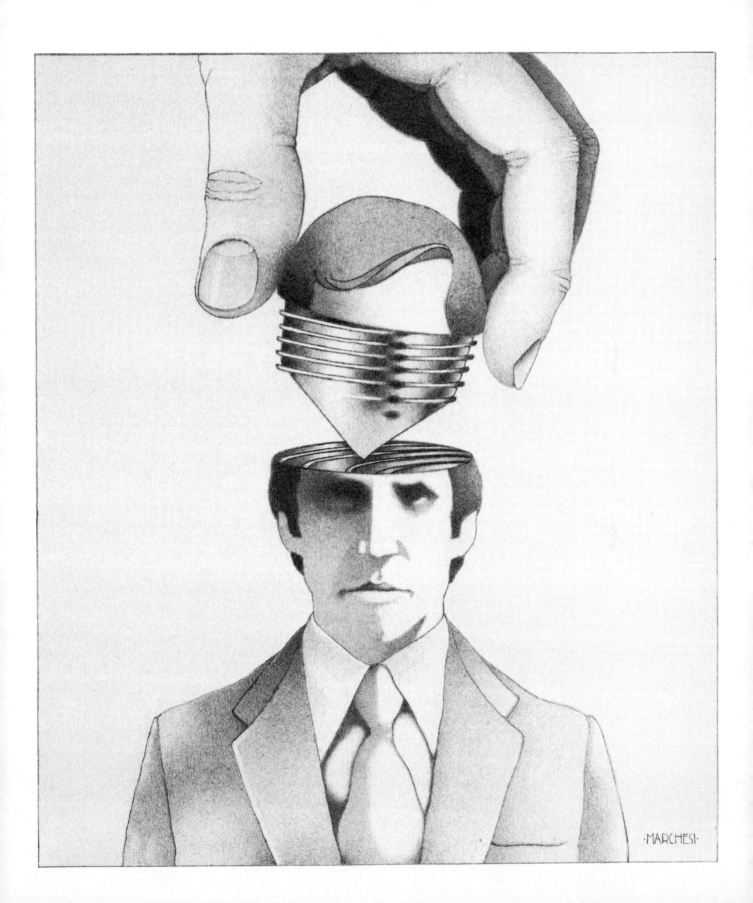

40

The Thin Edge is the title of a novel television series that has recently appeared on educational broadcasting networks. The "thin edge" refers to the narrow line that all of us walk between mental health and mental illness. It is hoped that this type of programming will help to eliminate some of the misunderstandings that people have concerning mental health and mental illness.

This series examined five subjects in hour-long programs devoted to each. The subjects explored included depression, aggression, guilt, anxiety, and sexuality. Each of the programs delved into the genetic, biochemical, and environmental aspects of certain mental disorders in an attempt to "demystify" these highly emotional states. Current knowledge, treatment, and prevention were also examined. In addition, hotlines to answer questions and community outreach and public education projects in cooperation with local mental health groups were provided and planned.

Programs such as the *Thin Edge* are desperately needed so that people can better understand and learn how to cope with their mental and emotional problems. Many millions of Americans suffer from mental health problems and few know how or where to seek help. Many individuals think that "they are the only ones" suffering from certain symptoms. Programs, such as this one, allow people to see that many others share a similar problem. For example, it has been estimated that more than 60 million Americans suffer from depression and more than six million of these individuals need medical help in overcoming severe depression symptoms.

In the first section of the chapter, the "thin edge" between mental health and mental illness is explored. Neither is an absolute, definitive term, but, instead, a matter of degree. The key to mental health is the ability to cope and keep one's balance along this "thin edge."

mental health versus mental illness

Sigmund Freud defined mental health in his writings some 50 years ago. His definition was simple: The ability to work and the ability to love. This definition is, perhaps, too simple for the complex world we live in today. One can have both of these abilities (to love and to work) and still not be mentally healthy. Certainly these two factors are important to mental health, but there are other factors of equal importance.

As previously mentioned, mental health and mental illness are not absolute terms. Both are dependent on the degree to which a person exhibits certain behavior patterns. What is considered normal or abnormal differs from society to society and even among groups within the same society. What one society approves as normal behavior, another society might be shocked at. For example, some cultures used to kill deformed children at birth, while other cultures helped such children to live useful lives.

Normality and abnormality are also related to how often and when one does something rather than to what someone does. If one cries occasionally—that is considered normal. If you cry many times a day then that may be considered abnormal behavior (except, if one is a small child). If you are neat about your home and yourself that is considered a normal trait. However, if your neatness is carried to extremes where everything is wrapped in plastic, stacked, and labeled, then you might be considered abnormal.

"Normal" and "abnormal" may not be scientific terms, but they serve to suggest a *range* of behavior. People who exhibit abnormal behavior are not necessarily hopelessly mentally ill. However, they may benefit from mental health therapy to help them better adjust to life and cope with its problems. Individuals who are thought of as abnormal in our society may be eccentric and enjoy being "abnormal." However, the majority of individuals who suffer from abnormal behavior are unhappy with themselves and find it difficult to relate to others. Mental health therapy is not interested in making everyone the "same," but in helping each individual to live his or her own life to its fullest potential.

In general mental illness is not an inherited disorder. Most mentally ill persons are normal at birth but are exposed to "mentally unhealthy" environments. The expression "in general" was used at the beginning of this paragraph because some research has indicated that schizophrenia may be linked to a genetic defect that predisposes a person to this disorder. However, according to this theory, the environmental factors are still thought to determine the onset of the disorder. This theory is discussed in greater detail in the section concerning schizophrenia.

Another general misunderstanding about mental illness is that it is synonymous with

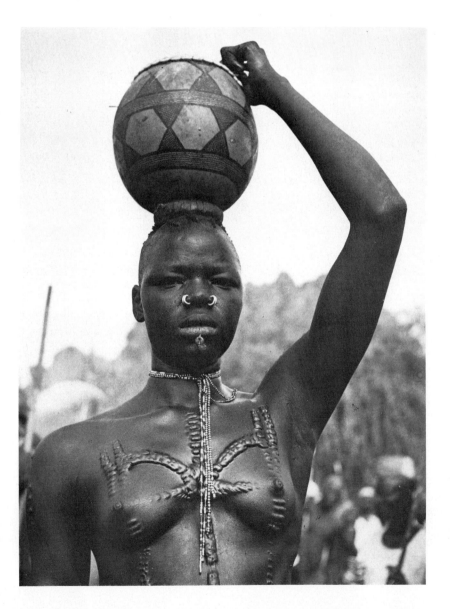

Body scarring is not considered to be normal behavior in our society, but among the Korongo tribe the beauty of this woman is enhanced by the scar-tissue design on her chest.

mental retardation. True mental retardation occurs for a variety of reasons that are physical in origin. A child may be born as a mongoloid as a result of having an extra chromosome. Brain damage resulting in mental retardation may occur prior to birth or during the birth process. Metabolic insufficiencies may also result in retardation. However, this is not mental illness. The mentally retarded individual has an inability to learn to varying degrees; the mentally ill individual is intellectually able, but has an inability to cope and adjust to the world around him.

Some mental health authorities prefer to describe mental illness as an emotional illness rather than a mental one. In this way they avoid any misunderstanding concerning mental retardation and mental illness.

Mental health can best be understood as a complete understanding of one's motivations and behavior. The mentally healthy person, therefore, knows what he is doing and why he is doing it. According to authorities in this area, mental health can only be achieved by the recognition and prevention of emotional disorders before they have become serious threats to one's mental well-being. Once these emotional disorders have gotten out of hand, mental health can be restored in most cases through early detection, treatment, and rehabilitation.

the nature of mental disorders

There are classifications of mental disorders as there are classifications in other scientific areas. However, it is most difficult to assign certain characteristics to one disorder and not to another. Many mental disorders have overlapping symptoms and once again it becomes a matter of degree. Throughout the years, mental health personnel have tried to change or drop completely the terminology associated with mental disorders. But classification does have some merits because it establishes basic definitions of symptoms that authorities throughout the world can recognize and understand. It helps to establish certain guidelines by which an individual with a certain disorder can be treated. Perhaps some day a better method will be proposed, but for now we will explore the nature of mental disorders through the established classification symptom.

PSYCHOSES

Psychosis is the classification term used to describe a mental disorder where the individual is no longer able to cope with the outside world. Individuals suffering from this disorder are referred to as psychotic.

There are both organic and functional or situational psychoses. Organic psychoses have a physical origin such as a head injury, a disease, or a congenital defect. Organic psychoses occur, in some cases, as a result of advanced, untreated syphilis (a venereal disease discussed in Chapter 16). Advanced alcoholism may, too, result in psychoses. This is explored in Chapter 5. Functional or situational psychoses occur from no known physical cause. They are considered to be learned behavior patterns.

SCHIZOPHRENIA

Schizophrenia is a psychoses that means "split" personality. Schizophrenics suffer from personality changes that may be quite abrupt. They may be alternately depressed and elated. There are many symptoms associated with this disorder. Few people fall into the category of abrupt emotional change; in fact many schizophrenics are extremely difficult to diagnose.

It is estimated that more than one-half of all mental patients are schizophrenic. This disorder afflicts one out of every 100 Americans. It usually affects people between the ages of 15 and 45. Young people are often diagnosed as having this disorder in their late teens and early twenties. Schizophrenia is considered a chronic disease that is of long rather than short duration.

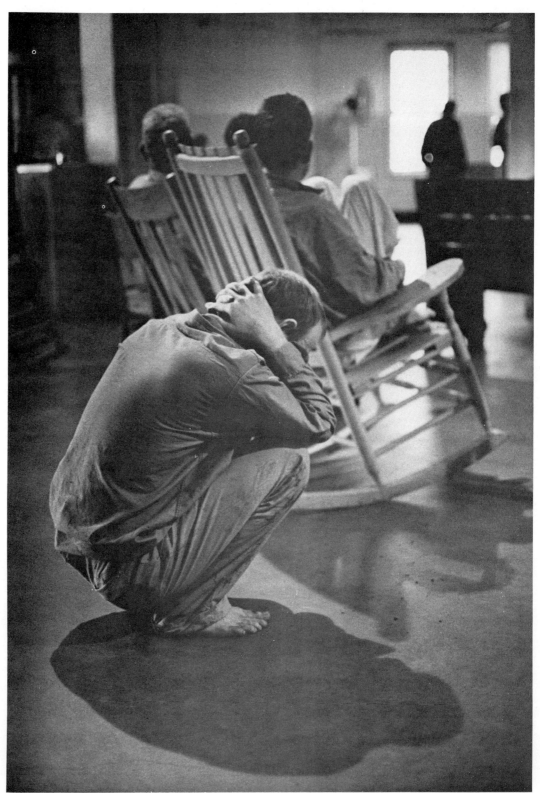

A catatonic schizophrenic.

As previously mentioned, there are numerous symptoms associated with this disorder. Some of the more common symptoms are given here:

1. Marked behavior change; one may be quiet one moment and very restless the next.
2. Severe depressed periods where one may not be able to associate at all with the outside world.
3. Withdrawal and loss of emotion.
4. Conversational change—rapid chatter followed by periods of silence.
5. Delusions and hallucinations (hearing and seeing things that are not really there); schizophrenics may feel that they are being followed or are the victim of some type of plan or plot.
6. Disinterest in personal appearance.

Schizophrenia may have a gradual onset where the patient realizes something is wrong, but is not quite sure what it it. Hospitalization may be required for short periods throughout his lifetime. Treatment is available in the form of therapy and with certain drugs. The problem that still remains is that no one has found the cause of the illness. Many people in this field have found evidence of a biochemical cause of schizophrenia, but research in this area is still in its early stages.

A simple test developed by Dr. Philip Holzman at the University of Chicago may help to identify those susceptible to the disorder. The test consists of following a person's eyes as he watches a swinging pendulum. The eyes of a normal individual move smoothly from side to side, but those of a schizophrenic stop and start or jerk back and forth as he watches the pendulum. Dr. Holzman has also found that close relatives of schizophrenics have eye-tracking problems although they may not have any other symptoms of the disorder.

This test has led Dr. Holzman to theorize that a genetic defect may make certain people susceptible to schizophrenia. However, environmental factors will determine if the disorder will actually develop. Certain drugs can overcome this eye-tracking problem and also alleviate other symptoms of the disorder. This leads researchers to believe that the condition of schizophrenia is related to a chemical imbalance in the brain. This imbalance probably affects the substances that transmit impulses from the central nervous system to the muscles.

SEVERE DEPRESSION

Severe or clinical depression is different from the usual situational depression that many people experience sometime in their lives. Depression in the usual sense is defined as feeling "down," "out-of-it," or just moody. There are real reasons or situations that result in these feelings of depression. One usually comes out of his depression after the situation has passed or has become less important. Typical, normal bouts of depression are short-lived and do not affect all aspects of one's life.

Severe or clinical depression, on the other hand, is a much more serious and long-lasting condition than generalized depression. Clinical depression is defined as a lack of energy and interest in life. This feeling may last for weeks or even months. Routine responsibilities are difficult to accomplish. Getting dressed, eating, or cleaning one's home become impossible tasks. Other physical symptoms appear and the individual may suffer from insomnia and extreme fatigue.

Some severely depressed individuals have alterations of mood and behavior. They may be manic-depressive; that is, they experience periods of elation and depression. These feelings are extreme and may occur within weeks or months of each other. Severely depressed individuals may also exhibit superficial happiness, excessive talking, periods of uncontrollable crying, and unusual mannerisms.

In a recent interview, Dr. Bertram S. Brown (Director of National Institute of Mental Health) estimated that between four and eight million Americans suffer from causes of depression serious enough to keep them home from work and in need of medical treat-

National Institute of
Mental Health (NIMH)
is a government agency
in the Department of
Health, Education and
Welfare. Its goals are the
promotion of mental
health, the prevention
and treatment of mental
illness, and the rehabil-
itation of mentally ill
persons. The institute
conducts research in all
aspects of mental health
and illness—biological,
psychological, and socio-
logical—and sometimes
funds private institutions'
research. The institute
also supports state and
community mental health
programs.

ment. Studies have indicated that about 15 percent of the adult American population suffers from significant symptoms of depression. Symptoms of the disorder also seem to be increasing among younger people in the 15 to 35 age group.

Quite often cases of depression are wrongly diagnosed as schizophrenia. Recent research indicates that in one major city, 20 percent of the patients admitted to mental hospitals as schizophrenics were actually severely depressed individuals. Severely depressed individuals may suffer from illogical thought processes, paranoid feelings, and severe mood changes that are similar to the symptoms of schizophrenics.

Many older individuals have been diagnosed as senile in the past. Today, these people are being identified as suffering from severe depression. Dr. Brown has defined the severely depressed individual as having feelings of "helplessness, haplessness, and hopelessness."

Who becomes severely depressed? Is there a genetic predisposition? According to the research in this area, the answer is "yes" to a certain degree. In some individuals, the genetic factor seems heavy, if not predominant. In others it may be minimal, depending on the type of depression and its severity.

Statistics also reveal that the majority of patients who seek treatment for depression are women, about 2 to 1 in all age categories. Certain parents fall into a pattern of depression when their last child leaves home and they feel unable to do anything more with their lives. This type of depression pattern is similar to that of the person who retires and is unprepared for their future in terms of what to do with their time.

Another interesting factor concerning mental illness is that "single" individuals—whether they are divorced, widowed, or never married—are treated or hospitalized for psychiatric reasons twice as often as married people. Why do you think this is so?

There have been some effective breakthroughs in the treatment of severe depression. Some

of these treatment methods have also been successfully used in the treatment of schizophrenia. One method involves the use of electroshock or electroconvulsive therapy (ECT). The usual course of ECT is between four and ten treatments over a period of approximately two to three weeks. Chemicals are used along with the treatment to control muscular and convulsive body movements. Most people only need one course of treatments and it is a rapid form of release for many severely depressed individuals.

There are, however, some problems concerning the use of ECT. Civil liberty and consumer rights groups have protested the use of this treatment on the grounds that it can cause brain damage and memory loss. These groups have found that in many cases the individual who is being treated has not been informed of the possible side-effects of the treatment. If they have been informed, doctors have told them that the side-effects are minimal. They are considered minimal in most cases, but not in all cases.

A law that imposes severe restrictions on the use of ECT was passed in 1975 by the state of California. This law requires that there must be the consent of a relative or guardian (even if the patient has requested the treatment) and there must be prior written approval by a panel of three doctors. ECT must not be used unless all other types of treatment have been exhausted. How do you feel about such a law? Do you think that the use of ECT therapy violates the civil rights of an individual?

Another breakthrough is the use of antidepressant drugs, which have a direct effect on the nervous system and show remarkable results. Another type of chemical used to *prevent* the onset of severe episodes of depression is lithium chloride. This simple salt is helpful in warding off depression, especially the manic-depressive type of depression.

Like insulin, which diabetics take to avoid the effects of the disease, lithium chloride is taken regularly as preventive medication. Presently, it is estimated that more than 30,000 individuals are taking lithium chloride and researchers suspect that several hundred thousand individuals could benefit from this course of treatment. Drug therapy is discussed later in this chapter under "Treatment of Mental Disorders."

LOSS OF TOUCH WITH REALITY

The severely psychotic individual may lose contact with reality. A severely depressed or otherwise psychotic individual may sit in a corner, unable to move or show emotion, and stare into space. He has no idea of what is going on about him, may not talk at all, or, if he does talk, makes little sense.

There are fewer cases of psychotic loss of reality today because of early diagnosis and new methods of treatment. Most psychotic individuals can be helped to some degree if the disorder is recognized in enough time. If an individual can be helped before he becomes psychotic then his chances of future mental health are greatly improved. For example, there are a number of signs of general depression that appear before a person becomes severely depressed. If early depression is recognized and treated then psychotic depression would not have a chance to occur.

NEUROSES

Neuroses are another major classification of mental disorders. Neuroses are less severe than psychoses, but they do affect the lives of many thousands of individuals. A person with a neurosis is referred to as being neurotic. A neurotic individual may suffer from a variety of emotional and physical symptoms. The cause of a neurosis is psychological, but may also produce physical symptoms.

The major difference between a neurotic and a psychotic individual is that the former does not lose touch with reality. Other symptoms of neuroses may include: (1) tension; (2) fear; (3) extreme nervousness; (4) compulsiveness; (5) physical symptoms with psychological causes; (6) depression; (7)

hysterical reactions; and (7) anxiety and indecision.

PSYCHOSOMATIC DISEASES

The neurotic often suffers from physical symptoms that have a psychological origin. This type of disorder is called a psychosomatic disease. Psychosomatic diseases are real and the neurotic person feels physically ill. Some psychosomatic disorders include high blood pressure, ulcers, asthma, headaches, and diarrhea. This is not to say that the *only* cause of these illnesses is psychological, but this is the case for many individuals.

How do psychosomatic disorders develop? A simplified pattern of development would start with an emotional pressure with which the individual could not cope. Eventually, the emotional pressure is "absorbed" by another part of the body. If an individual, for example, was tense and anxious at work this might result in severe headaches. The headaches are real and have a psychological origin and a physical cause. What other psychosomatic illnesses are you familiar with?

Many individuals suffer from physical symptoms that are related to distress and nervousness. In some people, the result is a "lump in the throat;" for others it is diarrhea and a nervous stomach. In many cases, ulcers have been shown to flare up under tension and stress. The acidity of the stomach is increased under stress and may cause further erosion of the stomach lining. The subject of stress will be explored in greater detail in Chapter 4.

ANXIETY

Anxiety may be defined as an emotional reaction to a fear of someone or something. This type of anxiety becomes a neurosis when the fear is: (1) intense and out of perspective; (2) affects one's behavior; and (3) cannot be controlled by the individual. Another type of anxiety involves feelings of guilt. This is when one's "guilty conscience" overcomes all of his other actions. Have you ever suffered from an anxiety neurosis?

DEPRESSION

The type of depression that is neurotic in character was touched on in the section concerning psychotic depression. Neurotic depression is milder than psychotic depression and is often situational. One becomes depressed because of someone or something that has seriously affected his life. In this type of depression, the individual does not usually feel that he is hopeless as a person. However, he may experience great fatigue, inability to concentrate, and a loss of appetite. Neurotic depressions can turn into severe depressions if not recognized and treated. In many cases, however, neurotic depressions can improve with time and a change in the original situation. Think about

a time when you were depressed. Was it a neurotic depression or too fleeting to be called anything but a "bad mood?"

PHOBIAS

A phobia is a strong fear that completely dominates a person's life. Almost everyone is afraid of certain things. One may be afraid of dogs or elevators. However, a "normal" fear would not keep you in the house because there might be a dog on the street. A "normal" fear would also not keep you from using an elevator when there was no other form of transportation available. However, a neurotic phobia would affect you in this way. There are many thousands of individuals who will not leave their homes because of an intense fear. In many cases, such fears completely dominate people's lives.

A recent television program spotlighted a

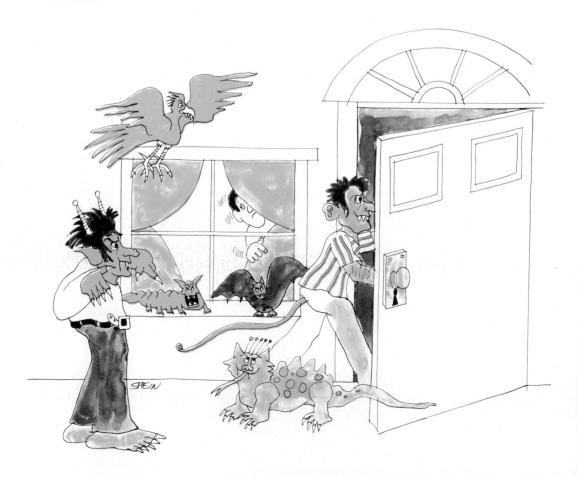

group of individuals who had not left their homes in months and in some cases, years, because of a fear of crime on the city streets. The therapist who worked with these people had made numerous short trips with them into the city. These trips helped them to begin to feel comfortable in the city environment. The trips began after weeks of intense therapy and resulted in success for many of these patients.

HYSTERIA

Hysteria is a neurosis that is not well understood. It involves the conversion of an emotional problem into an hysterical reaction. These reactions may take the form of paralysis, blindness, deafness, loss of sense of touch, or complete unconsciousness. The person suffering such a reaction is not pretending. His limbs are really paralyzed, although there is no physical cause. Reactions such as this were known to occur during wartime when frightened soldiers or committed pacifists found themselves paralyzed. Recovery depends on treatment and recognition by the patient of what caused this reaction.

Hysteria is not to be confused with the commonly used expression, "he's hysterical." This expression refers to someone who cries or screams and sometimes to an individual who laughs in an "hysterical" or uncontrollable manner. Have you ever used this expression, if so, what were you referring to?

PERSONALITY DISORDERS

Personality or character disorders are another classification of mental illness. People who have personality disorders deviate from the "norm" to an extent where it affects both the individual and the society in which he lives.

One type of personality disorder is that of drug dependency. Both the drug addict and the alcoholic fit into this category. These individuals have difficulty in coping with

life without these drugs, and their addictions, in many cases, affect the family as well as society. Both drug dependency and alcoholism are discussed in detail later in this book.

Delinquency is another type of personality disorder. The delinquent individual is one who has antisocial reactions. Such reactions include: all types of crime, cheating, lying, and fighting. The delinquent has little regard for the person or property of others and tends to do what he wants to do when he wants to do it.

SUICIDE

Suicide or attempted suicide is a definitive sign of mental illness. Suicide may be simply defined as the taking of one's own life. In many communities, suicides are not reported, which leads many authorities to estimate that the actual American suicide rate may be double that of the reported rate.

Today, suicide is the third leading cause of death among young people between 15 and 19 years of age. It has been estimated by Yale University School of Medicine that suicide accounts for 8 to 12 percent of deaths among college students. Teenage suicides in this country are estimated at 30 a day and this number reflects a tripling of the rate of ten years ago.

People who commit suicide often exhibit self-destructive symptoms prior to the suicide. Deeply depressed individuals often become suicidal. Many authorities feel that the life-style of the suicide victim involves a continuous movement toward self-destruction. Symptoms of self-destructive behavior include overeating, overwork, heavy smoking, dangerous driving, and numerous other "fate-tempting" situations.

Other reasons for suicide are linked with finances, position, and marital status. Studies have indicated that wealthier individuals are more prone to suicide than those who are less affluent. One explanation for this may be that wealthy people are not used

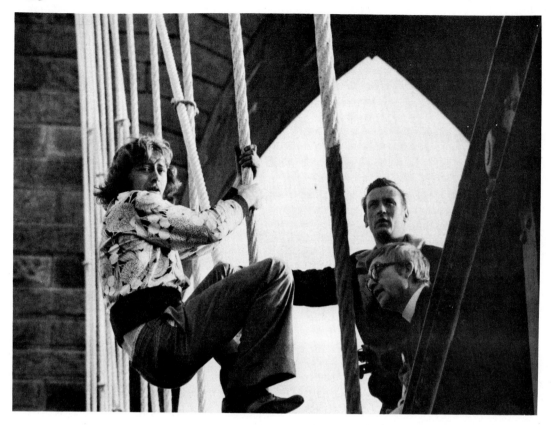

This young man, clinging to a cable of the Brooklyn Bridge, was ambivalent about suicide. He was eventually persuaded to climb down by a clergyman and friend.

to failure and financial setbacks. Also, successful people often tend to lose interest in what they are doing because there is no longer an incentive to do more or better.

More men than women commit suicide, and of the men and women who do, more are divorced, widowed, or single. Many women who do commit suicide do so because of family and societal pressure to be married. Single women often see their nonmarried state as personal failure and some react to it by committing suicide. It can be hoped that this cause of suicide in women will be decreased as the use of the "old maid" label declines in our society.

Suicide prevention has been growing in recent years. Most of you have probably seen an advertisement for a "Suicide Hot-Line," where a person who is depressed can call in and receive help at any time during the day or night. Other groups, such as the Save-a-Life League, also exist for

the purpose of aiding potentially suicidal individuals.

Joseph Hirsch in his article, "Suicide: Predictability and Prevention," discussed the LAD (Loss, Aggression, and Depression) syndrome which often points to a presuicidal person. Hirsch lists the following points that may characterize a potential victim of suicide:

1. The LAD syndrome.
2. Previous history of emotional and physical illness.
3. A preoccupation with death and a desire to die.
4. Increase in age is linked to increase in suicide.
5. Recognition of certain age and sex patterns.
6. Suicide rates are higher among the unmarried, divorced, and widowed.
7. Time, season, and weather may have some influence.

8. The "anniversary" syndrome (anniversary of some important event) may trigger suicide in an already depressed person.[1]

Do you agree with these points and the LAD syndrome? Do you think there are any other factors that might precipitate suicide? What factors do you think may lead to suicide among college students?

[1]Hirsch, Joseph, "Suicide, Part 4: Predictability and Prevention," *Mental Hygiene* (July 1960), 382-389.

Many individuals face similar problems— what do you think enables certain people to cope while others take their lives?

treatment of mental disorders

There are many types of treatment available to people suffering from mental disorders. Some of these methods of treatment

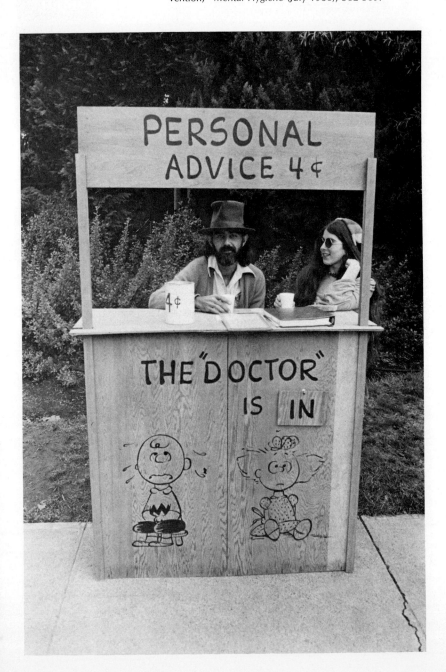

are briefly discussed in the following sections of this chapter.

PSYCHOTHERAPY

The term psychotherapy comes from the word *psyche* or mind and *therapy* or treatment. There are many different types of psychotherapy and new types seem to appear every few years. Some of the major areas of psychotherapy are briefly discussed here.

Psychoanalysis is a type of therapy developed by Sigmund Freud. It involves the in-depth study of a patient from the time of his earliest memories until the present. This type of therapy often takes many years of intensive work by the psychiatrist and patient. The patient is helped to better understand and cope with his personality through these sessions.

Group therapy is based on the concept that people find it easier to relate to others who have similar problems. In group therapy, a psychiatrist, psychologist, or other trained leader guides the group in talking openly about their problems.

Family therapy involves an entire family unit being treated at the same time. Often, when one member of the family suffers from a mental disorder it affects the entire family. Also, the way the family reacts to this person may be helpful in the treatment of the individual. Family therapy is often led by marriage counselors, psychiatric social workers, psychiatrists, or psychologists.

Psychodrama is a method of acting out one's feelings through scenes, plays, or other relevant material. The "players" act out hostility, aggression, and other problems. They are better able to cope with these problems once they are out in the open.

Other forms of therapy are numerous and include hypnosis, transcendental meditation, screaming, encounter groups, behavior modification, and a variety of other "therapies." Some are legitimate and have experienced leaders. Others are money-making

schemes that take advantage of the "therapy craze." Be sure you have checked into any therapy program completely before signing up for it. Check out the credentials of the therapist, persons who have already been through the program, therapy methods, and supposed results. You may also want to check with the state consumer agency for any fraudulent groups that may have been exposed.

drug therapy

There has been much research in recent years with drugs that can affect mentally ill patients. The drugs that are used today with the greatest success are tranquilizers and antidepressants. The tranquilizers are used to quiet extremely disturbed patients so that other forms of therapy can be utilized. They help to relieve symptoms of anxiety and tension and have been successful in relieving psychosomatic symptoms.

Antidepressants are drugs that help to elevate the mood of a severely depressed individual. These drugs enable the therapists to work with the individual once he is free from some symptoms of depression.

There has been controversy in certain localities concerning drug therapy. Many mental institutions have been accused of "overdrugging" and not discriminating carefully enough concerning who should or should not be given these drugs. Institutions have been charged, for example, with using tranquilizers in place of personnel, in order to keep patients under control. Reports of patients in a constant stupor have been released. What do you think about the use of drug therapy? Can you suggest a way in which its use would be controlled to a greater extent?

HOSPITALIZATION

Today psychiatric patients may be treated in state, local, or private hospitals. The large state mental institutions have been on the decline in recent years. They have been replaced, to a certain degree, by the

Psychoanalysis is a method of treatment introduced by Sigmund Freud. It is based on the theory that the reasons for many of our actions are unconscious. Psychoanalysis tries to make these hidden motives conscious, so that we can deal with them sensibly. One technique for doing this is free association, where the person being analyzed is encouraged to say whatever comes into his mind. Another method is dream analysis; according to psychoanalysts, dreams tell a symbolic story about the wishes and fears of the unconscious mind.

Group Therapy, which originated shortly after World War I, is a form of psychological treatment in which several people are treated at the same time, thus saving money for the patient and time for the therapist. For many people the experience of expressing their feelings in the group situation is valuable; feedback from other group members may help them see themselves as others see them.

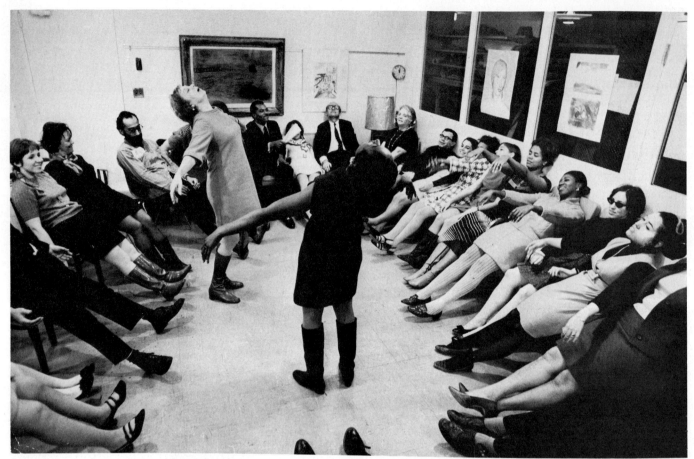

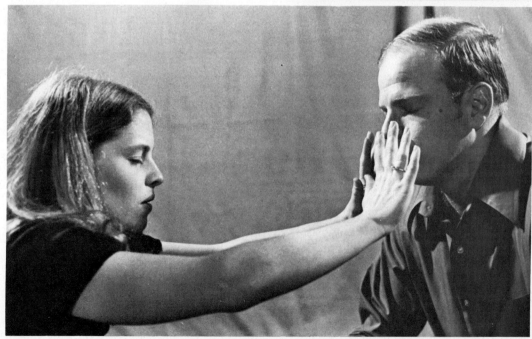

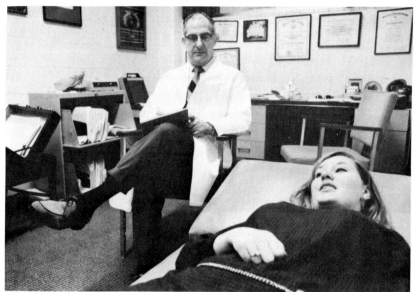

A variety of therapy methods: group therapy, at far left; sensitivity training, at left below; psychoanalysis, at right; and psychodrama, below (Mrs. Moreno of the Moreno Psychodrama Institute directing a session).

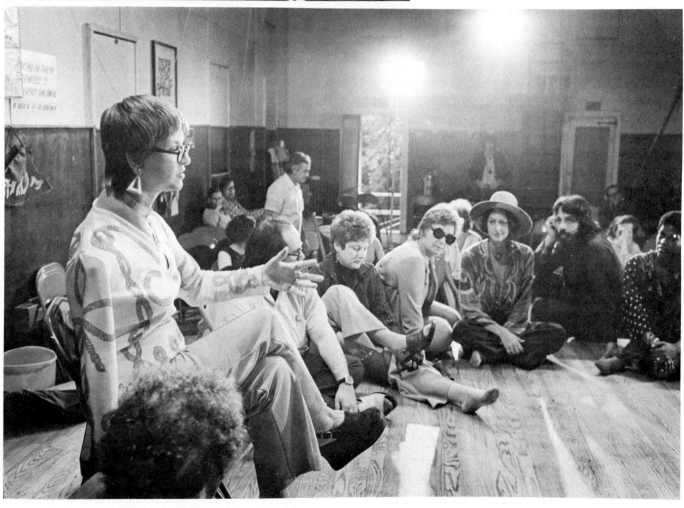

54

Community Mental Health Center. This center involves the treatment of patients in community-based residential or halfway houses. Other patients are encouraged to live at home and come to mental health centers for outpatient treatment.

The concept behind this is to break up the large state hospital and bring the patient in closer touch with his family and community. Nonresidential centers also provide needed community mental health services and are staffed by people experienced in the area of mental health.

Is this approach working? In theory, most people would agree that it is an excellent idea. However, when theory is put into practice certain problems do appear. For example, neighborhood groups have refused to allow mental health centers into their communities because they feared the mentally ill patients. Sometimes outpatients themselves are the victims of crimes, as in a recent case, when a youth gang entered a halfway house and raped several young women.

How do you feel about this approach to mental treatment? Do you think that most people would tend to oppose such a facility in their neighborhood? Would you oppose it? If so, why would you oppose it?

prevention of mental illness

Can mental illness be prevented? "Yes," many symptoms of mental illness are easily recognizable in their early stages. Too many people overlook these symptoms in themselves and others—until it is too late.

Dr. Brown, the Director of the National Institute of Mental Health, feels that friends and relatives can play a vital role in helping a disturbed individual. He advises that one should not continually criticize another person or tell him that he will "snap out of it." Instead, offer approval to friends and relatives and help them to feel secure when they are in a depressed mood. He also advised individuals to listen to others and

take their suicide threats seriously. People who talk this way usually mean it, and can be helped with appropriate treatment.

The prevention of mental illness is related to some of the factors discussed in Chapters 1 and 2 concerning personality development and emotional growth and health. Security and love are essential to the prevention of mental illness.

THINKING IT OVER

1. Explain why mental health and mental illness cannot be defined in absolute terms.
2. Discuss the terms "normality" and "abnormality" and how they are related to mental health.
3. What is the difference between mental illness and mental retardation?
4. Discuss the differences between psychoses and neuroses.
5. What is meant by an *organic* as opposed to a *functional* psychosis?
6. What is a *personality disorder*? Discuss some personality or character disorders.
7. Discuss some of the reasons why people commit suicide.
8. Discuss your feelings as to why teenage and college-age suicides have been increasing in recent years.
9. Discuss a few forms of psychotherapy and how they treat the mentally disturbed individual.
10. What is drug therapy? Are you in favor of drug therapy?
11. What is a community-based health center? What are some of its assets and liabilities?
12. Do you think that people are better off in a community residential center than in a state hospital? Explain your answer.
13. How can mental illness be prevented?

KEY WORDS

Anxiety. An intense, internalized fear.

Depression. May be psychotic or neurotic depending on severity of symptoms; characterized by despondency, insomnia, loss of appetite, and other symptoms.

Drug therapy. The use of drugs in the treatment of mental disorders.

Hysteria. A neurotic reaction where a physical sensation or ability is lost due to a psychological cause.

Mental health. A feeling of total mental and physical well-being.

Mental illness. Numerous symptoms that result in a general inability to cope with life's problems.

Mental retardation. An inability to learn in varying degrees.

Neuroses. A milder form of mental disorder (as compared to psychoses); no loss of touch with reality.

Personality disorder. A classification of mental illness that includes delinquency, alcoholism, and drug addiction.

Phobia. An intense fear of something that completely dominates one's life.

Psychoses. Severe mental disorders characterized by a loss of touch with reality.

Psychosomatic disease. A physical symptom that has a psychological origin.

Psychotherapy. A term that includes many different methods of treatment for mental disorders.

GETTING INVOLVED

Books and Periodicals

Green, Hannah. *I Never Promised You a Rose Garden.* New York: Holt, Rinehart and Winston, 1964. A young girl's struggle with emotional illness.

Plath, Sylvia. *The Bell Jar.* New York: Bantam Paperbacks, 1972. The feelings of a young woman who suffers from a mental breakdown.

Schreiber, Flora. *Sybil.* New York: Warner Paperback Library, 1974. The true story of a split personality involving 16 male and female selves.

Slavson, S.R. *Introduction to Group Therapy.* New York: International Universities Press, 1970. A description of group therapy by one of the leaders in the field.

Waelder, Robert. *Basic Theory of Psychoanalysis.* New York: International Universities Press, 1960. An introduction to psychoanalysis.

"What You Should Know About Mental Depression," *U.S. News & World Report,* September 9, 1974. An interview with Dr. Bertram Brown, the Director of National Institute of Mental Health, concerning the growing problem of mental depression.

Movies

Made for Each Other, with Renee Taylor, Joseph Bologna, 1971. A couple meet and fall in love at a group therapy session. Distributed by Budget, Macmillan, Mogull's, Films Incorporated.

One Flew over the Cuckoo's Nest, with Jack Nicholson, 1975. Comic-tragic look at life in a mental hospital. Distributed by United Artists.

Three Faces of Eve, with Joanne Woodward, 1957. True case history of a woman with three personalities. Distributed by Films Incorporated.

Wednesday's Child, with Sandy Ratcliff, 1972. Based on the work of controversial British psychiatrist R.D. Laing. Distributed by Cinema V.

What Is Gestalt? with Dr. Fritz Perls, 1969. The founder of the Gestalt movement in psychotherapy leads an unrehearsed group therapy session. Distributed by Films Incorporated.

4
COPING SKILLS

Stress is all around us each day. Most of us are subjected to more stress than we can easily handle. This chapter discusses some of the stresses that we experience daily and some methods of coping with these stresses. You will explore such topics as environmental stress, physical reactions to stress, and the stress involved in dealing with death and dying.

Defense mechanisms, as a method of coping with stress, are also examined. You will read about the most commonly used defense mechanisms and why we use them. Other methods of coping with stress are also discussed. The use of drugs in the form of alcohol, tobacco, and illicit drugs is discussed. Physical reactions to stress are also examined.

How can one relax and relieve stress? Various forms of relaxation are cited. Guidelines are listed to help you recognize methods of coping with the stresses of daily life. After reading this chapter, you will have a better understanding of the stresses that you are subject to and ways of coping with these stresses.

While reading this chapter, think about the following concepts:

■ A state of good mental health is only possible when one is able to cope with daily problems.

■ The inability to cope with stressful situations may lead to mental and emotional disturbances.

■ The death of friends and loved ones is inevitable.

■ One must be able to recover from the sadness of a death.

■ Defense mechanisms can be helpful in coping with stress but are potentially dangerous to mental health when overused.

■ When individuals are relaxed and rested, they are better able to cope with daily stress.

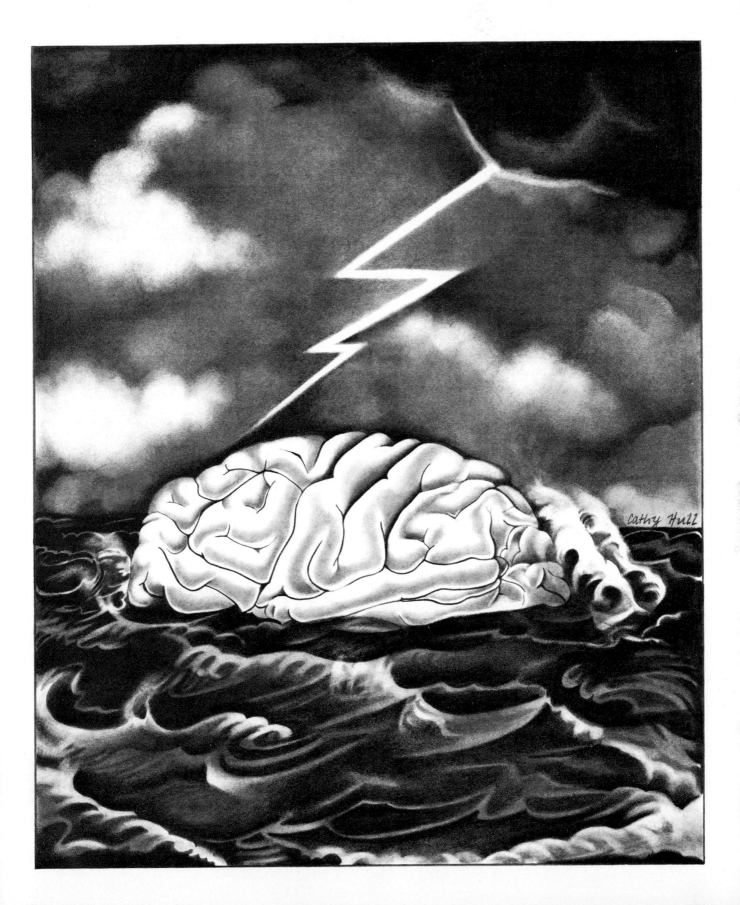

58

A state of good mental health is only possible when one is able to cope with everyday problems, both big and little. Stress is one of the factors in daily life to which people are constantly subjected. The dictionary definition of stress is "emotional or intellectual strain or tension." We know it better as a car overheating in the middle of a long tunnel, a divorce, or sickness in the family. You can probably provide your own examples of stress-producing situations.

In 1967, Dr. Thomas Holmes published his "Social Readjustment Rating Scale"[1] which was developed as a means of rating the stress a person may be subjected to over a period of time. The "stress test" listed a number of events and assigned numerical values to these stress-inducing events. For example, death of a spouse was valued at 100 stress points (the highest possible stress rating). Other stress factors included divorce, pregnancy, change in job, and financial difficulties.

In order to take the test, you check any of the events listed that has occurred in your life that year. By adding up the number of stress points assigned to each event, you will have a total of the amount of stress you have been exposed to during that period of time. This total can be used to predict your chance of suffering serious illness within the next two years. Dr. Holmes believes that there is a strong relationship between stress and physical illness. This is not to say that a high score will guarantee sickness, but it is an indication that one could become ill as a result of this stress.

Take the stress test on page 59 and add up your score. Do you think that emotional stress can result in physical illness? Have you had this happen to you? If so, think about how it could have happened.

Hans Selye (1907-   ), a Viennese-born doctor, now lives in Canada, where he is associated with the University of Montreal. Dr. Selye's research is mainly concerned with how the body adapts to various conditions. He has shown that stress—both mental and physical—can cause actual bodily changes.

stress and stressful situations

In his book, *The Stress of Life,* Dr. Hans Selye discusses in detail how stress can result in physical illness and what one can do to control this to some extent. Dr. Selye defines stress as "essentially the rate of wear and tear caused by life." Most people are aware of the effects of stressful situations. However, *all* stress is not bad; some stress conditions can be an invaluable experience and can leave people feeling very good about themselves. For example, if one is under stress to get a good grade in a subject and does, the stress may have played a role in the studying that one did. Can you think of any other examples where stress has played a positive role in a particular situation? What were they?

Selye developed the concept of the stress syndrome or the general adaptation syndrome (G.A.S.) The stress syndrome develops in three stages. The first stage is the *alarm reaction,* wherein the body sounds an alarm as a reaction to stress. The second or resistance stage is when the body attempts to return to the steady-state or homeostasis. In the final or *exhaustion stage,* there is little resistance to infectious organisms and there may be a generalized breakdown of adaptation.

Some individuals are better able than others to release the tension associated with stress. They may have an ability to cope by using certain defense mechanisms (discussed in a later section) or methods of relaxation. Others, who have difficulty in coping, may develop psychosomatic disorders (refer to Chapter 3). According to Selye, high blood pressure, heart disease, allergies, ulcers, and migraine headaches are only a few of the physical problems that people can develop from being subjected to excess stress.

If you are interested in learning more about G.A.S., read *The Stress of Life.* This book has become one of the classic references on the subject of stress and its effects on the physical self.

[1] With the permission of the copyright holder, Pergamon Press Ltd., Oxford, England.

STRESS TEST

Event	Value	Your Score	Event	Value	Your Score
Death of spouse	100	_____	Trouble with in-laws	29	_____
Divorce	73	_____	Outstanding personal achievement	28	_____
Marital separation	65	_____	Spouse begins or stops work	26	_____
Jail term	63	_____	Starting or finishing school	26	_____
Death of close family member	63	_____	Change in living conditions	25	_____
Personal injury or illness	53	_____	Revision of personal habits	24	_____
Marriage	50	_____	Trouble with boss	23	_____
Fired from work	47	_____	Change in work hours, conditions	20	_____
Marital reconciliation	45	_____	Change in residence	20	_____
Retirement	45	_____	Change in schools	20	_____
Change in family member's health	44	_____	Change in recreational habits	19	_____
Pregnancy	40	_____	Change in church activities	19	_____
Sex difficulties	39	_____	Change in social activities	18	_____
Addition to family	39	_____	Mortgage or loan under $10,000	17	_____
Business readjustment	39	_____	Change in sleeping habits	16	_____
Change in financial status	38	_____	Change in number of family gatherings	15	_____
Death of close friend	37	_____	Change in eating habits	15	_____
Change to different line of work	36	_____	Vacation	13	_____
Change in number of marital arguments	35	_____	Christmas season	12	_____
Mortgage or loan over $10,000	31	_____	Minor violation of the law	11	_____
Foreclosure of mortgage or loan	30	_____	Total		_____
Change in work responsibilities	29	_____			
Son or daughter leaving home	29	_____			

environmental stress

Stress is a part of daily life. Environmental stress exists in the form of pollution (to be discussed in detail in Chapter 21). Environmental stress may be caused by noise, crowds, living conditions, and numerous other factors encountered in the environment. What other stressful factors exist in your environment?

Mental and emotional stress are other forms of stresses that can result in anxiety. These stresses may be related to one's job, family, or social pressures. Most people experience some type of stress reaction from their jobs. Whatever work one does, there are usually other people who must also be satisfied by that work. For example, an artist may feel that he only has to satisfy himself, but in order to make a living from his art his work must also be appreciated by others. There are few people who do not have to "report" to someone else for approval in their work. In which situations would one not have a certain degree of job stress?

There are other factors that may add to job stress. One's co-workers, schedules, boredom, hours, pay, and numerous other factors may result in stress on the job. Think about some of the stressful aspects of a job you have now or have had in the past. How did these factors affect your functioning?

If you refer to the "stress test" on this page, you will see that divorce is given a stress value of 73. This high stress value indicates one way in which family stress can affect the individual. There are numerous ways

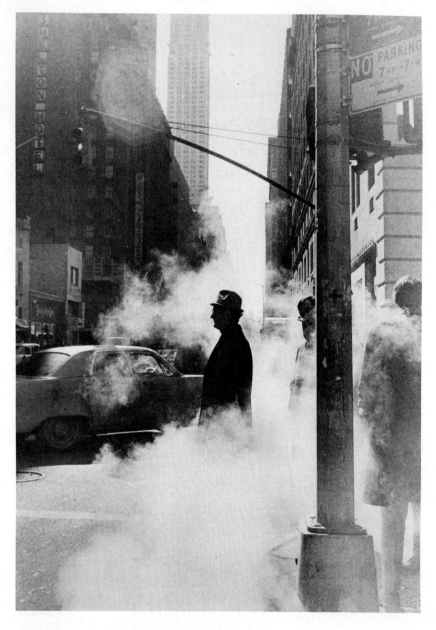

in which interactions among family members can result in stress. Fighting among family members, responsibilities to family members, and interference by relatives are only a few of the day-to-day stress factors. You can probably add to this list.

Another frequently mentioned cause of environmental stress is social pressure. Social pressure differs for everyone but can range from "keeping up with the Joneses" to drug taking. In the former example, many people feel pressured into bigger and better "everything" because their friends "expect" it of them. The latter example is really not much different. People in certain groups are "expected" to take drugs in order to be accepted by the group. This brings us back to *peer* or *group pressure* discussed in Chapter 1.

Many people who suffer from these pressures and who experience the resulting stress have not come to terms with themselves. They are often too preoccupied with what other people expect of them to be concerned about what they both want and expect for themselves.

We are living in an era when change is rapid and stress on the individual drastically increased. Life styles have changed and many people wonder if they are missing out by not also changing. To consider only a few ways in which change has affected us, think about how life can be ended by pulling a plug on a resuscitator and about who is in a position to make that decision. Think about the status of the family today and the fact that the divorce rate is at its all-time high. Other *change* factors include women's liberation, expanding technology, lack of respect for older people, and the virtual end of the extended family. A list of such changes could go on "forever."

How do people react to the fast pace around them? Alvin Toffler explores this subject in his best-seller of a few years ago, *Future Shock.* Toffler defines future shock as "the distress, both physical and psychological, that arises from an overload of the human organisms' physical adaptive systems and its decision-making processes." He feels that there are limits to the amount of change that the human being can absorb and that by endlessly speeding up change, without determining human limits, we run the risk of submitting people to demands they cannot tolerate.

Toffler finds that people react to future shock in different ways. Symptoms include anxiety, hostility to authority, violence, physical illness, and apathy. Some individuals exhibit a rapid swing in life style, while others withdraw and try desperately to reduce the number of decisions to be made.

Future Shock is a fascinating, informative book that will give you a better understanding of the world you live in and how you react to that world. Think about some examples from your own experience that are concerned with change and one's reactions to change. Do you think that the world around you is changing too rapidly and are you experiencing a kind of "future shock?"

The inability to cope with stressful situations may lead to mental and emotional disturbances. Any prolonged difficulty in coping may be a warning sign of mental illness. If people are experiencing psychosomatic illness, depression, or a feeling that "everything is going wrong," they should seek professional help.

DEALING WITH DEATH AND DYING

One of the most stressful situations is the death of a family member or close friend. According to Holmes' "stress test," the death of a spouse had a value of 100 points—the highest on the rating scale. Studies have indicated that during the first year following the loss of a spouse, death rates among widows and widowers are higher than average. In one study conducted at the Institute of Community Studies in London, the mortality rate of widowers was found to be about 40

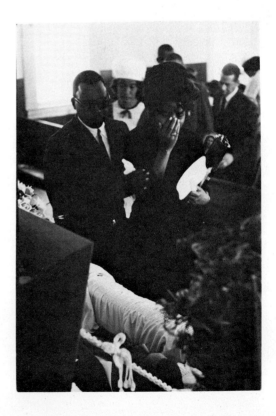

62

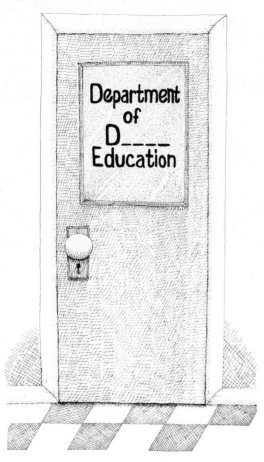

Death is a dirty word.

transplants, <u>euthanasia</u> (so-called mercy killing), and abortion are discussed on the news daily. Death is also discussed through the media in reference to war casualties, crime victims, assassinations, and drug-related deaths. Death is no longer thought of as something that happens only to the old or very sick. It is a subject that should be openly discussed so that people can *learn* how to cope with it and what to expect when they learn that they are dying.

Professional people who face death, often on a daily basis, are frequently unprepared to cope with it. Because of this, some hospitals have formed therapy sessions to help doctors and nurses cope with the death of their patients. Grady Memorial Hospital in Atlanta, Georgia, has formed a weekly therapy group for staff members who regularly care for the terminally ill.

Many of the nurses in attendance reported that there is often a tendency to avoid contact or conversation with the dying patient. Many nurses are ashamed of their feelings of revulsion evoked by patients who had been seriously disfigured by their ailments. The therapy sessions taught the importance of recognizing one's feelings about death and facing the reasons for those feelings.

Many professional people in medicine take a patient's death as their own personal failure. Others feel that they cannot make progress with terminally ill patients and therefore are frustrated in their daily routines. The nurses in the therapy group at the Atlanta hospital were urged to talk to their patients and to learn to feel comfortable with the fact that this patient may die.

How does one cope with death? Of course, one cannot answer this question with a few platitudes. Anyone who has suffered the loss of a loved one knows this only too well. Grief is a normal aspect of death. As in the other aspects of mental health discussed, it is the amount of time spent grieving, not grief itself, that is a cause for concern. In order to better cope with death, one must be able to recognize that the death of friends and loved ones is inevitable. One must also be able to recover from the sadness of death.

percent in the first six months following the death of their spouses.

Various reasons are given for such statistics. Some people feel that excess grief is the major reason. However, others have speculated that the survivor must make a multitude of decisions in a short period of time. These decisions and the life changes that occur following death could and frequently do cause great stress and resultant physiological effects.

Death is a subject that few people like to talk about. Until recently, the topic was rarely discussed. However, today there are more and more courses dealing with the subject of <u>thanatology</u> (study of death). There are many reasons given for the increase in such courses. Medical discussions involving

Elisabeth Kübler-Ross (1926-), a Swiss-born psychiatrist, initiated the current interest in studying death and dying with a seminar that she started in 1965 at the University of Chicago's Billings Hospital. Dr. Kübler-Ross found that terminally ill people go through five stages: (1) denial of the facts; (2) anger; (3) bargaining with death; (4) depression; and (5) finally, acceptance. It helps if relatives and friends are truly understanding rather than patronizing or falsely cheerful.

How does one relate to a person who has recently had a close friend or relative die? In David Hendin's book, *Death as a Fact of Life*, he quotes the chief social worker of Montefiore Hospital's (New York City) bereavement project: "We try to encourage them to talk about all kinds of details from their lives starting with courtship, marriage, family events to cover the entire relationship through life with the departed." Most experts in the area of death education feel that it is very important for the bereaved person to talk about the departed individual. This allows the bereaved to go over some of the experiences shared with the departed person. Many people feel that this will cause the bereaved to break down and cry, but this is often what is most needed at this time.

Bereaved individuals often suffer from a combination of anger, guilt, and acute loneliness. They may feel angry that the person who has died has left them. They may also feel anger that they could not prevent the death. Many people who are bereaved direct their anger at the physician, clergyman, or a close relative. It is important not to suppress the anger of bereavement. Such individuals desperately need to express this anger as an outlet for their frustration.

Guilt may take the form of the bereaved person feeling guilty that he has survived while the loved one has died. A parent who witnesses the death of his child, even if that child is an adult, is especially prone to this type of guilt. Helping a bereaved person to understand these feelings may help him to better cope with the situation.

Loneliness is another common feeling of the bereaved person. Many people feel abandoned and unable to exist on their own. Friends and relatives should try to visit the bereaved person often for many months following the death. The bereaved individual should be encouraged to "get out" and join in activities. Friends should not wait for the bereaved person to call them, but should take the initiative to visit and invite the person out.

We have discussed ways of coping with the death of others, but what about one's own death? This is a question that few people think about until the eventuality faces them. In her book, *On Death and Dying*, Elisabeth Kübler-Ross refers to five stages or coping mechanisms that people go through who are facing their own death. The first stage is *denial and isolation*. The person refuses to accept the possibility of his death. Later in this stage, the person may admit to the possibility of his death but tends to withdraw and remain isolated.

The second stage is usually that of *anger*. The person wonders why he was chosen for this fate and why others were not chosen. This stage is usually replaced by the third or *bargaining* stage. Here the individual hopes that a chance exists that good behavior and cooperation will be rewarded by recovery and a longer life. The fourth stage is often *depression* that is concerned with the loss one will experience by dying. The final or *acceptance* stage is one that involves a realization of one's death. However, this acceptance is not necessarily that of contentment. This stage may be surrounded by fear, anger, hatred, or other emotions, depending on the individual.

For many people, coping with the death of a loved one or the possibility of their own death is made easier by a strong belief in something. This "something" may be God, religion, or an inner faith that some people are able to acquire. For others, death is easier to cope with if they have lived a full and rewarding life. Some people, after having narrowly escaped death, look at life in a very different way. They tend to appreciate every minute of every day and enjoy the simple pleasures around them. You may have heard the question, "What would you do if you only had six months to live?" How would you answer this question?

Death education is helping to bring the word *death* out of the shadows that have kept it hidden too long. Death is a problem that everyone will encounter sometime and therefore the knowledge of how to cope with one's feelings is essential to mental health. It is important to recognize that, as Elisabeth

64

Kübler-Ross points out, "death is a part of a life, a very important part."

the defense mechanism

Defense mechanisms are methods that people employ to help them to better cope with daily tensions. The use of defense mechanisms helps individuals to maintain a certain level of self-respect. By using these coping devices, one is able to unconsciously protect himself from threatening situations. Some of these mechanisms are discussed in the following paragraphs.

REPRESSION

Repression is a defense mechanism that you have probably used often. Have you ever *forgotten* an unpleasant experience or "pushed" it out of your mind? For example, if you applied for a job that you didn't get, you might tell a friend that you had yet to hear from that company. This would satisfy the need of not being refused for the job. You had *repressed* the experience. There are many examples of repression. Can you think of one?

RATIONALIZATION

Rationalization is one of the most commonly used words in the English language. How many times today did you say, "you are rationalizing" or "don't rationalize"? What did you mean when you said this? When a person rationalizes, he deceives himself so that he can cope with a failure or disappointment. For example, if there is a very popular person in your class, you may say, "Is that the only reason to go to college"? By this remark, you have made yourself feel better by insinuating that this person is only interested in a social life—not in books. This helps one to avoid a loss of self-esteem by *rationalizing* the situation to fit one's own needs.

PROJECTION

Projection is the mechanism of blaming something or someone else for one's own failure. Projection may occur when we blame an inanimate object for our failure. An example of projection is when one has a terrible game of tennis and comes off the court saying, "I've got to get a new racquet—this one is awful!" How many times have you used this mechanism?

When projection is used to blame someone else, it usually takes the form of having another person accept the responsibility for one's failure. For example, if you were to fail an exam then blame the professor for failing to teach the material, this would be projection.

SUBSTITUTION

Substitution or compensation are methods of replacing one goal with another. If a person is having difficulty in one area of his life, he often directs all his efforts toward another area. For example, a man who is having problems at work may come home and devote all his time to a community project where he can gain personal satisfaction. Substitution can be most valuable in helping people to gain respect for themselves that is not forthcoming from certain areas of their life.

IDENTIFICATION

Have you ever known someone who idolized a certain "star" and tried to look and act like that person? This individual was *identifying* with that personality. Identification is a defense mechanism whereby the individual gains self-esteem from identifying with another person or group of people. This often occurs when teenagers join groups and identify with the other members. Their self-worth is raised by just being a part of a group. Can you think of any examples of identification from your own experience?

FANTASIZING

Through fantasy, individuals are able to work out solutions to problems. By imagining certain outcomes, the situations that are bothering them become temporarily solved. For example, if you were concerned about the grade you got on an exam, you could think about how well you did. You would feel better—but, of course, the solution would only be temporary.

Daydreaming is a part of the fantasy defense mechanism. Daydreaming can be extremely therapeutic and can help people to relax and feel good about themselves. However, daydreaming can become a problem if one depends on it too often. If one daydreams to the point where one's sense of reality is lost, then he has a serious emotional problem.

DISPLACED AGGRESSION

Have you ever had a tense day and "chewed out" the first person you met upon coming home? This is typical of the mechanism of *displaced aggression.* The anger you felt

Regression in the extreme.

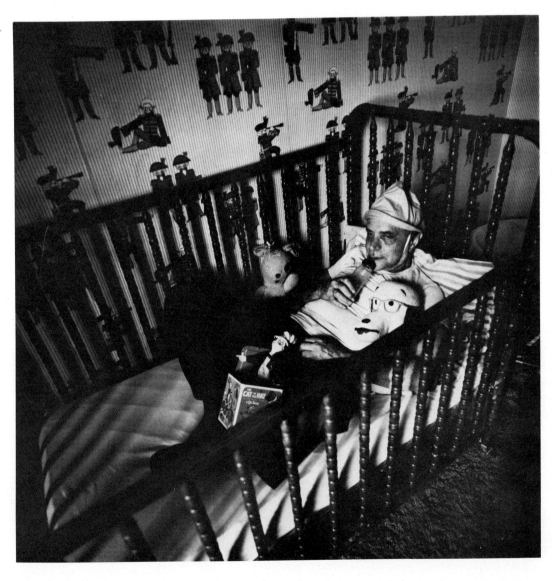

toward your friend or boss is displaced to your roommate, parent, spouse, or child. This is a commonly used defense mechanism. When and how did you last use it?

REGRESSION

Regression, like rationalization, has become a much-used expression. "You are regressing" is often aimed at someone with whom you are angry. Regression is defined as a desire to rid one's self of tensions and return to those "carefree" days of childhood. Men or women may expect their spouses to care for them as their mothers did when they were children. Regressive behavior can be a very difficult type of behavior to have to live with.

EVALUATING DEFENSE MECHANISMS

As you can see from the examples given, defense mechanisms only serve as temporary solutions to problems. In some cases, the problem still remains, only the solution has has been postponed. Defense mechanisms can be most helpful in helping people to adjust to certain life situations; however, if used to excess they can be dangerous to one's mental health.

Think about the mechanisms we have discussed. Take each mechanism individually and try to think about whether or not you use it and if so, how often do you use it? Are you consciously aware of using certain mechanisms? Also, think about how the use of these mechanisms is affecting you and the people close to you.

The use of defense mechanisms to the point where they are destructive to the personality can result in mental illness. For the most part, people depend on these mechanisms only occasionally to help them to cope with particularly difficult situations. Many people are quite aware of what they are doing, but doing it helps them retain their self-assurance and enables them to function better for that moment. It is the overdependence on such mechanisms that presents the

problem, not the occasional need and use of such coping devices.

other methods of coping

How do you cope with stress? There may be things that you do that you never thought were coping mechanisms. Do you drink alcoholic beverages or smoke? Most people who smoke or drink an appreciable amount are using these substances to help them cope. Drinking can be a form of relaxation (in moderation) or a temporary escape from reality (drunkenness). Alcoholism would be considered a total escape from reality and an extreme form of coping with stress.

The same is true for smoking. It provides both a drug reaction and oral gratification. It also gives a person something to do with his hands. Just as the small child copes with stress by thumb-sucking, the adult may cope by lighting up a cigarette.

Some people cope through drug-taking in the form of pills, marijuana, or the so-called hard drugs. They may not feel that this behavior is a way of coping but the ultimate goal is "to feel good" or "feel peaceful." These feelings are associated with nonstressful situations. Can you think of other ways that people have of coping with their environments?

How many of you work out every morning or jog for a half hour or an hour? Some people are exhilarated by these activities and feel a great release of tension through physical exercise. Refer to Chapter 11 for more information about how important physical exercise can be to the relief of stress.

Other physical reactions to stress include floor pacing, finger tapping, ear-pulling, head scratching, and knuckle-cracking. Look around you sometime when you can easily observe others. How many are exhibiting physical reactions of coping? Can you add any other activities to this list?

An extreme form of coping is a nervous breakdown. A person who suffers a breakdown is escaping and in his own way adjusting to a very stressful situation. With the therapy available today, most people who suffer from nervous breakdowns can look forward to a restoration of their mental health.

How do you cope with stress? Do you have certain methods that you find work well for you? Are you consciously aware that many of your activities are attempts at coping with stress? Think about this question. You might find the answer somewhat surprising!

the art of relaxation

Much has been written about how to relax. It is an individual matter. Some people relax in an active way, while others choose passive methods of relaxation. Do you relax by watching a baseball game or by playing baseball? That is the difference between active and passive relaxation.

There are various forms of relaxation avail-

Yoga has been practiced for centuries by Easterners and is becoming more popular today in the West. It enables a person to achieve relaxation of mind and body through meditation and exercise.

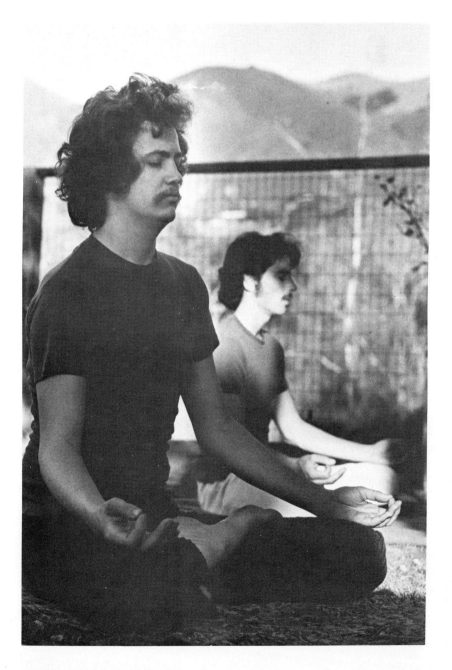

68

Transcendental meditation (TM) is a technique of meditation taught by the International Meditation Society, which was founded by the Maharishi Mahesh Yogi. Meditation, it has been found, slows down the body's metabolism and brings some relief from tension. But many researchers feel that other meditation techniques work as well as the fairly high-priced TM.

able. Some people are active in sports, others have hobbies, still others prefer to read or listen to music. Some people have found relaxation through meditation. Through a system of thought, breathing, and muscle relaxation, some people are able to achieve a state of complete tension release. If you wish to find out more about meditation, refer to the "Getting Involved" section on page 69. Other articles and books on the subject are available at your library.

HOW TO COPE WITH STRESS

As you have read in this chapter, there is no one formula for coping with stress. However, there are a few suggestions that can be used as guidelines to help you handle stressful situations. Consider the following:

1. Develop a priority system. This is helpful in delegating time. A great deal of stress results from poor planning and lack of time in which to accomplish certain tasks.
2. Think about certain stressful situations that may occur. Plan your reactions to these situations in advance, so that you are not taken by surprise when they occur.
3. Try to react as unemotionally as possible to stressful situations. This is difficult, but can be accomplished if one is willing to work on it.
4. Take time out for relaxation. Nothing is so important that it cannot wait a few minutes, while you do something that you enjoy. Usually when individuals are relaxed and rested (mentally, emotionally, and physically), they are better able to cope with the day's problems.

Can you add any other points to this list? Make a list of additional guidelines in handling stress and then discuss them in class.

THINKING IT OVER

1. Discuss Hans Selye's *general adaptation syndrome.*
2. Discuss ways in which the environment subjects individuals to stress.
3. Define the term, *future shock.* How has future shock affected your life?
4. In what ways can the inability to cope with stress lead to mental and emotional disturbances?
5. Discuss some ways of helping others to cope with death.
6. What elements of grief does the bereaved person experience?
7. Discuss reasons why thanatology is an important subject to study.
8. Discuss four defense mechanisms and give original examples of each.
9. Discuss some other methods that people use to help them cope with stress.
10. Discuss some methods of relaxation. Briefly discuss how you relax.
11. Discuss the stress-relief guidelines that are listed in the chapter.
12. Write a list of ways in which you think people can best cope with stress.

KEY WORDS

Defense mechanisms. Methods of coping with stress that allow an individual to protect himself and retain his self-esteem.

Fantasizing. An escape from reality by imagining a solution to a problem.

Future shock. Distress that arises from an overload of the human organism's physical adaptive systems and its decision-making processes.

General adaptation syndrome. The method by which stress affects one's physical health.

Identification. The gain of self-esteem by association with an individual or group.

Projection. The shifting of blame from oneself to another person or inanimate object.

Rationalization. Self-deception by the use of a socially acceptable reason for one's failure.

Regression. Returning to behavior of a younger age.

Repression. The "forgetting" or repressing of an unpleasant experience.

Substitution (compensation). The direction of energies into an area in order to offset one's failure in a different area.

Thanatology. Death education; the subject of death and how to cope with it.

69

GETTING INVOLVED

Books and Periodicals

Benson, Herbert. *The Relaxation Response.* New York: Morrow, 1975. Reducing tension through relaxation and meditation (not transcendental meditation).

Bloomfield, Harold H., Cain, Michael Peter, and Jaffe, Dennis T. *TM.* New York: Delacorte, 1975. What transcendental meditation can do for you (but not how you can do it).

Caine, Lynn. *Widow.* New York: Morrow, 1974. A woman's reaction to her husband's death.

Denniston, Denise, and McWilliams, Peter. *The TM Book.* Los Angeles: Price/Stearn/Sloan-Three Rivers, 1975. More about transcendental meditation (but not how to do it).

Gould, Lois. *Such Good Friends.* New York: Random House, 1970. A fictionalized account of a man's fatal illness and its effects on his wife.

Hendin, David, *Death As a Fact of Life,* New York, Warner Paperback Library Edition, 1974. The legal, medical, and emotional aspects of death.

Kübler-Ross, Elisabeth. *Questions and Answers on Death and Dying.* New York: Macmillan, 1974. The pioneer death therapist gives honest answers to some frequently asked questions.

McQuade, Walter. *Stress.* New York: Dutton, 1974. What stress is, and what you can do about it.

Selye, Hans. *The Stress of Life.* New York: McGraw-Hill, 1956. The noted researcher into the effects of stress, explains his theories.

Toffler, Alvin. *Future Shock.* New York: Bantam Books, 1971. The best-seller that explores the shock caused to people by our rapidly changing society.

Movies

All the Way Home, with Jean Simmons, Robert Preston, 1963. The impact of death on a family. Distributed by Films Incorporated.

Bang the Drum Slowly, with Michael Moriarty, Robert de Niro, 1973. About a dying baseball player. Distributed by Films Incorporated.

But Is This Progress? Documentary, 1973. The effects of technology on people. Distributed by NBC, Films Incorporated.

What Man Shall Live and Not See Death, documentary, 1971. Doctors, clergymen, and the dying talk about death. Distributed by NBC, Films Incorporated.

PART II
DRUG DEPENDENCIES

5
ALCOHOLISM AND ALCOHOL

Who are the consumers of alcoholic beverages? Who is an alcoholic and how does a person become one? These and other questions concerning alcohol, its use, and dependence are discussed in this chapter. You will learn how alcoholic beverages are produced and about the alcohol industry. Alcohol as a drug is also discussed. You may be surprised to learn that alcohol is a socially accepted drug that is often called a "social beverage." How the body uses alcohol is discussed in relation to its effect on the body, how it is taken into the cells of the body, and how its consumption may result in drunkenness or intoxication. You will also learn about the problems caused by excessive drinking. Questions are posed that, depending on your answer, may indicate a drinking problem. Treatment for alcoholics and members of their families is also discussed. You will learn about diseases that may result from excessive drinking. After reading this chapter you will have a better understanding of the subject of alcohol and you will be able to participate in alcohol-related discussions in a more informed manner.

While reading this chapter, think about the following concepts:

■ Many people drink alcoholic beverages to be sociable or because of peer pressure.

■ Alcohol is defined as a drug but it is a socially acceptable drug.

■ You can drink and stay sober.

■ Anyone can become an alcoholic.

■ Alcoholism is a treatable disease.

■ The families of alcoholics should be involved in their treatment.

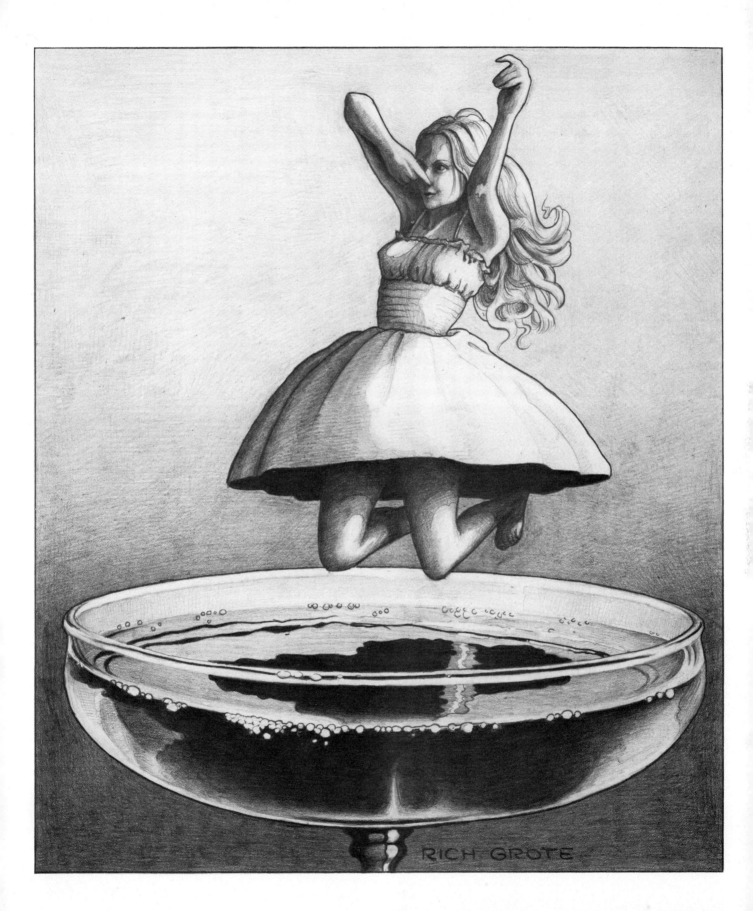

RICH GROTE

An article in *Time* Magazine (April 22, 1974) was entitled "Alcoholism, New Victims, New Treatment." The new victims that the article referred to are young people ranging in age from 13 to the mid-20s. Drinking in this age group has sharply increased in recent years. Reports of young people drinking at parties, in school yards, and at sporting events continue to increase around the country. Why are young people drinking more today than five years ago? One reason is that drinking is in fashion—it is often accepted by one's age peers. Another reason is that it is also frequently accepted by one's parents and other adults. Because many adults drink,

they find it difficult to object to the drinking habits of their teenage sons and daughters. They also feel less threatened by drinking than by the taking of drugs. A story that has been told many times and in many different ways points up this particular problem. *A 16-year-old boy was brought to the local station house charged with drunken driving. His parents arrived moments later and his father, after hearing the charge, said to the policeman, "drunken driving—is that what all this fuss is about—he could be stoned on marijuana or worse—and you bring him in because he had a little too much to drink!"* How would your parents react in this situa-

Many teenagers think that it's being clever when they drink, but fooling around with liquor can lead to accidents or alcoholism.

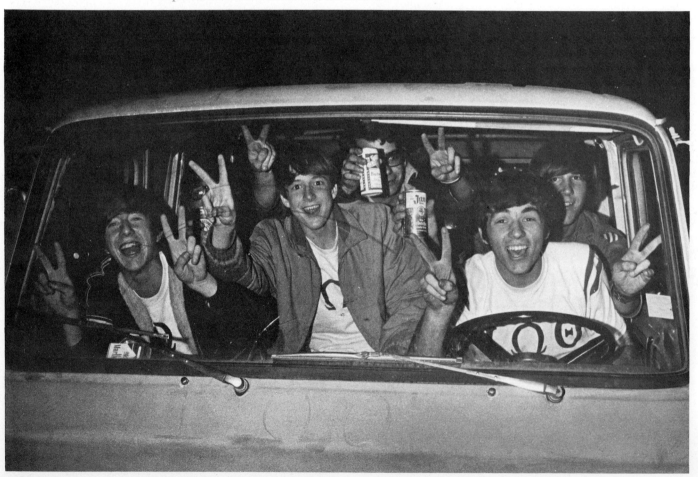

tion? What do you think would be some of the reasons for their reaction?

Many people of all ages, religions, and ethnic groups drink for a variety of reasons. In the next section of this chapter the alcohol industry and consumer are discussed.

the alcohol industry and the consumer

The alcohol industry is a very "big business," employing more than two million people in 1970. In that same year, the payroll for the industry exceeded $8.5 billion. Retail sales of alcoholic beverages amounted to $12 billion, with $3 billion going to tax revenues. In the same year, the beer industry had retail sales in excess of $7 billion a year ($1 billion going to tax revenues) and employed more than 60,000 people. According to the industry, adult Americans consumed more than 367 million gallons of alcoholic beverages and 115 million gallons of beer in 1970. In addition, the industry also reports a consumption of over 200 million gallons of wine and 100 million gallons of illegally produced alcholic beverages for the same year.

There are more than 500,000 firms involved in the production of alcoholic beverages. Bottles, labels, cans, and transportation services are all involved in getting the product bottled and delivered to the consumer. In 1970, it was estimated that more than $100 was spent for every man, woman, and child in the United States on all types of alcoholic beverages as compared to approximately $70 per person in 1960.

The consumption of alcohol per person has increased 26 percent during the years from 1960 to 1970. It is estimated that Americans consume 2.6 gallons of alcohol per adult every year. According to recent statistics, there are 95 million Americans who drink to some degree. Of the 95 million reported drinkers, one out of every ten or roughly 9 percent are considered problem drinkers or alcoholics. Alcohol abuse is discussed later in this chapter.

WHO ARE THE CONSUMERS OF ALCOHOLIC BEVERAGES?

As you can see by the statistics, more than 95 million persons in the United States drink to some degree. Who are these 95 million Americans? They are teenagers, young men and women, and adults. They come from many different social and economic backgrounds as well as religious and *ethnic* (a group of people having a common language or customs) groups. They drink infrequently, moderately, and heavily. Of the people who drink, 25 percent are moderate to heavy drinkers and 45 percent are light or occasional drinkers. Men and women in the 45 to 49 age group are the heaviest drinkers. Men, however, drink more heavily than women. Statistics also show that heavy alcohol consumers are more likely to be single, divorced, or separated persons rather than married or widowed individuals.

Surveys in recent years indicate that about 90 percent of all college students and 65 to 75 percent of high school students drink alcoholic beverages. A study conducted in San Mateo, California, indicated that drinking has increased among that city's high school students between the years 1970 to 1973. This study identified a drinker as anyone who used alcohol on 50 or more occasions during the year. The results of the study indicated a 12 percent increase of drinkers among ninth grade boys (11 percent in 1970 to 23 percent in 1973) and a 13 percent increase among senior boys (27 percent in 1970 to 40 percent in 1973). The increase in drinking among senior girls was 15 percent (14 percent in 1970 to 29 percent in 1973). Think about these statistics in relation to the number of persons who drank in your high school class or among your close friends. How do these statistics agree with your own experience? If they differ greatly, try to explain why.

People may differ in their drinking habits according to their social and economic levels. It is interesting to note that higher socioeconomic groups include a greater

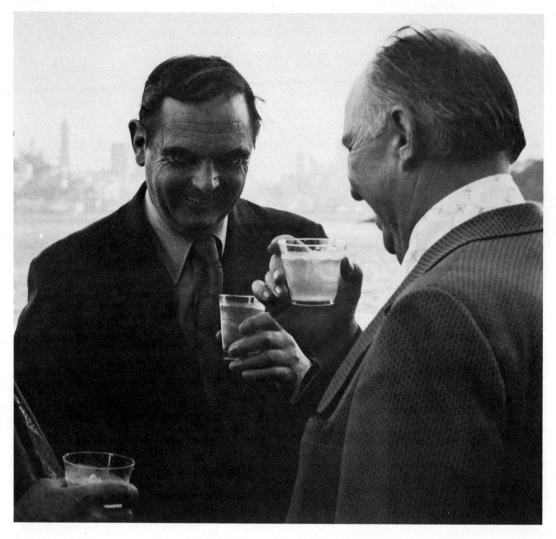

number of drinkers, but they drink less heavily than lower socioeconomic groups. More persons drink in the above $5,000 income level than those in lower income groups. However, heavy drinkers are most commonly found in the $4,000 or lower income level. The largest number of alcohol consumers are middle-management people, professionals, and salespeople.

Where people live also affects their drinking habits. People who live in large cities tend to drink more frequently, and alcohol is an important part of urban entertaining. Cocktail parties, pool parties, and business luncheons all involve some drinking. In fact, some people claim that more business is accom-

plished over two or three martinis at lunch than in two or three days of meetings. Persons who live in rural areas or in small towns usually drink less than their urban counterparts. Some of the reasons for this include the church and the type of social events that take place in rural areas. Many rural people depend on the church for social activities, and parties and dances are often community events where entire families are involved.

Drinking among ethnic and religious groups has been studied by many people in many different ways. It has been found that first generation or foreign-born citizens of the United States include a higher percentage of moderate drinkers than do second or third generation Americans. There are more Irish, Italian, Polish, or Russian Americans who drink than people from other ethnic backgrounds. Drinking, for example, among the Irish is a friendly experience rather than a ritual connected with a religious event. Persons of Scottish and English backgrounds have the greatest number of abstainers from alcohol. Episcopalians, Jews, and Catholics drink more than other religious groups. However, a greater percentage of Catholics are heavy drinkers. Among the people that you know, do drinking patterns break down by any socioeconomic, religious, or ethnic group?

Persons who consume alcohol do so for a variety of reasons. One of the more obvious reasons is the example of parents and friends. If children are brought up in a home where alcohol is consumed on an everyday basis, then the children also tend to consume alcohol in their teenage years or as adults. In one study of teenage drinking, half of the teenagers polled said they had had their first drink in the presence of their parents. Parents sometimes think it's "cute" to give a youngster a taste of a drink or some beer. If the parent is permissive with alcoholic beverages then the children will most likely follow this established pattern. Did your parents or their friends ever offer you a drink before you were eighteen? Think about the time you had your first drink and the circumstances surrounding it. What are your feelings concerning alcohol permissiveness on the part of parents?

WHY DO PEOPLE DRINK?

We have briefly discussed the alcohol consumer and some of the reasons why he drinks. In this section, we will explore some of the underlying reasons that generally motivate people to drink.

One reason why most people drink is because of peer pressure. Peer pressure exists in all age groups and is certainly not limited to teenagers or young people. In an earlier discussion, you were asked to think about the circumstances surrounding your first

drink. If you weren't in the presence of parents or family, most likely you were with your friends. Most of us have been through the scene where a friend has a bottle of liquor at a party and says something like, "a little never hurt anyone—try it, you'll like it!" When college students have been interviewed about their first drink, most answered that it took place between the ages of 15 and 19 (closer to 15 for boys) and that they often hated the taste of the drink and became sick. But these experiences did not keep them from drinking again, shortly after the first experience. Many college girls who were asked to reveal their first drinking experience remember having that first drink with their parents. Many girls reported that their parents gave them the "first" drink as a ritual in preparation for what they might experience at college.

Peer pressure exists in all age groups but is particularly strong among teenagers. As you may recall from Chapter 1, belonging to a group and feeling accepted is essential to the teenager. Being a part of a crowd that drinks will entice many teenagers to drink. In some peer groups, the avoidance of liquor keeps the group together. Young people frequently have the option to become a part of a drinking or a nondrinking group. However, the drinking group may be considered to be the "in" or "swinging" group while the nondrinking group may be less popular and looked down upon by the majority of teenagers.

In one study, teenagers were asked to give their personal reasons for drinking. Approximately half of the boys and girls polled responded that they drank because they liked it. Less than a quarter of the teenagers polled said they drank to be with the crowd. About the same number responded that they drank to celebrate an occasion. Very few stated that they drank because they were unhappy.

Another reason why many teenagers drink is because it is illegal (today most teenagers can drink at age 18) and therefore drinking remains both a forbidden and desired experience for young teenagers. The human mind

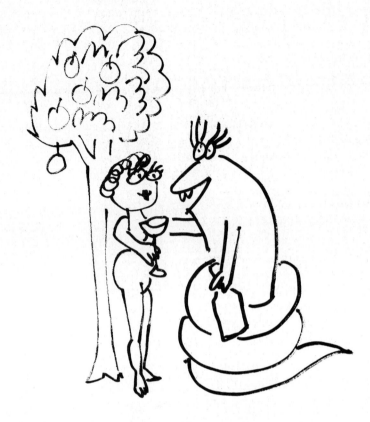

Forbidden fruit.

often sees that which is forbidden as more tempting than that which is free for it to have. There is also a certain excitement attached to drinking and keeping it from one's parents or others who might disapprove. Why do you think that the illegality of drinking at a certain age is an inducement to drink? Have you personally found this to be true?

When teenagers drink many persons say it is for peer group approval. However, when adults drink, the term frequently heard is that they drink to be "sociable." One drinks in the company of others for relaxation and to alleviate the tensions of the day. Adult parties are often judged by the kind and amount of liquor consumed. Peer pressure is strong in adult groups and the abstainer or light drinker is often teased or put down because of his drinking habits. Drinkers tend to want everyone to join them so *"they can have as much fun as us!"*

Drinking leaves many people with a very pleasant effect. Shy people may speak more openly, and persons with small nagging problems may forget them temporarily. Many people enjoy the feeling they get from a few drinks and drink to achieve that "high." It is not a feeling they desperately "need" to have, but rather a pleasant feeling that may add to sociability. These people are social drinkers who drink lightly or moderately and are able to enjoy the drinking experience, feel good at having a few drinks, and know how to drink and how much to drink. These are not dependent drinkers who *must* have a drink in order to get through a social encounter with others.

People may also begin to drink because they do not feel a part of any group. This is a bit more complex than peer group pressure. It involves a feeling of despair by many people concerning family, friends, or the church. Many families no longer have the close-knit ties of years ago. Young couples are often living many miles from parents or other relatives. Young mothers have no one to help them care for their children or to talk to about their problems. Families are breaking up more frequently, and divorce is much more common today than ever before. Many people find themselves living alone and having to make difficult adjustments without any help from others. In addition, we live in a very mobile time when a person may live in many areas of the country before his retirement. A new job, a new home, and new friends all mean adjustments that are often most difficult. Many people no longer have church affiliations as they did in the past. They attend church with less frequency, and social activities are usually separate from the church. All of these factors result in people feeling that they do not belong. They may turn to drinking in order to help them adjust to these life experiences and tolerate changes in a less tension-producing manner. If drinking is kept to a minimum, the result may be helpful under certain circumstances. However, if one finds himself dependent on alcohol to cope with every problematic situation, then he is probably headed toward alcohol dependency, which is discussed later in this chapter.

People also drink liquor because it is readily available and widely advertized. Millions of dollars are spent each year on advertising, packaging, and generally "pushing" alcohol into every conceivable outlet. It is sold at drugstores, grocery store counters, liquor stores, cocktail lounges, bars, and restaurants. It is displayed as a gift and packaged for holiday giving. More people probably give and receive alcohol at Christmas than any other type of gift, and large quantities of alcoholic beverages are consumed at the many traditional holiday parties. In fact, it is reported that one-half of all yearly sales of packaged liquor occur during December. Alcohol, as was discussed earlier in this chapter, is big business, with large tax revenues going to the government. It may be harmful to the general public in some cases,

but it is beneficial to its producers, their employees, and the Internal Revenue Service.

Think about an advertisement for an alcoholic beverage that you may have seen in a recent magazine. What type of image was presented by the "ad"? Was romance, glamour, or pleasure one of the themes? You can refresh your memory by looking through a number of magazines and forming your own opinion about the image of the product being sold. The masculine, athletic, adventure image is the one often seen in television ads about beer. The advertising of "hard or distilled" liquor is banned by radio and television broadcasting. However, beer ads are common and beer companies often sponsor football games where the audience is largely male and considered to be beer drinkers.

We have discussed a few of the major reasons why people drink. However, one reason often overlooked is religious, ceremonial, or traditional drinking. In the Catholic church wine is an integral part of the service, and in the Jewish religion holidays are celebrated by the drinking of wine. For example, during the Jewish Passover dinner, the drinking of wine is called for in the written service and prayers are said prior to drinking the wine. Brides and grooms are toasted with champagne, and drinking is a way of celebrating happy occasions. Boats are christened by breaking a bottle of champagne over their bows. As you can see, liquor and occasions to drink it are all around us. It is most difficult to remain a teetotaler in a time when liquor is socially accepted and easy to get.

AN ATTEMPT TO CONTROL DRINKING

Over the years there have been many attempts to control drinking. Organizations such as the Women's Christian Temperance Union and the Anti-Saloon League were highly organized, powerful groups that fought for liquor control. Due to the efforts of these and other organizations, the Eighteenth amendment was passed by the Senate in December 1917. The amendment introduced the era of prohibition (the forbidding of production, transportation, or sale of alcohol in the form of alcoholic beverages). The Volstead Act, passed in 1919, clearly defined all the conditions of prohibition.

The new era of prohibition was also a new era of lawlessness where illegal liquor was plentiful. In spite of the hiring of a few thousand prohibition agents, a very small percentage of smuggled liquor was seized. You have probably heard of "speakeasies," where illegal alcohol was sold. In the mid-twenties, more than 30,000 speakeasies were reportedly operating in New York City. Organized crime was heavily involved in profiteering from prohibition, and the gangster, Al Capone, had control over more than 10,000 speakeasies in Chicago. Prohibition

had begun as an effort to control alcohol and crime resulting from its use and abuse and had actually encouraged crime and gangsterism.

After 13 years of failure to gain compliance with the Eighteenth Amendment and the Volstead Act, the Twenty-first Amendment was passed in 1933. This amendment repealed the prohibition laws. Following the repeal of the prohibition amendment, liquor became widely available and general safeguards concerning alcoholic beverage sale and consumption were not stringently enforced. This trend has continued into the present, where liquor of all types is both available, widely advertised, and socially accepted.

Federal agents enforcing the Volstead Act, pose with hundreds of gallons of confiscated liquor.

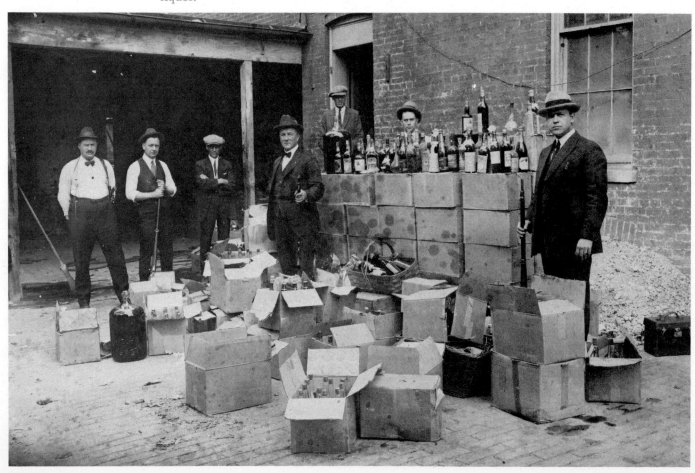

81

alcoholic beverages

What is alcohol? We have discussed the people who produce *it,* the people who drink *it,* and why they drink *it*—but we have yet to discuss "it." The "it" is a chemical combination of carbon, hydrogen, and oxygen. There are many different kinds of alcohols, but the one that is most often found in alcoholic beverages is ethyl alcohol or ethanol. The chemical compound for ethanol is C_2H_5OH.

Many of you have probably heard the term "wood alcohol." Wood alcohol or methyl alcohol is a basic ingredient of rubbing alcohol, antifreeze, and bay rum products. Chronic alcoholics may drink these products because they are inexpensive, but they are also dangerous. Methyl alcohol stays in the body longer than ethyl alcohol and produces a poisonous chemical that is stored in the body. Of course, one would have to drink it in sufficient quantity (about a quart in a week) to produce the highly poisonous effect that may result in death.

HOW IS WINE MADE?

When you think of wine making, a picture of barefoot peasant girls crushing grapes may come to mind. However, wine making today is big business with no time for this traditional grape crushing procedure. Wine is made by taking grapes containing 15 to 30 percent sugar and releasing their juices. When white wine is produced, only the juice is used. However, in the production of red wine, the entire grape is used and the red pigment of the grape skin gives the characteristic rose or red coloring to the wine. Yeast is added to the grape juice and the fermentation process (changing sugar to alcohol) begins. This process takes four to ten days and then the wine is stored in casks or tanks for periods ranging from a few months to many years. Flavor usually improves according to the length of the aging period. The quality of the wine is also dependent on the grapes used in a particular type of wine. The grape quality may change from year to year and that is why you may hear people say, "'69 or '71 was a good year." The more expensive wines are aged longer, while cheaper wines are sold after a few months of aging. The next time you go to a restaurant that serves wine, ask for the wine list. Though you may not be familiar with all of the names, you will see a year printed after most of the wines. This date indicates the year that the wine was made. See if the year the wine was made bears any relation to the price of the wine.

Wine usually has an alcohol concentration of 10 to 22 percent; the majority of wines fall in the 12 to 14 percent range. *Dry wine* is less sweet than other wines, while sparkling wines (champagne, burgundy) contain dissolved carbon dioxide that makes them fizz like soda. These wines usually have a 12 percent alcohol content. Fortified wines such as sherry often have brandy added to increase the alcohol content of the wine.

Wine has become a very popular drink in recent years. More young people are drinking "pop" wines (inexpensive carbonated wines) and "jug" wines (wine packaged in gallon jugs). Wine-tasting parties, often hosted privately or run by civic organizations, are popular with some age groups. Wine sales have steadily increased and more people than ever before are drinking some type of wine product.

HOW IS BEER MADE?

Beer has always been a popular alcoholic beverage. Beer drinking is considered a sociable activity and is an integral part of college fraternity parties, Friday night poker games, and family picnics. Beer is made from cereals through a process called malting (converting starch to sugar). Malt is made from moist barley grains. When the barley grains are dried, they produce a substance that breaks starch into a simple sugar called *maltose.* Cereal is ground and boiled with water to produce a mixture called mash. The mixture is cooled and left standing for four to five hours at a controlled temperature. The substance remaining is called *wort* and it is carefully strained. *Dried hops* (a bitter herb)

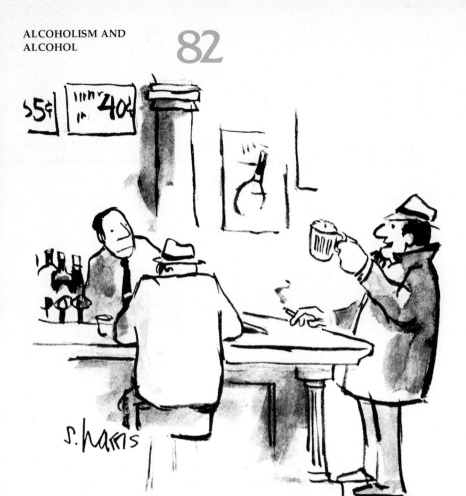

"TO LOUIS PASTEUR, A GREAT HUMANITARIAN— THE MAN WHO KEPT BEER FROM TURNING SOUR."

is added to give beer its bitter taste. The resulting mixture is boiled, filtered, and cooled. Brewer's yeast is added to induce fermentation, and a few weeks later the fermented liquid is separated, cleared, carbonated, bottled, and pasteurized. Ale, porter, and stout are produced in a similar manner, but usually have a higher alcohol content than beer. Their color and flavor also differ from beer. Why do you think beer is usually considered a man's drink? How do you think this attitude came about?

WHAT IS A DISTILLED BEVERAGE?

Wine and beer are undistilled beverages, which simply means they need not go through the process of distillation (the separation of substances by evaporation and condensation) in order to be produced. Distillation is essen-

tial in the production of alcoholic beverages containing more than 15 percent alcohol content.

Whiskey is manufactured from the starch in cereal grains. The starch is changed to sugar by adding malt to the substance. Yeast and molasses are sometimes added, and most of the starch is turned into alcohol in about three days. The alcohol product is then distilled in an apparatus that first vaporizes the liquid alcohol by heat and then condenses the vapor into a liquid again. This apparatus is called a still. The result of this first process is raw whiskey which has a 60 to 80 percent alcohol concentration. However, the flavor of raw whiskey is of a poor quality so the whiskey is diluted to reduce the alcohol content to about 52 percent. The whiskey is then aged in charred oak barrels from two to eight years. As the whiskey ages, its flavor improves. This occurs as a result of the barrels it is aged in and the production of congeners (byproducts of the alcohol manufacturing process). Some of the congeners are toxic or poisonous products, but the amount present in alcoholic beverages is insufficient to be dangerous. Congeners are anything in the beverage other than alcohol or water. Vodka has few congeners; scotch and bourbon have more.

Different types of whiskey get their name from the cereal from which they are made. Bourbon is made from approximately 50 percent corn; rye, 50 percent rye; and corn whiskey, 80 percent corn. Imported scotch whiskey is made from malt and roasted in peat barrels.

You have probably heard the term proof used in discussions about alcohol. The term proof tells you the percentage of alcohol found in an alcoholic beverage. The percentage of alcohol is equal to half the proof. Therefore, if a whiskey is 100 proof, then it is made up of about 50 percent alcohol. Most American whiskey ranges from 80 to 100 proof.

Other distilled beverages include brandy, rum, gin, vodka, and liqueurs. Brandy is distilled wine and has a 40 to 50 percent alcohol content. Molasses is the major ingredient in rum, and rum is usually 80 to 100 proof. Gin is usually 80 to 100 proof and combines alcohol, water, and flavoring. Vodka is 90 to 100 proof and contains alcohol and water. The lack of odor in vokda is due to the absence of congeners. Liqueurs are usually made by adding sugar syrup and different types of flavoring to brandy.

ALCOHOL AS A DRUG

Alcohol is considered a drug (any chemical substance that alters the state of the organism either physiologically, psychologically, or emotionally). Most of you probably never think of alcohol in this sense. When you think about a drug, pills or heroin may come to mind—but not alcohol. Caffeine and nicotine are also considered drugs because they alter the body in some way. Alcohol, caffeine, and nicotine may be termed socially acceptable drugs.

Alcohol is a depressant (a substance that slows certain body functions). If you are one of the people who becomes very excited or happy after a few drinks, you may be wondering how alcohol can be a depressant. The answer is that excited forms of behavior result from a slowing of certain brain functions. The area of the brain that controls this type of behavior is affected by alcohol and the brain "loses control" to a certain degree. An increased consumption of alcohol results in a greater slowing of brain function until a stupor or drunken state may be induced. Studies have shown that alcohol can be detected in the brain within a half-minute after swallowing an alcoholic beverage. Alcohol acts as a depressant to the entire central nervous system (the brain, spinal cord, and nerves that rise from each). However, studies have not been able to prove exactly how the central nervous system is affected by the alcohol. Some scientists believe that alcohol interferes with the chemical transfer involved in the communications system of the central nervous system. The alcohol may block transmission of "messages" from the brain to the rest of the body. Large amounts of alcohol have resulted in the paralysis of the central nervous system. This paralysis is not a permanent condition because the nerves are not physically injured or damaged in any way. When the alcohol in the system diminishes, the paralysis will disappear. You may have heard reports of chronic alcoholics suffering from paralysis of a permanent nature. This type of paralysis may result from dietary deficiencies that often accompany cases of chronic alcoholism.

If you recall the definition of the word drug given earlier in this section, you will remember that a drug affects one psychologically and emotionally. Alcohol tends to be a disinhibitor (a substance that releases inhibition or control). The action of alcohol on the brain cells alters behavior that is frequently controlled by one's inhibitions. A quiet person may become very talkative after a few drinks. A shy person may become more aggressive and be less concerned about what other people may think about his behavior. As the alcohol concentration in the blood increases, loss of judgment, concentration, and understanding may also increase. A person may have difficulty recognizing people in the room or show poor judgment in the way he speaks to others. It is interesting to note that the individual who is drinking is usually not aware that his behavior has been affected. He may believe he has complete control over his senses and body. The next time you are at a party where someone has had too much to drink, try to observe if he is aware that his judgment has been impaired. You will probably discover that he has no idea that he is any different than before he took those drinks. If you have ever been in this situation, recall how you felt about your actions.

In addition to psychological and emotional changes, the person who is drinking may encounter muscular and sensory changes. One's ability to perform tasks requiring *skill* (such as driving) is diminished. Muscular coordination is often reduced, resulting in a shuffling of feet and a slurring of words. Skill tests have been given to people when they have been drinking and when they are sober. In all cases, the drinking individuals showed a decrease in their ability to perform certain skills as compared to their ability in the sober state. However, almost all the people tested thought they were able to perform the skill better after having a few drinks. They were unable to recognize the effect the alcohol had on their ability to function both mentally and physically.

Have you ever heard the term "Mickey Finn?" This does not refer to a cartoon character but to an alcoholic beverage that has been drugged to render the victim unconscious. A "Mickey Finn" may make the drinker unconscious, but a far more dangerous practice is the combining of alcohol and another depressant drug. Alcohol and barbituates (a drug used in medicine to induce sleep or quiet an individual) taken together can cause unconsciousness and death. Respiration and heart function are so

reduced that death may result in a fairly short time. If one takes alcohol and a tranquilizer (a drug used medically to quiet an overexcited individual) at the same time, sleep will become prolonged. Coordination and judgment are usually depressed and coma and death may result if sufficient quantities of both drugs are taken within a short period of time.

Stimulants (drugs that stimulate the central nervous system) combined with alcohol often result in a loss of judgment that might lead to impulsive and dangerous acts or cause serious accidents.

alcohol and the human body

According to our previous definition, alcohol is a drug. However, alcohol is also considered to be a food. It is low in nutritive value but high in caloric and energy value. The effect of alcohol on the body is unlike the effect of other foods. In this section of the chapter, you will learn about what happens to alcohol from the time it is taken into the body until it is eliminated.

ABSORPTION

Absorption (the taking in of a substance through the blood vessels) takes place in the stomach and the small intestine. Because alcohol is a chemically simple substance, it can be absorbed almost immediately by the blood vessels — it does not have to be digested before it can be absorbed. Approximately 20 percent of a drink of alcohol is absorbed directly from the stomach into the bloodstream. The remaining 80 percent is absorbed through the blood vessels of the small intestine.

Many factors influence the rate of alcohol absorption in the stomach and small intestines. The amount of alcohol consumed determines how long it will take for all of it to be absorbed. The blood vessels can only absorb a certain amount of alcohol at a time. Therefore, the more alcohol consumed, the greater amount of time necessary for complete absorption. Another factor involved in the rate of absorption is the amount of other types of food substances present in the stomach. You have probably heard the saying, "don't drink on an empty stomach." It happens to be a scientifically accurate warning. All foods contain a certain amount of water. The water in these foods acts to dilute the alcohol and slow down its absorption rate.

All food substances act in this manner. However, certain foods are more effective in slowing absorption. Foods that are high in protein (fish, meat, milk, cheese) have a complex chemical makeup and remain in the stomach longer than other foods. If alcohol is combined with high-protein foods, its absorption is delayed. Foods with a high pulp content (potatoes and celery) also delay the absorption of alcohol. The importance of absorption delay is that alcohol cannot affect behavior until it is absorbed into the bloodstream and reaches the brain cells. The body has the ability to break down small quantities of alcohol in the liver. The heat and energy produced by this process is then used by the body. However, the liver can only break down a limited amount of alcohol in a specified amount of time. Alcohol that is not broken down continues to travel in the bloodstream to all parts of the body. If enough of it reaches the brain cells, behavior will be affected.

Another factor that affects the rate of absorption is a condition known as pylorospasm or "dumping." The pylorus valve controls the passage of stomach contents into the small intestine. If a person is experiencing pylorospasm, the valve opens before the small intestine is ready to receive the stomach contents. As you may recall, the small intestine absorbs a greater amount of alcohol than does the stomach. When the "dumping" effect occurs, absorption of alcohol into the bloodstream is much greater than if the alcohol had remained in the stomach. The person may become nauseous or have to vomit, or suddenly seem to be drunk.

What you drink also affects the absorption rate. The greater the concentration of alcohol in a beverage, the more rapid the absorption. If an alcoholic beverage is heavily diluted with water (such as beer), then absorption of pure alcohol is delayed. It is interesting to note that carbonated alcoholic beverages (champagne and other carbonated wines) are absorbed more rapidly because the carbonation tends to speed up absorption. For the same reason, alcohol mixed with a carbonated beverages is also absorbed more rapidly than other drinks. Drinks that are mixed with water or nutrient substances (tomato juice, orange juice, or milk) are absorbed more slowly than carbonated mixed drinks. What type of drink should you order if you want to remain in control of your behavior? How is this drink different from what you thought you should drink in order to remain sober?

In addition to the type of alcoholic beverage you drink, you should also consider how quickly you drink it. The speed of drinking an alcoholic beverage is an important factor that affects the rate of absorption. If one slowly sips a drink, then less alcohol is being taken into the stomach and subsequently absorption can take place at a slower rate. If one "downs" or "chug-a-lugs" the whole drink in a few minutes, then the concentration of alcohol in the stomach is more than the body can handle at one time. If you drink too rapidly, behavior will probably be affected and you may also feel sick to your stomach.

DISTRIBUTION

Distribution (the way in which alcohol travels from the blood vessels to the cells of the body) of alcohol occurs throughout the body via the bloodstream. If more alcohol is absorbed than can be broken down by the liver, then intoxication (drunkenness, loss of control, behavior change) takes place. Intoxication is the depressant effect that alcohol has on the brain. This effect results in a loss of judgment, concentration, muscular controls, and other symptoms, depending on the degree of intoxication. Intoxication in relation to chronic alcoholism is discussed later in this chapter.

OXIDATION

The oxidation (release of heat and energy from dissolved food substances) of alcohol takes place in the liver. It is here that alcohol is combined with oxygen and energy is released. The waste products of this process are carbon dioxide and water. The burning of alcohol to produce energy takes place in three separate steps. Alcohol is acted upon by an enzyme (a substance that speeds up chemical reactions). This enzyme, alcohol dehydrogenase, converts the alcohol into a substance called acetaldehyde. This is a poisonous substance. However, it is then further oxidized into acetic acid (a harmless substance). The acetic acid is then further oxidized to release heat, energy, and waste products. The first step takes place in the liver, but the remaining steps may occur elsewhere in the body. This reaction can best be shown by the following diagram:

alcohol + alcohol dehydrogenase → acetaldehyde → acetic acid → carbon dioxide + water.

The rate at which oxidation takes place depends on the amount of enzyme present in the liver to initiate oxidation. The average person can usually oxidize one drink per hour or the equivalent of about one-half ounce of alcohol every hour. However, there are other factors that may affect this rate of oxidation. If a man weighs 200 pounds, his liver is most likely larger than that of a man weighing 150 pounds. The 200 pound man probably has more of the oxidation enzyme present in his liver than does the person of lighter body weight. A heavier person tends to absorb alcohol more slowly and oxidize it more rapidly. The slower rate of absorption is due to the presence of a greater amount of fluid in the body of the heavier person. The fluid serves to dilute the alcohol content. In most cases, heavier people are able to drink greater quantities of alcohol and experience fewer side effects. In your

own experience, have you found this to be true?

Other conditions that may retard the oxidation of alcohol include liver disease, malnutrition, sickness, and the abuse of other drugs. It should be stressed here that alcohol is burned at different rates according to an individual's metabolism (all the chemical processes of the body). Although general rules can be stated, people do react on an individual basis and that may account for differences in oxidation rates of alcohol. You probably know people of normal or light weight that can drink more than two or three drinks in an hour and show no behavioral or physical changes. Their alcohol absorbtion rate may be slower than average, while their oxidation rate may be faster.

You may be wondering if there is any way that you can increase your rate of oxidation so that your body can burn alcohol more rapidly. People have suggested jogging, drinking black coffee (sometimes with a raw egg in it), or tomato juice, and taking cold showers. None of these remedies will have any lasting effect on speeding up the oxidation or "sobering" process. The best advice is waiting it out and sleeping it off!

ELIMINATION

A very small amount of alcohol is eliminated through the body in the form of carbon dioxide and in the urine. Approximately 10 per cent of the alcohol taken into the body is eliminated in this manner. The bulk of the consumed alcoholic beverage (90 percent) is absorbed, distributed, and oxidized.

CAN YOU DRINK AND STAY SOBER?

The answer is yes! Anyone who consciously wants to "stay in control" and remain sober can do so if he follows some simple rules. Never drink on an empty stomach. If you aren't able to eat a meal before drinking, then try to snack or at least eat something while you drink. Stick to diluted drinks and try to avoid carbonated mixers in your alcoholic beverages. As you may recall, carbonated beverages speed up the absorption of alcohol into the blood vessels. Always sip your drink slowly and avoid having more than two very diluted drinks in an hour. If you follow these rules, the body will be able to keep up with your alcohol consumption and you will remain sober. Do you presently consume alcohol in this manner? If not, do you think you could follow these guidelines to controlled drinking?

WHAT IS A HANGOVER?

If you have never experienced a hangover, you probably cannot describe it. Everyone has heard the horror tales of someone else's hangover. The symptoms often include headaches, nausea, depression, and a general feeling of fatigue. Chronic alcoholics may experience intense physical discomfort and emotional anxiety. Some studies have shown that fatigue prior to drinking is often a contributing factor to the discomforts of a hangover. Many of the same treatments that people prescribe for sobering up (coffee, tomato juice, fresh air) are recommended for hangovers. The best remedy for a hangover is to take something for the headache (if you have one) and try to sleep or at least rest.

problems that accompany drinking

The abuse or misuse of alcohol may result in a variety of problems to the drinker, his family, and society in general. The excessive use of alcohol may not be the only cause of family disruption, but it may compound existing problems. In this section of the chapter you will learn more about the abuse of alcohol and how it affects all of our lives.

ALCOHOL AND SOCIETY

How can an entire society of people be affected by those who drink excessively? Society is affected by family disruption, accidents, crime, and dollar losses in our major indus-tries. All of these factors are frequently alcohol-related problems.

Excessive drinkers have high arrest rates for such charges as vagrancy, disorderly conduct, and crimes against other people. It has been reported that more than 75 percent of police time is spent on alcohol-related crimes. Of those persons who are serving prison time for serious crimes, between 20 and 40 percent have been drinking excessively for years. In one study, approximately 90 percent of prisoners who were intoxicated at the time of their arrest reported that their criminal behavior was due to excessive drinking. The National Institute on Alcohol Abuse and Alcoholism (NIAAA) recently reported that in about half of all murders in the United States, either the victim or the murderer, or both, had been drinking. In addition, they reported that in approximately one-quarter of all suicides, alcohol was found in the bloodstream of the victim. As you can readily see, excessive drinking does affect crime rates and in turn society is directly affected.

Another way in which alcohol abuse directly affects society is reflected in dollar losses due to job absenteeism, inferior quality of products produced, and related health, unemployment, and welfare benefits paid to excessive drinkers. An estimated 15 billion dollars is lost annually by American business as a result of excessive and chronic alcohol consumption. This breaks down to about $10 billion in lost work time, $2 billion in health and welfare services, and $3 billion in property damage, medical expenses, and insurance claims. A recent survey of a number of corporations identified the following profile of the employee who drinks to excess: (1) between 35 and 50 years old; (2) about half are women; (3) largest numbers are professional and middle management personnel (about 45 percent); (4) 50 percent have graduated from or attended college; (5) absenteeism is approximately 15 times greater than that of the nondrinker or social drinker; and (6) the accident rate is 3.6 times greater than that of other employees. These losses affect the economy and in turn each of us is affected by the excessive drinker.

ALCOHOL AND FAMILY

Alcohol abuse may not be the primary cause of family disruption, but it is a contributing factor in many cases. The NIAAA recently reported that people who abuse alcohol are seven times more likely to be separated or divorced than the general population. Some of the factors that contribute to family disruption include inadequate income because of job absence and unemployment, fighting over money spent on alcohol, aggressive behavior, loss of patience with children and spouse, and difficulties in communication. In addition, friendships are often lost because of alcohol abuse, and children feel both frightened and embarrassed by the drinking parent's behavior. When alcohol abuse becomes a chronic problem, the family situation will usually further disintegrate. Help for families of chronic drinkers is discussed later in this chapter.

DRINKING AND DRIVING

Alcohol combined with driving results in thousands of deaths and injuries each year. The NIAAA recently reported that nearly half of the one million major injuries suffered in automobile accidents are caused by drivers or pedestrians who are intoxicated to some degree. More than one-half of automobile

deaths may also be traced to excessive alcohol consumption. Most of the drivers involved in these accidents are social drinkers who either are unaware of their condition or are unwilling to admit that their driving skills may be impaired by alcohol. A person who has had only a few drinks will exhibit a loss of concentration, perception, and coordination. His reaction time (the time it takes for a muscle to respond to a stimulus) is increased by about one-third after two or three drinks have been consumed. Any delay in reaction time can cause an accident. Imagine what would happen if you reacted too slowly to brake at a stop sign or red light signal. The person who has had too much to drink will tend to take more chances. This tendency, combined with a decrease in reaction time, often results in highway deaths and injuries. Many of these deaths and injuries involve young people in the under-21 group. Arrests for drunken driving in this age group has increased dramatically since many states have lowered the drinking age to 18. Michigan reported a 141 percent increase in drunken driving arrests in the year following the lowering of the drinking age.

If you refer to Table 5-2, you can see the time you should wait before driving after a specified number of drinks, based on your blood alcohol concentration. In Table 5-1

Table 5-1

Accident probability chart

[a]*Reprinted with permission of Alcohol Countermeasure Project, New Jersey Division of Motor Vehicles.*

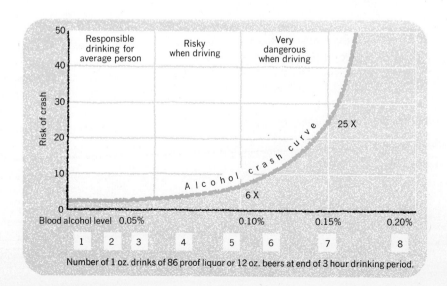

Don't drive over POINT·Z̲E̲RO·FIVE

.05 stands for a specific percentage of alcohol in the bloodstream, commonly referred to as blood alcohol concentration (BAC). At slightly above .05% BAC, the risk of causing a crash doubles. Some persons (especially inexperienced drinkers and inexperienced drivers) cannot drive safely even below .05%.

BAC is determined by the amount of alcohol consumed, the time required by the body to destroy alcohol, and the person's weight. The body eliminates alcohol at a constant rate that cannot be changed. A heavier person has more blood in his system to dilute alcohol. Therefore, a lighter person will be more affected if he drinks the same amount as the heavier person.

If you think you might drink beyond .05%, let someone else drive, or take a cab or bus. It may be the most important thing you ever did.

Here's how to use the chart:
1. **Look** up your weight. If it falls between two figures on the chart, take the lower weight.
2. **Note** the number of drinks you've already had, or plan to have.
3. **Find** the number of hours you need to wait between the start of drinking and the start of driving.
4. Then — **make yourself wait the proper amount of time before you drive.**

NEW JERSEY DIVISION OF MOTOR VEHICLES
Alcohol Countermeasures Project

POINT·Z̲E̲RO·FIVE
Drinking/Driving Chart

Number of Drinks* Consumed

BODY WEIGHT	1	2	3	4	5	6
	Hours to wait after start of drinking and before driving					
100 lb.	0	3	6	9½	12½	15½
120 lb.	0	2	4½	7½	9½	12
140 lb.	0	1½	3½	5½	8	10
160 lb.	0	½	2½	4½	6½	8½
180 lb.	0	0	2	3½	5½	7
200 lb.	0	0	1½	3	4½	6
220 lb.	0	0	1	2½	3½	5½

*1 Drink = 86 proof 1½ oz. of whiskey, gin, vodka, etc. 1 bottle beer (12 oz.) 3 oz. wine (20%) or 5 oz. wine (12%).

Table 5-2
[a] Reprinted with permission of Alcohol Countermeasure Project, New Jersey Division of Motor Vehicles.

you will see the increasing risk of accident if you drive before waiting long enough for your blood alcohol concentration to lessen.

In most states, a person with a blood alcohol concentration of 0.1% is considered intoxicated. How many drinks would a 160 pound man have to take to be considered intoxicated? Refer to Table 5-2, to help you in your calculations.

The most accurate method of determining intoxication is through analysis of the blood, urine, saliva, breath, and spinal fluids. One method that utilizes a machine called a breathalyzer analyzes the alcohol content of the air that one breathes out. Other tests are also used that are designed to determine one's mental and motor ability. If a person is intoxicated, his performance on these tests will vary from the established norm. However, many of these tests do not give a clear indication of drunkenness, as each individual differs as to the amount of alcohol he can consume and still be able to function normally behind the wheel of a car or elsewhere. Have you or a friend ever been subjected to a test for intoxication? If so, what type of test was used and do you think it was an accurate determination of the individual's condition?

alcoholism

Until this section of the chapter, alcohol has been discussed as an industry, a product, and how it affects the body. Alcohol dependence or alcoholism is the subject of the remainder of this chapter.

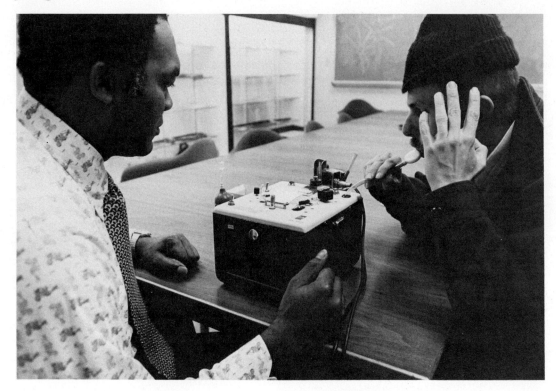

A breathalyser machine determines intoxication levels by measuring the amount of alcohol in the exhaled breath of the person being tested. This individual is being tested at the Charlotte, North Carolina police department.

ALCOHOLISM IS A DISEASE

Alcoholism differs from social drinking and problem drinking in that it implies a need or dependence on alcohol.

The social or moderate drinker makes up 90 percent of the drinking population. The social drinker is able to relax when drinking and usually confines his drinking to certain occasions such as parties or when he is out to dinner. The moderate drinker, as the name implies, usually drinks only one or two drinks and is almost always "controlled" in his drinking habits. Of course, this is not to say that the social drinker never drinks more than he should. Even controlled drinkers can overstep their limits at certain times. One always remembers that favorite uncle who "never" drinks but at certain weddings and parties he seems to "feel no pain!"

The problem drinker is the individual who drinks excessively without control or moderation. He often engages in drinking bouts with his friends and boasts of how much he can drink without showing any ill-effects.

Problem drinkers do not need an occasion to drink, but frequently drink at home and in bars or cocktail lounges. The problem drinker may go on alcoholic binges and then stop drinking for a period of time. It is estimated that one out of every 17 problem drinkers will become an alcoholic. The chronic alcoholic is a sick person both emotionally and physically. His dependence or need for alcohol separates him from social and problem drinkers.

There are an estimated 9 to 10 million alcoholics in the United States, and this number continues to increase every year. Alcoholics come from every walk of life and almost every age group. There are teenage alcoholics and this number continues to increase every year. Alcoholics are wealthy as well as poor and may be executives as well as skid-row "down and outers." In fact, only about 5 percent of the nation's alcoholics fit into the skid-row or derelict group. The rest hold jobs and are estimated at making up 4 to 8 percent of the total work force. Many alcoholics hold executive positions. Because of the tension of their jobs and the many opportunities available for drinking, many of these people may first become problem drinkers and some may end up as alcoholics.

There are many different definitions of an alcoholic. Some definitions are based on amount of consumption, others on physical or emotional symptoms. One definition offered by the Rutgers University Center of Alcohol Studies is "an alcoholic is one who is unable to consistently choose whether he shall drink or not, and who if he drinks, is unable to consistently choose if he shall stop or not." There is no sharp distinction between the problem drinker and the alcoholic, and most alcoholics do not even realize that they are alcoholics. They may drink at lunch, before dinner, and in the evening, but they still feel that they are very much in control of their drinking. Facing the reality of alcoholism may not come about until they have caused injury to themselves or others or have exhibited some serious physical problems.

The National Council on Alcoholism has drawn up a list of 26 items that indicate possible alcoholism if one answers "yes" to any of the questions. Some of the items include: Do you ever have a few drinks when others will not know about it? Have you ever woken up after drinking unable to recall many of the events of the previous evening? Do you get angry when others discuss your drinking habits? You may want to write for the complete list and other information concerning alcoholism. This information can be obtained from the National Council on Alcoholism, Inc., 2 Park Avenue, New York, N. Y. 10016.

There are certain warning signals that indicate possible or impending alcoholism. The most important signal is that the drinker begins to look at alcohol as if it were a drug rather than a beverage. The drinker begins to drink to obtain a feeling of genuine release of tension. He no longer drinks because it is the social thing to do, but because he feels he cannot get through the evening if he does

not drink. Other warnings include a change in drinking habits to a more frequent and more alcoholic pattern. The drinker begins to drink more often during the day and increases his consumption of drinks.

The person who experiences many of the previously mentioned danger signs may be an alcoholic or may be about to become one. Other signs, however, are far more dangerous and usually indicate chronic alcoholism. These signs include the drinker who has occasional *blackouts*. These are periods of time that the drinker is unable to recall. He may have appeared under control while drinking; however, the next day he cannot remember the events of a certain period of time when he was drinking. The chronic alcoholic usually sneaks drinks and attempts to keep his drinking habits a secret from those who are close to him. He may drink at the office and keep a bottle in his briefcase or desk drawer. Though he may feel guilty about his drinking habits, he tends to cover them up by lying and rationalizing his behavior.

How would you answer the following questions: Does one drink make you want many more? Do you drink when you wake up in the morning? Do you spend much of your money and time on liquor and related activities? Do you constantly rationalize your drinking behavior and deny that it has become a problem? Do you find yourself eating little or going for days without any food? Have you lost your old friends and find your new friends are also interested in drinking? Do you stay home from work more often than before? Do you hide your liquor supply? How did you answer these questions? Any "yes" answers indicate probable alcoholism. Try the test out on others (do not tell them what you are trying to find out). You may find that people who do answer "yes" to some of these questions will completely deny any possibility of alcoholism.

The probable or definite alcoholic differs from the chronic alcoholic in the extent of his sickness. Chronic alcoholics are frequently intoxicated for hours or even days at a time. They will do anything to get liquor.

They will drink any and all types of alcohol as long as they become intoxicated. Such liquids as rubbing alcohol, vanilla extract, and bay rum are often consumed. The chronic alcoholic is often weak as a result of poor nutrition and he may suffer from tremors and irrational fears. These and other symptoms are a serious indication that an individual is a chronic alcoholic and needs immediate treatment.

What are some of the general causes that result in a person becoming an alcoholic? Most research in this area groups the causes as physiological, psychological, and sociological.

The physiological cause of alcoholism has been linked to an abnormal craving by the body for alcohol. Some researchers have found that if an adequate vitamin supplement is provided, this craving for alcohol will be controlled. Other researchers refute such studies and present research that indicates a metabolic disturbance that results in a craving for alcohol. Other studies have shown that as a result of continued excessive drinking the brain and other organs of the body function better in an internal alcoholic environment. The person must therefore continue to drink because the body demands alcohol in order to function. Some research also supports the theory that alcohol may lessen the physical problems associated with the malfunction of the pituitary and adrenal glands. As you can see, all of these studies report possible reasons for the alcoholic's constant need for alcohol. None of these studies provides absolute proof of the alcoholic's need for alcohol and new research is being reported all of the time.

The psychological basis for alcoholism is thought to be a desire to relieve emotional problems. Researchers have found evidence to support the theory that alcoholics are emotionally or mentally ill individuals. Inferiority, insecurity, and a lack of love and affection during infancy are just a few of the psychological problems that are linked to alcoholism in the adult.

The sociological influences are those that are imposed by the environment. One's family, peer group, and business associates directly affect an individual's drinking habits. In addition, his tensions at home and at work may serve to foster alcoholism. Most persons who support the sociological causes of alcoholism believe that excessive drinking can only occur in a social climate that accepts drinking as a way to relieve tension and emotional problems.

Researches have also reported the possibility that alcoholism is linked to an hereditary factor. Dr. Donald Goodwin, a psychiatrist at Washington University in St. Louis, Missouri, has evidence that supports this theory. He has studied the case histories of 133 Scandinavian men who had been separated from their natural parents and raised by foster parents. The sons of alcoholic natural fathers were found to be four times more likely to become alcoholics than the sons of nonalcoholic natural fathers. Another study of twins who were separated from each other supports the same finding: that alcoholism may in part be linked to heredity.

There is no one clear-cut cause of alcoholism. There is evidence that supports the physiological, psychological, sociological, and hereditary factors, but no single factor has been proved to be the "absolute" cause. Most researchers think that alcoholism results from a variety of causes and conditions. There is no one type of alcoholic personality. Many persons who could potentially become alcoholics never do. Others, who appear to have few of the usual problems of excessive drinkers do become chronic alcoholics. It can only be said that, given certain combinations of hereditary, physical, and psychological conditions in a social setting where drinking is acceptable, anyone could become an alcoholic.

TREATMENT OF ALCOHOLISM

Many different types of treatment are available to alcoholics. A person has only to recognize that he needs help and help will be available to him and his family. This is the most difficult part of treatment: getting

Alcoholics Anonymous (A.A.) was founded in 1935 by two former alcoholics, William G. Wilson and Robert H. Smith, who noticed that when they talked about their experiences in trying to give up alcohol, their own desire to drink vanished. The method worked for other alcoholics too, and A.A. is now an international organization with more than 500,000 members. The only requirement for membership is an honest desire to stop drinking. A.A. members concentrate on keeping sober for only one day at a time. The main techniques for living up to this "twenty-four-hour plan" are self-analysis and group confession and discussion.
A.A. believes that alcoholics must learn to face life realistically. That's why members learn this prayer: "God grant me the serenity to accept the things I cannot change, courage to change the things I can, and wisdom to know the difference."

a person to admit that he is an alcoholic and to willingly seek help. The objectives of treatment include: (1) helping a person to accept the need for treatment; (2) helping him to stop drinking; and (3) helping him to cope with his problems and lead a relatively "normal" life. Treatment includes medical, psychological, and spiritual approaches and a combination of these. The best results are obtained when the alcoholic's family and friends are also involved in treatment to some extent.

Medical treatment involves a complete physical examination to determine possible conditions that result from excessive use of alcohol. These conditions are discussed in detail later in this chapter. Most alcoholics require dietary advice and treatment for nutritional disorders. Tranquilizers are often required if the person is experiencing body tremors. Certain physicians will administer drugs that offer temporary relief from alcohol dependency. One drug, *Antabuse,* causes severe discomfort if one drinks after taking the drug. Another drug causes vomiting when combined with alcohol. There drugs are used along with other treatment and they help to *condition* the alcoholic to stop drinking. This type of drug therapy is called *aversion therapy* because it produces an aversion or a dislike for alcohol. These methods are only used for temporary control of the problem. Other methods must be used to establish a permanent nondrinking condition.

Hospital treatment is widely available in the United States today. There are private and public hospital centers that run treatment programs which combine physical treatment with psychological approaches. One such program is conducted at Lutheran General Hospital near Chicago. The length of the treatment is 21 days and the cost is about $1,800. The patient is treated for medical symptoms for the first five days of his stay at the hospital. He is then assigned to one of three 25-patient teams. The teams meet three times a week and frequently invite wives, husbands, children, and employers to attend the meetings. The meetings include general discussions, films, and lectures concerning

alcoholism. In-depth psychological treatment is avoided as the treatment concentrates on the existing problem and how to control it.

Group therapy, where people talk with each other to help solve their problems, is a common practice in the treatment of alcoholism. It is used in almost all alcohol treatment programs but is probably best known for its use by Alcoholics Anonymous. Alcoholics Anonymous or A.A. was founded in 1935 by two alcoholics who were trying to help each other stop drinking. Today A.A. has between 650,000 and 750,000 members in the United States. It also has a large membership in foreign countries. There are no required dues or fees and no individual is allowed to contribute more than $300 a year. The local groups do not employ any professional people but rely on the alcoholics themselves to help each other to control their drinking. Each A.A. group runs itself and is not dependent on a national organization or community controls. Members of A.A. believe in taking each day as it comes and they attend meetings only when they feel the need.

There are *Twelve Steps* that form the core of the A.A. program of treatment. These steps are presented to members as a suggested approach to their own recovery. The steps are not mandatory in any way. Many members, however, feel that acceptance of these steps is necessary to maintain sobriety. The steps are as follows:

1. We admitted we were powerless over alcohol—that our lives had become unmanageable.
2. Came to believe that a power greater than ourselves could restore us to sanity.
3. Made a decision to turn our will and our lives over to the care of God as we understood Him.
4. Made a searching and fearless moral inventory of ourselves.
5. Admitted to God, to ourselves, and to another human being the exact nature of our wrongs.
6. Were entirely ready to have God remove all these defects of character.

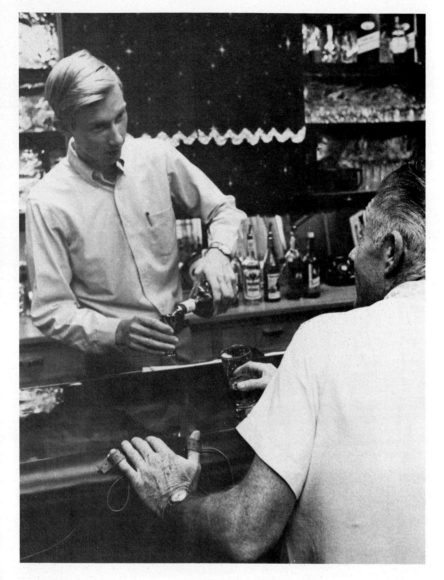

Aversion therapy methods in treating alcoholics include both administering electric shocks and nausea-producing drugs to deter the alcoholic from further drinking. Each time this man takes a drink, he receives an electric shock.

7. Humbly asked Him to remove our shortcomings.
8. Made a list of all persons we had harmed and became willing to make amends to them all.
9. Made direct amends to such people wherever possible, except when to do so would injure them or others.
10. Continued to take personal inventory and when we were wrong promptly admitted it.
11. Sought through prayer and meditation to improve our conscious contact with God as we understood Him, praying only for knowledge of His will for us and the power to carry that out.
12. Having had a spiritual awakening as the result of these steps, we tried to carry this message to alcoholics, and to practice these principles in all our affairs.

In addition to the *Twelve Steps*, A.A. also has *Twelve Traditions* which are suggestions to members to help maintain the growth of the organization or Followship (as it is often called). The *Traditions* stress the primary concern of A.A. as a group of individuals who want to remain sober and help others to do the same. The *Traditions* are as follows:

1. Our common welfare should come first; personal recovery depends upon A.A. unity.
2. For our group purpose there is but one ultimate authority—a loving God as He may express Himself in our group conscience. Our leaders are but trusted servants; they do not govern.
3. The only requirement for A.A. membership is a desire to stop drinking.
4. Each group should be autonomous except in matters affecting other groups or A.A. as a whole.
5. Each group has but one primary purpose—to carry its message to the alcoholic who still suffers.
6. An A.A. group ought never endorse, finance, or lend the A.A. name to any related facility or outside enterprise, lest problems of money, property, and prestige divert us from our primary purpose.
7. Every A.A. group ought to be fully self-supporting, declining outside contributions.
8. Alcoholics Anonymous should remain forever nonprofessional, but our service centers may employ special workers.
9. A.A., as such, ought never be organized; but we may create service boards or committees directly responsible to those they serve.
10. Alcoholics Anonymous has no opinion on outside issues; hence the A.A. name ought never be drawn into public controversy.
11. Our public relations policy is based on attraction rather than promotion; we need always maintain personal anonymity at the level of press, radio, and films.
12. Anonymity is the spiritual foundation of our traditions, ever reminding us to place principles before personalities.

Is A.A. for you or do you know someone who may need the type of help that A.A. provides? There are twelve questions that A.A. poses to help a person decide if he should seek help. The questions are given below for your consideration. How would you answer them?

1. Have you ever decided to stop drinking for a week or so, but only lasted for a couple of days?
2. Do you wish people would mind their own business about your drinking—stop telling you what to do?
3. Have you ever switched from one kind of drink to another in the hope that this would keep you from getting drunk?
4. Have you had a drink in the morning during the past year?
5. Do you envy people who can drink without getting into trouble?
6. Have you had problems connected with drinking during the past year?
7. Has your drinking caused trouble at home?
8. Do you ever try to get "extra" drinks at a party because you do not get enough?
9. Do you tell yourself you can stop drinking any time you want to, even though you keep getting drunk when you don't mean to?
10. Have you missed days of work because of drinking?
11. Do you have "blackouts"?
12. Have you ever felt that your life would be better if you did not drink?

If you answered "yes" four or more times, you are probably in need of some help. Remember that age is not necessarily a factor in being an alcoholic. Many alcoholics are in the teens or are young adults. Many members of A.A. are young people. In order to find out more about A.A. and how to get in touch with a local A.A. group write to: Alcoholics Anonymous World Service, Inc., P.O. Box 459, Grand Central Station, New York, N.Y. 10017.

Al-Anon is a family treatment group that helps to alleviate the problems of the 20 to 30 million people who are affected by the estimated nine million excessive drinkers in this country. Al-Anon began as an adjunct to A.A. but became a separate organization in 1954. It is known as Al-Anon Family

Al-Anon Family Groups and Alateen are offshoots of Alcoholics Anonymous. Al-Anon's members are the spouses and other relatives and friends of alcoholics; Alateen is for alcoholics' teenage sons and daughters. Both organizations have the same goals: to help the members of the alcoholic's family understand the nature of alcoholism, and to reduce family tensions by dealing with the problems of all family members. Like A.A., Al-Anon and Alateen rely on the techniques of self-analysis and group discussion. The exchange of ideas and experiences with people who have similar problems has been found very helpful.

Group Headquarters and its main offices are located at P.O. Box 182, Madison Square Station, New York, N.Y. 10010. Al-Anon had more than 9,000 groups in over 60 countries in 1973. The only membership requirement is that an individual has been or is being deeply affected by close contact with an alcoholic. As in A.A., members pay no dues and all contributions are voluntary. Al-Anon groups help relatives and friends of alcoholics to learn about alcoholism and its treatment. They help these people to benefit from talking with others in a similar situation. Al-Anon groups help nondrinking individuals to improve their attitudes and understanding of family members who are alcoholic.

Alateen is a fellowship of teenaged sons and daughters of alcoholics. It was founded to help those in the 12 to 20 age group who live in an alcoholic family situation. It is an outgrowth of Al-Anon and information concerning Alateen can be received from Al-Anon Headquarters. The major purposes of Alateen are: (1) to discuss problems that teenagers face in an alcoholic household; (2) to exchange experiences; (3) to help each other understand the principles of Alateen; and (4) to offer encouragement to each other and learn how to cope with their problems.

Alateen believes in the *Twelve Steps* that are basic to Alcoholics Anonymous. Alateen teaches its members the following basic concepts regarding themselves and their alcoholic parent:

1. That compulsive drinking is a disease; therefore, no one should condemn the alcoholic.
2. That the sick parent's loss of dignity should not be regarded with contempt but with compassion.
3. That some measure of emotional detachment must be acquired in order to cope with the situation.
4. That it is futile to try to force the addicted drinker into sobriety by reproaches, pleading, or defiance.
5. That it is stupid and self-defeating to resort to acts of reprisal or rebellion from which

they alone will suffer the consequences.
6. That they are endowed with spiritual and intellectual resources with which to develop their own potentials, no matter what happens at home.
7. That their chief concern must be to build satisfying and rewarding life experiences for themselves.

In addition to these groups there are also halfway houses that have been established to help the alcoholic remain sober and adjust to society. As the name implies, the halfway house helps to bridge the gap between hospitalization and an independent life. Many states have also established Local Alcoholism Reception Centers (LARC) where alcoholics are detoxified rather than placed in jail. Once the alcoholic is sober he graduates to a halfway house for treatment. Some of the houses operate on an outpatient basis; others provide a place for the alcoholic to return to for treatment, meals, and sleeping while he maintains his job.

There are five distinct types of halfway houses in existence today. The *voluntary* halfway house, as its name implies, is a self-supporting institution that is usually A.A.-oriented and managed by a former alcoholic. *Church-affiliated* halfway houses are organized by major religious denominations and are usually A.A.-oriented. They may be managed by former alcoholics or by interested ministers. *Partial-public* halfway houses are organized on a voluntary basis but may seek state or federal funding to aid in providing services. *Public* halfway houses are community organized and publicly sponsored. They are usually governed by public administrators. The *professional* halfway house is usually voluntary; however, it may only accept cases that are referred by hospitals, clinics, and social agencies.

In addition to the services offered by these halfway houses, there are also facilities available to skid-row derelicts. These facilities exist in skid-row areas and provide a place where the alcoholic can "dry out" and stay for a while. Many of these facilities are operated by the Salvation Army. In the Salvation

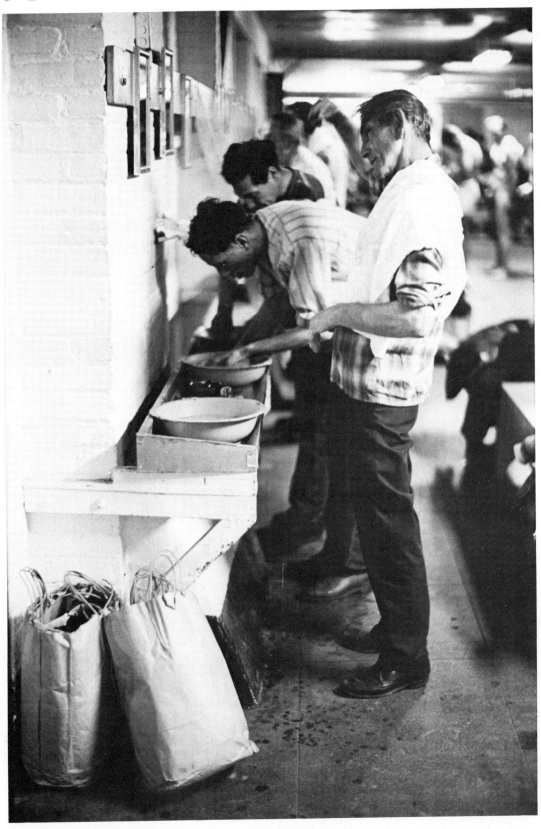

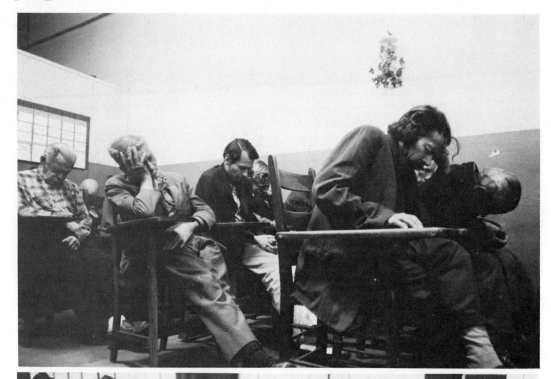

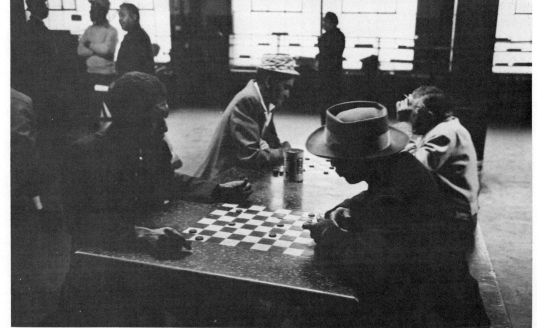

Rescue missions don't
offer a cure for alcoholism,
but they do provide
Skid-row alcoholics with
a place to rest, clean up
and socialize.

Army facilities, a person who drinks while
staying at the residence is immediately expelled. The Harbor Light program of the
Salvation Army provides alcoholics with
the opportunity for therapy as well as work.
Harbor Light offers an employment service

and residents are often hired by local people
to do such work as housecleaning or freight
handling. Skid-row community centers have
also been established in recent years. These
centers provide alcoholics with reading
rooms, laundry facilities, washrooms, cafete-

rias, and a place to stay overnight. All of these services are provided at a small fee. How would you feel about hiring an individual from a Harbor Light facility?

Private treatment centers also exist for those who can afford their services. These centers rely heavily on group therapy and try to stop an individual's drinking without looking into why one drinks. The Chit Chat Farms near Reading, Pennsylvania, is one such center that operates a 28-day program at a cost of $840. Are there any private treatment centers for alcoholics near your community? If there are, find out about their program and method of treatment.

An estimated business loss of $15 billion dollars a year is attributed to alcoholism. Industry, therefore, would be a good place to identify and treat alcoholics. Some companies have started extensive treatment programs that are successful. One such program was started in 1972 by the Firestone Tire and Rubber Company. At the end of the first year, about 300 alcoholics had been referred to the program by their supervisors. Since then, people often come voluntarily without referral. Another corporate program at Kennecott Copper Corporation places the responsibility for seeking help solely on the individual. Kennecott maintains a special hot line to the program headquarters. Once the person has voluntarily asked for help, he is referred to doctors and A.A.-type groups. Do you know of any corporate programs at work in local industries? Is there an alcohol hot line at your school or in your community?

ALCOHOL RELATED DISEASES

Alcoholics are prone to many diseases that are at least partly related to their alcoholism. Many of these diseases are related to nutritional disorders. Although large amounts of alcohol may satisfy an individual's caloric needs, one's nutritional needs are not met. Some of the diseases and physical conditions related to alcoholism are discussed in this section of the chapter.

Delirium tremens or "DTs" is a disease of the nervous system that may be related to a lack of proper nutrition. The disease may be fatal and occurs in about 5 percent of all alcoholics. The person with DTs may exhibit uncontrollable shaking, hallucinations, and convulsions. Delirium tremens is usually a disease of advanced alcoholism and is often temporary, lasting from two to five days. However, the attacks will repeat and are often triggered by injury, illness, or withdrawal from alcohol.

Cirrhosis of the liver results in a loss of liver function that may lead to death. Cirrhosis of the liver occurs in the general population but is six times more common in alcoholic patients. In cirrhosis, the liver swells with fatty tissue and becomes severely damaged. It is thought that damage results from both excessive alcohol intake and the malnutrition that usually accompanies alcoholism.

Wernicke's syndrome is a disease of the brain that results in mental dullness, paralysis of the eye muscles, poor muscular coordination, and brain hemorrhaging. An affected individual will find it difficult to answer questions and concentrate on a thought. This disease is also due in part to malnutrition, especially a vitamin B deficiency.

A recent study by Dr. K. L. Jones and associates at the University of Washington has shown evidence of physical abnormalities in children born to alcoholic mothers. The babies in the study all had mothers who were heavy drinkers and all of the babies showed low birth weight and stunted growth. In addition, the babies showed small head size, joint defects, heart defects, and other physical problems. The researchers believe that possible maternal malnutrition was not the cause, but that alcohol itself was somehow linked to the abnormalities of the infants.

A study issued in July 1974 by the National Institute on Alcohol Abuse and Alcoholism concerned itself with "Alcohol and Health." This study indicated that an excessive use of alcohol is related to certain cancers, including cancer of the mouth, pharynx, larynx, esophagus, and liver. When heavy drinking and heavy smoking are combined, the incidence of certain cancers increases dramat-

ically. If you want to read more about this
informative study, you can write for a copy
to the NIAAA in care of the U.S. Department
of Health, Education and Welfare,
Washington, D.C.

THINKING IT OVER

1. From your own experience do you think
there is much drinking among teenagers
and young adults today? Discuss your
answer giving some of the reasons why
you think there is more or less drinking
going on in these age groups.
2. Discuss the size of the alcohol industry.
Do some research concerning one type
of alcoholic beverage and its contribution to the total industry (such as wine,
beer, or whiskey).
3. Drinking is frequently linked to ethnic
or religious backgrounds. Take your own
survey and see if you can find any type
of drinking pattern (limit your survey to
between 15 and 25 people).
4. Give some of the reasons why people
drink. Have you found these reasons to
be the same as those of your friends?
5. Survey some magazines for advertisements concerning alcoholic beverages.
Briefly describe the aim of the "ad"
and who the "ad" is trying to reach.
6. Do you feel that anti-alcohol legislation
should be passed now or in the near
future? Explain your answer.
7. What is meant by the term *proof*? If you
have any alcoholic beverages at home,
write down their proof and the type
of beverage.
8. Why is alcohol defined as a drug? Do
you think that it should be defined in
this way?
9. What is a depressant drug and how does
a depressant drug affect your body?
10. Explain the meaning of a *disinhibitor*.
Have you found alcohol to be a
disinhibitor?
11. What can happen if alcohol is taken
with other depressant drugs? What is a
"Mickey Finn?"
12. Explain how one can drink and remain
sober.

13. How does alcoholism affect society in
general?
14. What is meant by the term *reaction time*
and how does alcohol affect reaction
time?
15. Discuss the signs of possible alcoholism.
How can one differentiate between a
problem drinker and a chronic alcoholic?
16. Discuss the physiological, psychological,
and sociological causes that result in
a person becoming an alcoholic.
17. How do you feel about the Alcoholics
Anonymous approach to treatment for
the alcoholic? Explain your answer.
18. Many people object to having a halfway
house in a residential section of a community. Do you agree with these people?
Explain your answer.

KEY WORDS

Absorption. The taking in of a substance
through the blood vessels.
Alcoholism. A disease exhibited by persons
who are dependent on alcohol.
Barbiturates. Drugs used to induce sleep or
to quiet an individual.
Breathalyzer. A device that analyzes the
alcohol content of an individual's breath
to determine the blood-alcohol ratio.
Central nervous system. The brain, spinal
cord, and nerves that rise from these
structures.
Congeners. The by-products of the alcohol
manufacturing process.
Depressant. A substance that slows down
body functioning.
Disinhibitor. A substance that releases inhibition or control.
Distillation. The process used in separating
substances by evaporation and
condensation.
Drug. Any chemical substance that alters
the state of the organism either physiologically, psychologically, or emotionally.
Enzyme. A substance that speeds up a
chemical reaction.
Ethnic group. A body of people who share
a common language or customs.
Fermentation. The process that changes sugar
into alcohol.

101

Intoxication. The state of drunkenness; showing loss of control and behavioral change following drinking.

Malting. The conversion of starch into sugar; a process used in the production of beer.

Mash. A mixture of ground cereal and boiled water.

Metabolism. The chemical processes of the body.

Oxidation. The release of heat energy from dissolved food substances.

Prohibition. Laws that forbid the production, transportation, or sale of alcohol in the form of alcoholic beverages.

Proof. The percentage of alcohol in an alcoholic beverage.

Pylorospasm. The uncontrolled opening of the pylorus valve into the small intestine.

Raw whiskey. Whiskey with a 60 to 80 percent alcohol concentration.

Reaction time. The time it takes to physically or mentally respond to a stimulus.

Stimulants. Drugs that stimulate the central nervous system.

Tranquilizers. Drugs used to quiet individuals.

GETTING INVOLVED

Books and Periodicals

"Rising Toll of Alcoholism: New Steps to Combat It," *U.S. News and World Report,* October 29, 1973. An informative article about alcoholism—the nation's number one drug problem.

This Is A.A. Alcoholics Anonymous Publishing, Inc., 1953. A pamphlet describing alcoholism and what A.A. does about it.

Wilsnack, S.C. "Femininity by the Bottle," *Psychology Today,* April, 1973. All about the woman drinker.

Movies

A Tree Grows in Brooklyn, with James Dunn, 1945. An alcoholic but charming father adds to the problems of growing up poor in Brooklyn. Distributed by Argosy Film Service, Budget Films, Clem Williams Films, Films Incorporated, Lewis Film Service, Macmillan Films, Modern Sound Pictures, Roa's Films, Select Film Library, Twyman Films, United Films, Westcoast Films, Wholesome Film Center, and Willoughby Peerless.

Days of Wine and Roses, with Jack Lemmon and Lee Remick, 1962. A man introduces his wife to alcohol, with disastrous results for both of them. Distributed by Budget Films, Cine-Craft, Clem Williams Films, Institutional Cinema Service, Macmillan Films, Modern Sound Pictures, Mottas Films, Roa's Films, Select Film Library, Swank Motion Pictures, "The" Film Center, The Movie Center, Trans-World Films, Twyman Films, United Films, Westcoast Films, Welling Motion Pictures, Wholesome Film Center, and Willoughby Peerless.

I'll Cry Tomorrow, with Susan Hayward, 1955. The biography of Lillian Roth, whose singing career was ruined by drink. Distributed by Films Incorporated.

Le Feu Follet (English title: *The Fire Within*), with Maurice Ronet, 1963. Alcoholism plays a part in a suicide. Distributed by New Yorker Films.

Long Day's Journey into Night, with Jason Robards, 1962. Eugene O'Neill's account of life with an alcoholic father. Distributed by Budget Films, Cine-Craft, Charand Motion Pictures, Institutional Cinema Service, Ivy Films/16, Kit Parker Films, Macmillan Films, Modern Sound Pictures, Mottas Films, Roa's Films, Select Film Library, "The" Film Center, The Movie Center, Twyman Films, United Films, Westcoast Films, Welling Motion Pictures, Wholesome Film Center, and Willoughby Peerless.

The Lost Weekend, with Ray Milland, 1945. The classic tale of three days in the life of an alcoholic. Distributed by Contemporary/McGraw-Hill Films, The Movie Center, and Universal 16.

Records

"Raised on Robbery," Joni Mitchell, *Court and Spark* album. Alcoholism and similar problems.

"Sweet Blindness," Laura Nero, *Eli and the Third Confession* album. About getting high on wine.

6
TOBACCO

Do you smoke? Have you recently "kicked the habit?" Many people are asked these questions every day by their friends and family. Why are so many people interested in smoking habits? One reason is that smoking is controversial because of the findings that indicate that smoking is a health hazard. People must decide for themselves, based on accurate information, whether they wish to smoke or not.

This chapter will provide you with most of the necessary knowledge to help you to make the right decision concerning smoking. You will learn about the history of tobacco, components of tobacco smoke, and the reasons why most people smoke. You will also learn why smoking is considered hazardous to one's health. If you want to "kick the habit," there are some easy steps to follow and information is provided concerning groups that will help you to stop smoking. If you are a nonsmoker, you will be interested in a current movement concerned with the rights of the nonsmoker. Once you have considered all of the information in this chapter, you will be able to make an informed decision concerning smoking.

While reading this chapter, think about the following concepts:

■ Tobacco is a drug.

■ Many people smoke for social reasons.

■ The components of tobacco are highly poisonous substances.

■ People can and do become psychologically dependent on smoking.

■ Cancer and other serious diseases have been definitely linked to smoking.

■ The nonsmoker has rights too!

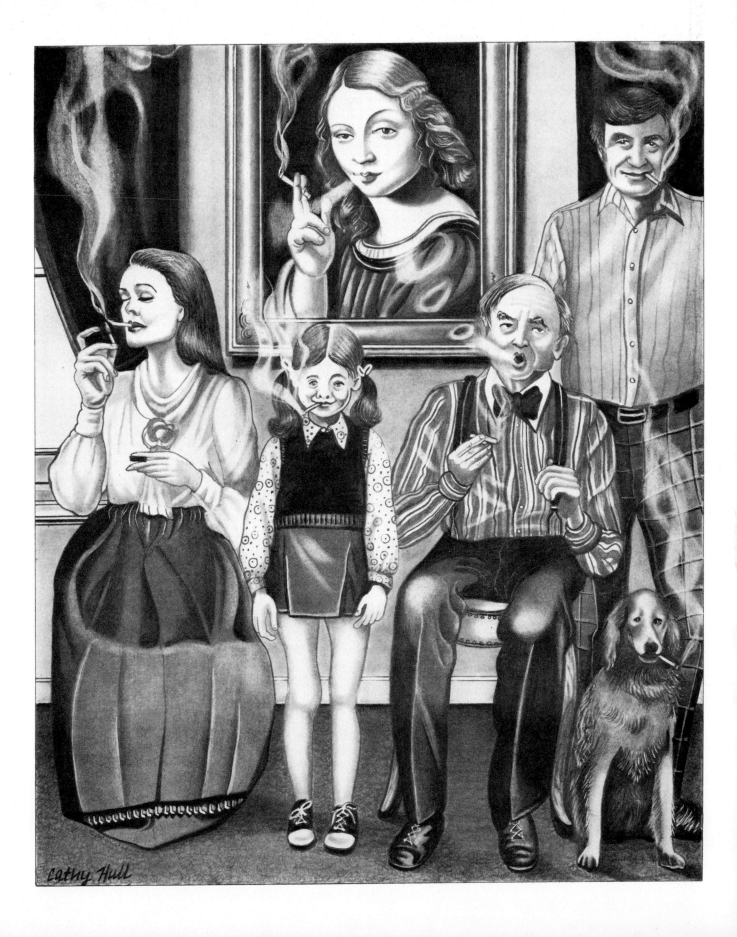

Cathy Hull

The history of tobacco can be traced back to Christopher Columbus who supposedly received a gift of tobacco leaves from the natives of San Salvador. The records seem to differ as to how "tobacco" received its name. Some stories indicate that the name was derived from a Y-shaped pipe called a *tobaco* that was used to smoke the substance through the nostrils. Other stories trace the words to the *Tobacos* province of Mexico where tobacco was widely used.

Tobacco was eventually introduced throughout Europe as a medicine that could cure all illnesses and conditions. A seventeenth century London doctor once described the virtues of tobacco as:

"to cure deafness, a drop of the juice in one ear; to cure headache, a green tobacco leaf on the head; for redness of the face, apply the juice of the ointment of a tobacco leaf; for a toothache, tie a tobacco leaf on the aching region..." (from A.E. Hamilton, *The Smoking World,* D. Appleton-Century Company, Inc., New York, 1927).

Tobacco use continued to spread throughout Europe as a "drug" and to be smoked by pipe. The American colonies exported great quantities of tobacco to England. Smoking of tobacco gradually decreased in Europe and the United States, but the chewing of tobacco grew in popularity. For example, in 1860 only seven of about 350 tobacco processing factories produced smoking tobacco. Spitoons were an accepted part of life in that era. It is estimated that by the end of the ninteenth century, one-half of all of the tobacco consumed in the United States was chewed, not smoked.

Although many individuals were still chewing tobacco, cigars and then cigarettes were introduced and continued to increase in popularity. By 1885, more than one billion cigarettes (584 billion were sold in 1973) were being sold annually and cigarette smoking continued to increase until the present. Although there have been periods in recent history when cigarette consumption has declined, the Federal Trade Commission reports a sales increase of 23 billion cigarettes in 1973 over the 1972 figure. This reflects an increase of over a million packs of cigarettes in one year. The impact on society of these and other relevant statistics is explored in this chapter.

what kind of drug is nicotine?

Nicotine is a naturally occurring stimulant drug. A stimulant is a substance that stimulates or speeds up body functioning through its action on the central nervous system. You will learn more about stimulants in Chapter 7.

Nicotine is an extremely potent drug that was first isolated as the active ingredient in tobacco in 1928. It is a highly poisonous substance; a relatively small dosage could kill a person. For example, one cigar contains enough nicotine to kill two people. However, this does not occur because all of the nicotine does not reach the smoker at the same time. Nicotine is only one component of tobacco smoke. The other components and nicotine are discussed in the following section.

COMPONENTS OF TOBACCO SMOKE

Tobacco smoke is composed of gases, vapors, and chemical compounds. The amount of each of these substances is determined by the type of tobacco being smoked and the temperature at which it is burned. The higher the temperature, the greater the amount of these substances in the smoke. Carbon monoxide gas, nicotine, and tars are the primary components of tobacco smoke.

As previously mentioned, nicotine is the active drug ingredient in tobacco smoke. It is a colorless, oily compound that is a deadly poison in concentrated form. An average man will die if injected with one drop (between 60 and 70 milligrams) of the substance. A typical filtered cigarette will contain between 20 and 30 milligrams of nicotine. However, a smoker who inhales cigarette smoke will absorb approximately 10 percent of the total nicotine content.

Nicotine affects the body in numerous ways. It stimulates the central nervous system and

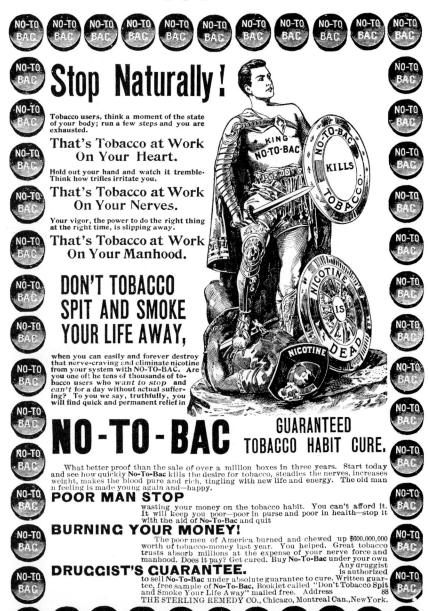

As early as 1895 there was an awareness of
the harmful effects of the use of tobacco and
a search for ways to break the habit.

seems to increase the electrical activity in the brain. However, very little conclusive evidence concerning human performance levels related to nicotine have been conducted. Nicotine does cause a constriction of blood vessels of the skin, decreased skin temperature, increased blood pressure and heart rate, and numbing of the taste receptors of the tongue. Nicotine is deactivated in the user and between 80 percent and 90 percent of the drug is rendered harmless before it is excreted by the kidneys.

Carbon monoxide gas is a deadly component of cigarette smoke and automobile exhausts. This substance is highly poisonous and can cause death if blood content levels exceed 60 percent of the gas. Carbon monoxide reduces the oxygen-carrying capacity of the blood, which results in an overall reduction of available oxygen. This is the primary reason that smokers complain of "shortness of breath" and an inability to participate in strenuous activities. Cigarette smoke has about 1 percent carbon monoxide while pipe smoke has 2 percent of the gas, and cigar smoke 6 percent.

Tobacco tar is a combination of chemicals that produce a brown, sticky mass when condensed from cigarette smoke. These tars contain nicotine and other chemicals—many of them cancer-producing or carcinogenic. These carcinogenic materials have been tested in research studies on animals and have been shown to induce the growth of different kinds of cancers. For example, in one such study a diluted solution of tobacco tar was painted on the backs of mice. Sixty percent of the animals tested developed skin cancer within a year. Tobacco-related cancers will be discussed separately later in this chapter.

TOBACCO DEPENDENCE

Do people develop a dependence on tobacco either physiologically, psychologically, or in both ways? Physical dependence and psychological dependence are terms used in discussing alcohol and other drugs as well as tobacco. *Physical dependence* is a physical need for a substance that may be characterized by increasing tolerance and withdrawal symptoms. *Tolerance* is defined as an increasing dosage of the substance required to obtain the same effects. Withdrawal symptoms are uncomfortable physical symptoms that result after one has stopped taking a drug. Tolerance and withdrawal symptoms are discussed in greater detail in relation to drugs in Chapter 7. *Psychological dependence* may be defined as a psychological need for a substance that results in an individual feeling that he or she could not function without that substance.

Can you develop a physical dependence on nicotine? It is known that people do develop a rapidly increasing tolerance for the drug;

however, physical dependence has not been specifically proven. There are research results that do point to the possibility that the smoker does receive certain physical rewards by smoking. Some research has indicated that the effect of nicotine on certain areas of the brain results in a tranquilizing or quieting effect on the individual. This effect would tie in with reports that many smokers increase their cigarette consumption in times of stress and anxiety. If you are a smoker, try to record the times of the day when you smoke the most. How do these times correlate with particularly anxious or stressful experiences?

Persons who have been tested with low-nicotine cigarettes (without their knowledge), smoked more of these cigarettes than they would normally have smoked. Physically these individuals craved the additional nicotine that was missing from the low-nicotine cigarettes. If you are a smoker, you can try this experiment yourself. Try smoking a very low-nicotine cigarette or cut down on the number of cigarettes you are presently smoking. Do you crave more cigarettes? Is the craving physical or psychological?

This last question leads us to the problem of psychological dependence. It is very difficult to separate the physical from the psychological in relation to smoking. An individual might crave more nicotine if he were to cut down on his smoking, but some of the craving is based on the psychological need or habit of smoking. A U.C.L.A. professor, Murray E. Jarvik, who has done much research in the area of nicotine dependence expresses the following viewpoint:

"Nicotine is the primary reinforcer (of smoking). But after you've been smoking heavily for many years, you have a powerful secondary reinforcer...with cigarettes, after all that association between tobacco and the smoke and the smell and the manipulating, all of these become reinforcing in themselves...."

This statement points to the close involvement of the physical and psychological dependencies. One fuses with the other and the smoker is probably unaware of why he enjoys smoking so much. It is a habit that is very difficult to "kick" because of the inter-relationship between these two dependencies. One can say that smoking is primarily a psychological dependence that is reinforced by the action of nicotine on the central nervous system.

Withdrawal symptoms of a severe physical type do not occur when someone stops smoking. There is no nausea, tremors, stomach discomforts, and other symptoms that are associated with drug withdrawal. However, there are psychological symptoms of withdrawal such as anxiety, restlessness, over-eating, and insomnia. Everyone who does withdraw from smoking does not exhibit these symptoms, but many individuals do depending to some degree on the strength of their own personalities. Have you ever withdrawn from smoking or watched a friend or relative go through this experience? Think about some of the symptoms that were experienced. Which symptoms would you probably exhibit if you were to become depressed or have difficulty in coping with certain problems?

COMMON AND
NOT SO COMMON USAGE

Tobacco has been used in a variety of forms throughout history. One commonly used form was snuff. You may have heard this term but were you quite sure of what it meant? Snuff is powdered tobacco that was sniffed for medicinal and social reasons throughout Europe in the seventeenth and eighteenth centuries. It is still used in Europe and the United States today, but to a much lesser degree. Consumption of tobacco in this form is less than half of what it was 50 years ago.

Chewing tobacco is a form of tobacco made from tobacco leaves mixed with molasses. It was developed in the United States and used primarily in this country. Chewing tobacco was so popular at one time that the amount of tobacco produced for smoking did

not equal the amount produced for chewing until around 1911.

Pipe smoking has been a popular method of smoking tobacco for many years. Between 1900 and 1940, the consumption of pipe tobacco remained relatively stable. However, since 1940 there has been a great drop in pipe tobacco consumption. Today, consumption is about one-fifth of what it was in 1940 or less than a half-pound per person per year.

Cigars are shaped, rolled tobacco leaves that people have smoked for centuries. Early cigars were hand-rolled but the modern variety is machine molded and rolled. Cigar manufacturing reached its height in 1920 when eight billion were sold. Between 1920 and 1930 cigar smoking decreased sharply and cigarette smoking began to increase. In 1920, the average cigar consumption was about 115 per person per year, but by 1940, this figure had dropped by about a third to 75 per person. This trend has continued until this day.

Cigarettes are small rolls of finely cut tobacco that are usually rolled in a thin paper. The history of cigarettes can be traced as far back as the early 1500s when tobacco-filled reeds were reportedly smoked in parts of Mexico. However, it wasn't until the mid-1800s that cigarette smoking began to take hold in Europe and the United States. As a note of interest, Philip Morris was an English tobacco merchant of the late 1850s who began producing hand-rolled cigarettes. Generally speaking, before World War I few people smoked cigarettes; those who did smoke usually rolled their own cigarettes. The recent history of cigarette smoking is discussed in the next section.

trends in
tobacco use

Cigarette smoking began to increase after World War I. Cigarettes were freely distributed to soldiers during the war and this practice resulted in a great increase in the number of cigarette smokers. The number of cigarette smokers increased again when women began to smoke. The first advertisement that showed

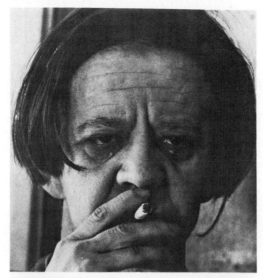

SMOKING IS VERY GLAMOROUS

AMERICAN CANCER SOCIETY

a woman smoking appeared in 1919. Advertising was crucial to making cigarette smoking acceptable to women and to society. Such influences as glamor, beauty, romance, and independence were stressed in cigarette ads.

In general, women have not smoked as much or for as long a time as men. But, they have begun to catch up in recent years. Since 1955, the number of women smokers has doubled, while the number of men smokers has declined. Statistics indicate that only 300,000 of the more than 4.5 million smokers who have quit since 1966 have been women. There has also been a greater increase in lung cancer among women than among men.

Another trend in cigarette smoking was the introduction of filter-tip cigarettes. The first filter-tips were manufactured in 1950 and less than 1 percent were sold in that year. By 1955, filter cigarettes had cornered about 19 percent of the market. The sales of filter-tips continued to rise, and today they are

smoked by more than 75 percent of all cigarette smokers. Much of this rise is related to findings that link cigarette smoking with cancer and other diseases, advertising bans, and tobacco education. All of these factors and their effects on smoking trends will be discussed in later sections of this chapter.

why do people smoke?

People smoke for many of the same reasons why they drink alcoholic beverages and take drugs. *Peer pressure* is a basic reason why many people, especially young people, begin to smoke. Smoking is a sign of acceptance among many groups of young people. Those who do not smoke are discouraged from joining "smoking" groups. Smoking allows these individuals to feel a part of the group and belong to something. In recent years, there seemed to be a "reverse acceptance." This term implies that many teenagers were rejecting cigarettes and were not accepting smokers into their group of friends. However, statistics do not seem to bear out this conclusion. A survey conducted by The National Clearinghouse for Smoking and Health indicated that between January 1968 and January 1970 cigarette smoking increased among teenage boys and girls. However, in 1972 smoking dropped back toward the 1968 level. Recent statistics (1974) indicate that the level had increased again and remained at the 1972 level. According to 1974 statistics, between 10 and 28 percent of American teenagers are currently smoking. What would you have guessed? Teenagers were asked this very question in a recent survey and 37 percent of them guessed 40 to 50 percent and another 37 percent guessed 60 to 100 percent. It is interesting to see that teenagers themselves think that more of them are smoking than the surveys actually indicate. See Table 6-1 for a comparison of teenage smokers between 1968 and 1969.

Another reason why many young people start to smoke has to do with independence.

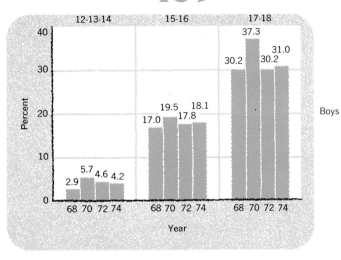

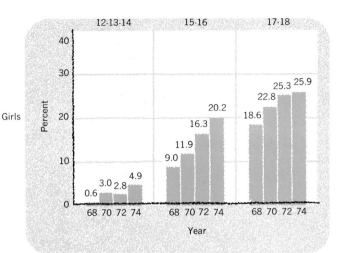

Table 6-1

Percent Regular Smokers — Teen Age, 1968–1974[a]
[a]With the permission of the National Interagency Council on Smoking and Health.

For many, smoking is an outward sign of being on their own and in many cases rebelling against parental authority. Do you remember when you had your first cigarette? Think about some of the feelings you had when you "lit up" for that first time.

Family influence is an essential factor in why people begin to smoke. The results of a national study conducted for the American Cancer Society are graphically illustrated in Figure 6-2. It is easy to recognize that the percentage of teenage smokers is directly related to whether one or both of their parents smoked. This is understandable, in that youngsters brought up in a home where the parents smoked came to take it for granted that this is an acceptable thing to do. Education will affect this group to some extent, but it is difficult to break down these established patterns. Many parents unknowingly condone

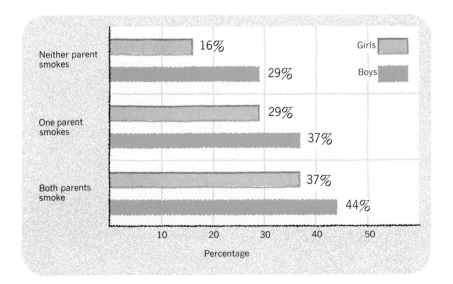

Figure 6-2

The smoking habits of parents has an effect on the likelihood of children's future smoking behavior.

Teenage smoking is
on the rise.

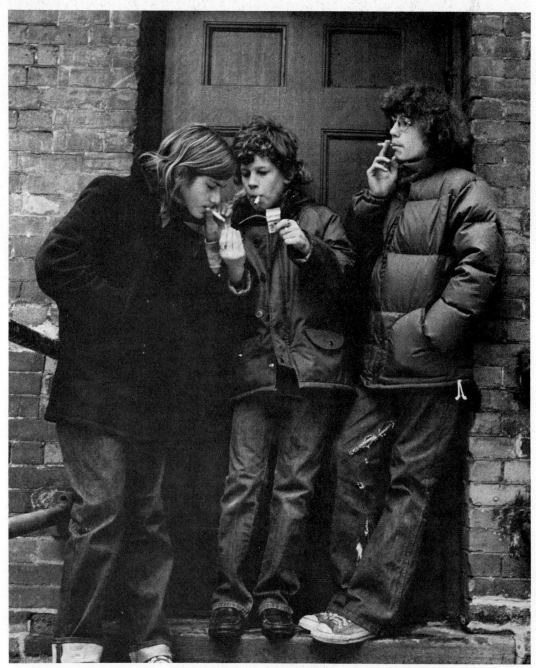

smoking among their teenagers. They feel that smoking cigarettes is certainly better than smoking "pot" or taking other drugs, and they tend not to get too upset about smoking.

There are many psychological theories that are proposed to explain why people smoke. These theories are often linked to oral gratification. Studies have indicated that smokers often have other oral habits such as excessive coffee drinking and alcohol consumption. Some statistics support the theory that the longer a smoker was breast-fed as an infant, the less he smoked and the easier it was for him to stop smoking. Do you or your friends that smoke tend to drink more coffee, chew on pencils or toothpicks, or walk around with unlit cigarettes in your mouths?

Some people say that they smoke to relieve nervous tension and to give them something to do. The relief of tension may have some physical basis in the effect of nicotine on the brain. However, this has not yet been proven. For many individuals, just having something to do allows them to become more relaxed.

Other individuals say that they smoke because it keeps them from eating. Although much of this is psychological, there are some physical effects of nicotine that could aid in appetite control. Inhaled nicotine from one cigarette has been shown to inhibit hunger contractions of the stomach for as long as

A 1930 ad for Lucky Strikes promoted smoking as an appetite control.

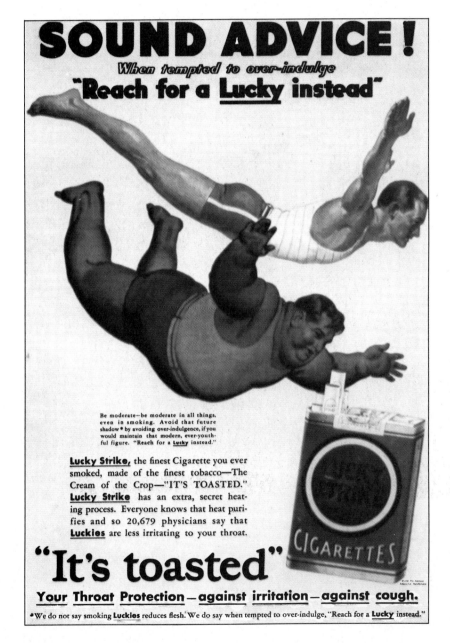

SOUND ADVICE!

When tempted to over-indulge
"Reach for a Lucky instead"

Be moderate—be moderate in all things, even in smoking. Avoid that future shadow * by avoiding over-indulgence, if you would maintain that modern, ever-youthful figure. "Reach for a Lucky instead."

Lucky Strike, the finest Cigarette you ever smoked, made of the finest tobacco—The Cream of the Crop—"IT'S TOASTED." **Lucky Strike** has an extra, secret heating process. Everyone knows that heat purifies and so 20,679 physicians say that **Luckies** are less irritating to your throat.

"It's toasted"

Your Throat Protection—against irritation—against cough.

* We do not say smoking **Luckies** reduces flesh. We do say when tempted to over-indulge, "Reach for a **Lucky** instead."

an hour. Nicotine inhalation also results in a slight increase in blood sugar and a numbing of the taste buds. Because of this numbing effect, many smokers say they cannot taste their food as well as they did before they smoked. One must, of course, consider the weight control factors of smoking (which are minimal) against the health hazards of the habit.

Report of the Surgeon General's Advisory Committee was published in January 1964, and received worldwide publicity. It stated that cigarette smoking can cause lung cancer and can play a part in heart disease, emphysema, bronchitis, and other diseases. Smokers seemed convinced that their habit was shortening their lives, for cigarette sales immediately dropped 15 to 20 percent. But, ironically, within a few months sales had climbed back almost to prereport levels.

Surgeon General's Advisory Committee – 1964

The Surgeon General's Advisory Committee on Smoking and Health published in 1964 the most comprehensive and authoritative report on this subject. After 15 months of intensive research and a study of more than 4,000 reports, the committee concluded that "cigarette smoking is a health hazard of sufficient importance in the United States to warrant remedial action." The committee states with certainty that "cigarette smoking is causally related to lung cancer in men; the magnitude of the effect of cigarette smoking far outweighs other factors." The data for women appeared to point in the same direction, though it was less conclusive at that time. Today, we know that the data for women in relation to lung cancer are as conclusive as the data for men.

The report also concluded that the death rate from heart disease is 70 percent higher in smokers than in nonsmokers. Cigarette smoking was also linked to deaths caused by chronic bronchitis and emphysema (these diseases are discussed later in this chapter).

The report additionally concluded that for cigar and pipe smokers combined there was a suggestion of high death rates for such diseases as mouth, esophagus, larynx, and lung cancer, and stomach and duodenal ulcers.

Following the release of the Surgeon General's Report on Smoking and Health, the Federal Trade Commission (FTC) concluded that

cigarette smoking advertisements were misleading and did not warn smokers of the possible hazardous effects of smoking. In 1965, the FTC proposed that all cigarette advertising must state the amount of tar and nicotine in the smoke of that brand of cigarettes. It further proposed that all packs of cigarettes and advertising must carry a warning statement such as: "Caution: Cigarette Smoking May Be Dangerous to Your Health." Today all cigarette packages and ads carry the following caution label (approved by Congress in 1970), "Warning: The Surgeon General Has Determined That Cigarette Smoking Is Dangerous to Your Health."

In January 1971, Congress prohibited the advertising of cigarettes on radio and television. This ban exists in eleven other countries including the Soviet Union. However, once the ban went into effect, magazine advertising doubled in the first three months following the ruling. Some countries are considering a total ban on any form of cigarette advertising. Some publications have already decided not to accept cigarette advertising of any type. This is in voluntary support of a controversial issue. Do you think that all cigarette advertisements should be banned? Some people have expressed the viewpoint that adults should not be treated as if they were children and should be allowed to decide about smoking on their own without intervention by government or other groups. How do you feel about this in relation to the advertising of cigarettes? How should other tobacco products be treated?

Many public agencies and private groups have taken up the cause of warning people about the hazardous effects of tobacco, particularly cigarettes. Such groups as the American Cancer Society, American Heart Association, and Tuberculosis and Respiratory Disease Associations all contribute time and money to vast educational programs concerning cigarette smoking. In addition, the National Clearinghouse for Smoking and Health, established in 1965 by the Public Health Service, provides a comprehensive educational program that includes pamphlets, studies, and plans to stimulate further cigarette controls.

effects of cigarette smoking

The immediate effects of cigarette smoking are noticeable in even the "beginning" smoker. Such symptoms as dizziness, nausea, upset stomach, clammy skin, diarrhea, and vomiting are often experienced. Habitual smokers may also experience some of the same effects. As mentioned earlier in this chapter, smoking tends to dull the senses of taste and smell and may depress appetite to a limited degree.

Smoking also contributes to numerous digestive disorders. Stomach and duodenal ulcers are much more common among smokers than among nonsmokers. Cancer of the stomach has been found to be 40 percent more common in smokers than among nonsmokers.

Nicotine acts as a stimulant to the central nervous system. It also acts to cause a discharge of a certain hormone that stimulates the release of stored sugar from the liver. This release of sugar may cause a temporary renewal of energy and lessening of fatigue. However, the sensation lasts for only a short time and is followed by depression and fatigue.

Smokers generally experience more respiratory diseases than nonsmokers. Such diseases as bronchitis, sore or scratchy throat, chronic cough, and hoarseness of the voice are more common among smokers. This is so because frequent smoking first slows down and then destroys the fragile <u>cilia</u> (hair-like structures that line the bronchial tubes and trap harmful substances such as soot and dust). When the cilia are destroyed, an individual is much more likely to become ill with a respiratory disease.

Smoking has a definite effect on the circulation. The heart-rate increases following smoking and blood pressure is elevated. The small, superficial arteries contract resulting in a lowering of body temperature. One study indicated that after smoking only one cigarette, the average skin temperature of the fingers and toes dropped more than five

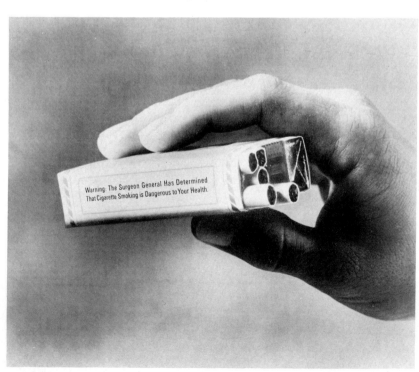

degrees. Abnormal electrocardiograms (a test that indicates the electrical activity of the heart) have also been noted during smoking. In some individuals, the heartbeat becomes irregular and chest pain may be experienced.

LONG-RANGE EFFECTS OF CIGARETTE SMOKING

The long-range effects of smoking include respiratory disorders, circulatory disease, and different forms of cancer. The fact that the serious effects of cigarette smoking are long-range makes it extremely difficult to convince students and others of the potential consequences of smoking. Most individuals tend to think of themselves as special or even immortal. They are the ones who will never get the disease, so they do not have to be concerned with controlling their smoking habit. To a young person, the thought of becoming ill many years from now is not enough of an impetus to make him stop smoking today.

BRONCHITIS AND EMPHYSEMA

Chronic bronchitis is an inflammation of the bronchial tubes that frequently recurs. Irritation of these tubes results in an excessive amount of mucus being secreted. Coughing occurs in an attempt to expel the mucus buildup.

Emphysema is a disease where the lungs lose their elasticity and are unable to expand and contract normally. This results in the eventual destruction of the tiny air sacs or alveoli where oxygen and carbon dioxide are exchanged. The lungs in chronic emphysema are unable to adequately exchange these gases and the heart must work harder to provide more oxygen for the body. Heart failure is the most common cause of death in emphysema patients.

The death rate due to emphysema and bronchitis is four times higher among those who smoke less than a pack a day as compared to those who have never smoked. If this is expanded to those who smoke more heavily, it is easy to see the relationship of cigarettes to death from these two diseases. Bronchitis and emphysema are discussed in greater detail in Chapter 15.

CIRCULATORY DISORDERS

Smoking has serious, often lethal effects on the body's circulation. Smoking has been known to cause the formation of a blood clot or thrombus within a blood vessel. Blood flow is first reduced and then may be blocked off in this vessel. This condition is known as Buerger's disease and often occurs in the feet. Gangrene poisoning may also set in and amputation of toes and fingers and sometimes the arms and legs is often required.

If you know anyone who smokes and has recently suffered from a heart attack, he probably does not smoke now! This is one of the first orders that a doctor will give a heart attack victim. Heart disease is closely linked to cigarette smoking and the death rate from this disease is one and one-half to two times higher among smokers than among nonsmokers. A man between the ages of 45 and 54 has a three times greater risk of a heart attack if he smokes more than a pack of cigarettes a day. Coronary heart disease kills more than 650,000 men and women each year and a large percentage of these individuals are smokers. Heart disease is discussed in more detail in Chapter 14.

CANCERS

When people discuss the effects of cigarette smoking, cancer is often the first thing that comes to mind. Cigarette smoke is thought to be a contributory factor in the cause of cancer. Cancers of different types have been statistically linked to heavy smoking for many years.

Cancers of the lip, tongue, pharynx, and larynx appear with much greater frequency among the smoking population. For example, cancer of the larynx is six times as frequent in male cigarette smokers in the 45 to 64 age group than among nonsmokers. These cancers are found more often in individuals who chew tobacco, smoke cigars, or use snuff than in the nonsmoking population.

Lung cancer is a deadly disease that is directly associated with heavy smoking. Of course, some nonsmokers do get the disease but statistics show that only 10 percent of all deaths from lung cancer occur in nonsmokers.

Lung cancer is a relatively new disease. Death from this disease was rare only 50 years ago. Today it is the most common cause of death due to cancer among American men and is rapidly increasing as a cause of death among American women. The increase of the disease is directly related to the increase of smoking during this century.

Lung cancer is identified as an abnormal growth of cells in the lungs. These cells destroy normal tissue and can eventually destroy the lung and cause death. The cancer-causing or carcinogenic substances in cigarette smoke have been shown to promote cancer production in animal tissue.

The symptoms of lung cancer include persistent cough, vague chest pain, increased coughing and spitting up of mucus, blood-streaked mucus, loss of weight and strength, and shortness of breath. There are a number of methods that can aid the physician in detecting this disease. A chest X-ray will help to diagnose an abnormality of the lungs. If the abnormality is thought to be cancer, a microscopic examination of a specimen of lung tissue can be performed with the aid of a bronchoscope (a tube through which a portion of the bronchial tubes can be seen.) Sometimes the mucus can be examined for the presence of cancerous cells. If cancer is discovered, the only treatment presently available is surgical removal of the cancerous growth. However, lung cancer is a deadly disease and only 7 to 10 percent of individuals who have this disease will survive more than five years following treatment. Approximately one-third of all lung cancer victims show a spread of the disease at the time of surgery. More than one-third of lung cancer victims cannot be helped by surgery because of the advanced stage of the disease.

This information paints a dismal picture of cancer recovery. However, lung cancer can be prevented or at least the chance of getting the disease can be reduced. The obvious way to prevent the disease is to never light another cigarette! If you cannot stop smoking, then at least try to cut down, smoke lower tar and nicotine cigarettes, take fewer puffs, and inhale less frequently. These and other methods of stopping smoking are discussed in the next section.

kicking the habit

This topic may best be introduced by the following poem written in 1915 by Graham Lee Hemminger:

"Tobacco is a dirty weed. I like it.
It satisfies no normal need. I like it.
It makes you thin, it makes you lean.
It takes the hair right off your bean.
It's the worst darn stuff I've ever seen.
I like it."

This poem expresses the difficulty that many people have in "kicking the habit." Many of them don't know why they like it, but they do!

There are many types of programs that concentrate on getting people to stop smoking. Some hospitals run antismoking clinics and many churches and other organizations sponsor programs and speakers to help people to stop smoking.

One of the largest withdrawal clinics is run by a group called *SmokEnders*. This is a profit-making organization that runs programs throughout the country. The organization was founded in 1969 and has treated thousands of individuals, many of whom have been successful in giving up the habit. The program consists of nine weekly meetings where participants are taught specifically prescribed activities, each of which is an essential ingredient in the entire pattern that relates to an individual's smoking, eating, recreation, and life style. Participants are taught to achieve withdrawal gradually and painlessly. If you are interested in finding out more about this program, you can write

SmokEnders, Inc., is a profit-making organization that conducts clinics to help people give up smoking. Their program involves breaking the habit patterns that go with smoking; for example, the smoker is encouraged to change his or her brand of cigarettes, to cut out cigarettes after meals, and so on. These methods are successful in many cases. SmokEnders won't give out information about their program, but they will tell you where clinics are held in your locale if you write to them in Phillipsburg, New Jersey 08865.

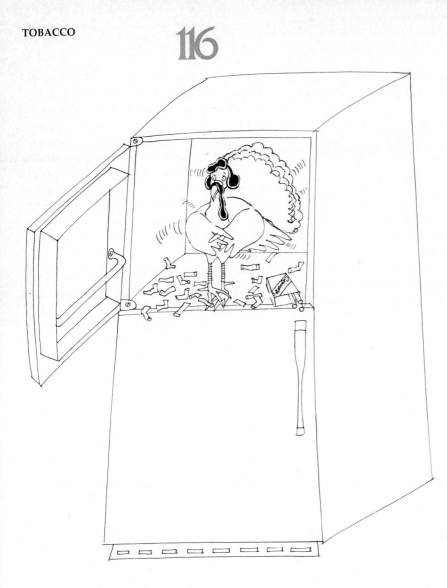

Cold turkey?

to: SmokEnders, Memorial Parkway, Phillipsburg, New Jersey, 08865.

There are also programs that are involved with hypnosis and self-hypnosis. Some of these programs are not legitimate and should be carefully examined prior to enrollment. Some individuals find help in psychological or psychiatric counseling. Each individual, depending on other influences in his life at that time, must seek the best program for himself.

Some people can "kick the habit" by themselves. In a great number of cases, individuals have "gone cold turkey" and have been successful. This approach, of course, will not work for everyone. If you desire to cut down or quit, here are some simple suggestions that will be helpful.

1. Be careful when choosing a cigarette. Choose one with minimum tar and nicotine content.
2. Smoke your cigarette only half-way down. If you do this, you will only get about 40 percent of the tar and nicotine instead of a possible 60 percent if you were to smoke to the end of the cigarette.
3. Take fewer draws on each cigarette and you will cut down without knowing it.
4. Inhale less deeply; take short, shallow puffs.
5. Smoke fewer cigarettes each day. Choose

a time of the day that you will not smoke at all. Don't think of it as cutting down, but as postponing.

6. By lengthening the period of time each day that you won't smoke, you can eventually stop smoking in a gradual manner.

Will you gain weight if you quit smoking? Many people will, because withdrawal from cigarettes results in improved appetite and sense of taste. In addition, many individuals will be restless and turn to food to replace their cigarettes. Weight gain in most cases is only temporary and if an individual had the self-control to stop smoking, he can use that willpower to control his eating habits. It all comes down to how important feeling good and being healthy is to you. If it is important, you will make the right decision.

It is interesting to note that higher education and fear of cancer are often not enough to make smokers stop smoking. A recent study indicated that the more-educated individuals also smoked more. Many of those interviewed seemed to express a definite attitude in that they were aware of the hazards but were unwilling to give up the pleasures of cigarettes. This defiance is also seen in cigarette advertising such as a recent ad that says: "I smoke, and I'm not going to apologize for it." Do you find that you or your friends express this kind of attitude toward smoking? How does such an attitude reflect maturity or immaturity?

Some of you may be thinking about the many smokers who are not adversely affected by their habit. Certainly this is true. Many individuals will smoke heavily and live long and healthy lives. However, based on the scientific evidence we have today, the majority of smokers will be adversely affected by their habit.

does the nonsmoker have rights?

Nonsmokers distressed about having to inhale the smoke from other people's cigarettes are fighting back by lobbying for laws that ban smoking in public places. According to *Action on Smoking and Health* (ASH), a Washington group devoted to the protection of nonsmokers, one-third of the states have passed legislation that prohibits smoking in certain public areas. On all airplanes and certain trains, no-smoking sections are already in effect. Nonsmokers would like to extend the legislation to all public meeting rooms, department stores, elevators, grocery stores, hospitals, theaters, and libraries. How do you feel about this type of legislation — should the nonsmoker have rights?

THINKING IT OVER

1. What type of a drug is nicotine? In what ways does it affect the body?
2. Can an individual become physically dependent on tobacco? Explain.
3. What is meant by psychological dependence on tobacco? Are you psychologically dependent on this drug? Explain.
4. Does cigarette smoking help people to relieve tension and restlessness? Explain your answer.
5. Give some of the reasons why people smoke.
6. Why has the number of women smokers increased in recent years?
7. Have you noticed a trend toward "reverse acceptance" of smoking? Explain your answer.
8. Does one's family influence his or her smoking habits? Did your family influence whether you smoked or did not smoke?
9. Give some of the major findings of the Surgeon General's Report on Smoking and Health.
10. Explain the various methods that the FTC has used to educate the public concerning the hazards of smoking.
11. List some of the ways that you can use to cut down or stop smoking.
12. How do you feel about the rights of the nonsmoker?

KEY WORDS

Alveoli. The air sacs of the lungs where carbon dioxide and oxygen are exchanged.

Action on Smoking and Health (ASH), a nonprofit organization based in Washington, D.C., was founded in 1967 by John Banzhaf III to protect the rights of the nonsmoker. Research has shown that, in a smoke-filled area, nonsmokers may inhale almost as many dangerous substances as the people who are smoking. So ASH works for legislation banning smoking—or at least separate smoking and no-smoking areas.

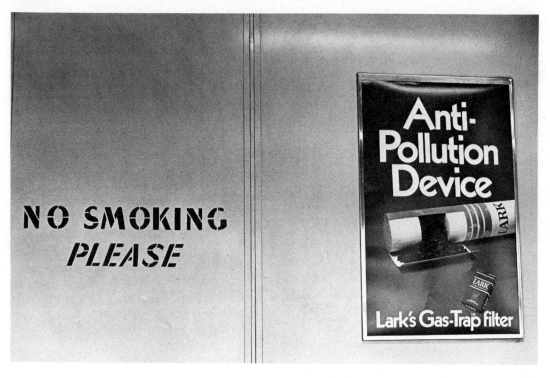

Bronchitis. A recurrent inflammation of the bronchial tubes.

Bronchoscope. An instrument used to examine the bronchial tubes.

Buerger's disease. A disease that develops from a blood clot in the fingers, toes, arms, or legs.

Cancer. Uncontrolled cellular growth that blocks normal growth and function.

Carbon monoxide. A highly poisonous gas found in car exhausts and cigarette smoke.

Carcinogenic. A substance that is cancer-producing.

Chewing tobacco. A form of tobacco made from tobacco leaves mixed with molasses.

Cigarettes. Finely ground tobacco wrapped in thin paper.

Cigars. Rolled, shaped tobacco leaves.

Cilia. Hair-like structures that line the bronchial tubes and trap harmful substances such as soot and dust.

Electrocardiogram. A device used to measure the electrical activity of the heart.

Emphysema. A loss of elasticity in the lung and eventual destruction of the air sacs.

Nicotine. A highly poisonous component of cigarette smoke.

Peer pressure. Doing something in order to please others and be accepted by the group.

Physical dependence. A physical need for a drug that is characterized by tolerance and withdrawal.

Psychological dependence. A psychological need for a substance that causes a person to think he needs the substance in order to function.

Snuff. A powdered form of tobacco.

Stimulant drug. A drug that speeds up the bodily functions by stimulating the central nervous system.

Tobacco tar. A combination of chemicals in tobacco smoke that have been found to cause cancer.

Tolerance. An increasing dosage of a substance in order to obtain the same effects.

Withdrawal symptoms. Physical and mental discomfort felt upon giving up a drug.

GETTING INVOLVED
Publications

If You Want to Give Up Cigarettes. The American Cancer Society. A booklet presenting suggestions from various experimental projects.

Danger. American Cancer Society. Persuasive pamphlet about the dangers of smoking.

The Dangers of Smoking: The Benefits of Quitting. American Cancer Society. A condensation of the history and research findings in health and cigarette smoking.

Smoking's Impact on Oral Health. The American Dental Association. A leaflet containing information on smoking and its effect on the oral cavity.

How to Stop Smoking. American Heart Association. A leaflet based on Dr. Donald T. Fredrickson's TV withdrawal program.

What Everyone Should Know about Smoking and Heart Disease. American Heart Association. Leaflet about smoking and the heart.

Me Quit Smoking, Why? American Lung Association. A booklet showing the health hazards of smoking.

Me Quit Smoking, How? American Lung Association. A booklet outlining the steps to quitting.

Smoking: Facts You Should Know. American Medical Association. A review of the effects of smoking.

Smoking and Health Newsletter. National Interagency Council on Smoking and Health. Quarterly publication about current news in smoking.

Chart Book on Smoking, Tobacco, and Health. U.S. Public Health Service. A booklet describing cigarettes and health, cigarettes and the economy, cigarette marketing, and cigarettes as a tax source.

Smoker's Self-Testing Kit. U.S. Public Health Service. Four tests to help the smoker understand his habit and decide what to do about it.

Public Exposure to Air Pollution from Tobacco Smoke. United States Public Health Service. How cigarettes contaminate the atmosphere.

The Health Consequences of Smoking. January 1973, United States Public Health Service. Seventh of the reports to Congress reviewing and assessing scientific evidence linking cigarettes to disease.

Posters

"We'll Miss Ya, Baby," (9 x 12 inches); "Life Is So Beautiful," (24 x 36 inches) Peter Max; and others, American Cancer Society.

"Thank You for Not Smoking," (8½ x 11 inches) American Heart Association.

"Listen Smokers . . ." (16 x 21 inches) United States Public Health Service.

No Smoking Signs, (8½ x 11 inches) American College of Chest Physicians.

Movies

The Embattled Cell, American Cancer Society, 1968. The working of living cells within the human lung.

Emphysema, the Facts, American Lung Association, 1973. The impact of this lung disease, its major cause—smoking—and prevention.

Is It Worth It?, American Lung Association, 1970. A dynamic film about the dangers of smoking.

The Mark Waters Story, United States Public Health Service. With Richard Boone. The true story of a newspaperman who wrote his own obituary while dying of lung cancer. (Available from the National Audiovisual Center, Washington, D.C. 20409.)

Quit, Quit, Again, United States Public Health Service. Geraldine Fitzgerald, Kevin McCarthy, and others tell why and how they quit smoking. (Available on free loan from National Audiovisual Center, Washington, D.C. 20409.)

Records

Smoke, Smoke, Smoke that Cigarette, Dan Hicks and His Hot Licks, Blue Thumb Label.

7
DRUGS–LICIT AND ILLICIT

Are you a drug user, misuser, or abuser? You may be surprised to find out that you might fit into one or more of these categories. In this chapter you will learn about all aspects of legal and illegal drug use. Basic drug terminology is explained so that you will have a better understanding of the chapter. The complex question of the "why" of drug abuse is explored. You will become familiar with the classification of common drugs, their accepted names and slang names, and their effects on the body and mind. You will learn why the word "dependence" has become widely used in place of the word "addiction." You will become familiar with the

terms "physical dependence" and "psychological dependence." These terms are essential to understanding drug abuse. In the final section of this chapter, treatment for drug abusers is explored through a discussion of therapeutic communities and methadone and heroin maintenance programs. After reading this chapter, you will have a better understanding of drugs and the drug problem. Familiarity with the subject will help you to have a more informed understanding of drugs, drug abusers, and the legal problems that they present.

While reading this chapter, think about the following concepts:

■ Drugs, like alcohol are "people problems."

■ Drugs are inert substances: substances that are harmless until taken by people.

■ We are all drug users.

■ Psychological dependence on a drug is usually a greater problem to kick than physical dependence.

■ Drugs are often taken for social reasons.

■ Drug treatment usually includes counseling and group therapy.

■ Methadone maintenance involves the substitution of one drug for another drug.

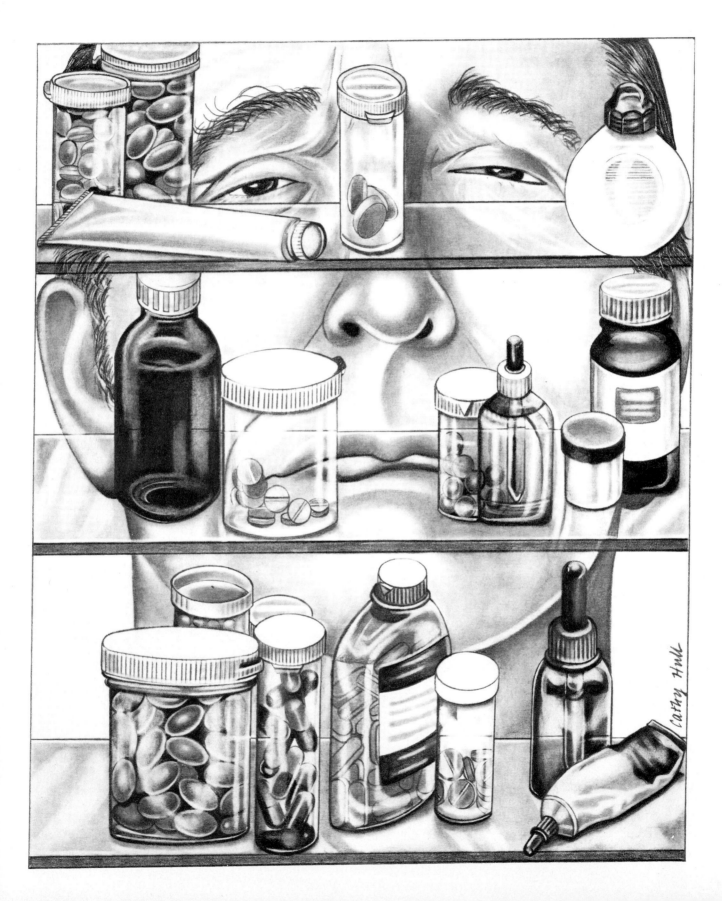

In the previous chapters alcohol and tobacco were defined as drugs. The definition of a drug is any chemical substance that alters the state of the organism either physiologically, psychologically, or emotionally. Like alcohol and tobacco, drugs are actually "people problems." Such substances are harmless (certain drugs taken for medical purposes are most useful) until they are combined with people. It is the abuse of alcohol and other drugs by individuals that results in dependency problems. For this reason, we should not label drugs as being "bad." This would lead us to believe that all drugs are harmful and there is nothing "good" to say about them. Drugs are inert substances: substances that are harmless unless taken. Even when taken, the danger of the drug is directly related to the dosage. In this chapter, we attempt to explore drugs and the drug problem from the "people" point of view. The "why" and "how" of people and drugs are essential to understanding drug misuse and abuse.

why do people abuse drugs?

People abuse drugs for many of the same reasons that they abuse alcohol. Drugs, like alcohol, are often taken under the influence of strong peer pressure. Peer pressure operates at every age level but is somewhat stronger among teenagers. Teenagers are constantly having new demands put on them. They are going through a transitional stage in their lives when uncertainty and feelings of inadequacy are common. Drugs fill the gap for many of these young people who are looking for an answer to the problems they have at that moment. The social pressure of friends is often all that is needed to turn a young person on to drugs. Most young people are introduced to drugs through their friends, frequently at a party or other social gathering. It is interesting to note here that most young people are *not* introduced to drugs by the stereotyped "shifty-eyed gangster pusher" that we all have read about. In most cases, friends offer pills and "pot" to each other.

Many people turn to drugs out of boredom. This is true of every age group. The teenager who has nothing to do and few interests is looking for a new form of excitement. Drugs often seem to be the answer. Older persons who feel that they are in a "rut" in their jobs or in their everyday lives may also look for an outlet for their boredom. Drugs provide that outlet and add an extra bit of excitement because of their illegality (in most cases) and because of the secrecy that often surrounds the taking of drugs.

This generation has often been called the "NOW" generation. This simply means that people want things to happen to them "now"—at this very moment. They want to experience life now and not have to wait 30 or 40 years to taste everything. Drugs are one aspect of trying life on and seeing what it's all about. It's an experience for today, a way of getting a different look at the world. One doesn't have to be very young to be a member of this "NOW" generation. We often read about or may know people who are trading in their old life styles for new ones. Executives are leaving lucrative positions to do what they really want to do. Their new life styles may mean a great loss of income but they feel the experience is worth it. This attitude of living for today has encouraged the use of drugs.

Drugs also provide an escape for many people. Persons who escape through drugs are trying to forget about their problems. We live in a "pill society" where people come to believe that all the answers lie in pills of different sizes and colors. Pills help to alleviate our headaches, calm us down, put us to sleep, and solve our birth control problems. We are sold on the beneficial effects of pills through the media and in many cases by our doctors. A society literally brought up on pills sees drugs as a panacea or cure-all for its problems and finds it to be a relatively easy transition from taking pills to misusing and abusing drugs.

Many people take drugs just for the fun of it. There is a good feeling that one gets from being high and some drugs have a very relaxing effect on the individual. Many people feel more at ease among strangers when they are high. The high they receive from certain drugs is similar to a high you get from drinking. The motivation of fun and enjoyment is the same for both drugs.

Of the people you know who use some form of drug, what is their motivation for taking it?

One major reason why people use drugs is more difficult to understand because of its complexity. It has to do with a feeling of purposefulness that many people in today's society have lost. By purposefulness, we mean a reason to exist, a feeling that something is worthwhile attaining. For some people this goal was the betterment of their family, community, or country. However, in recent years many of these goals have ceased to exist. Families have tended to disintegrate and people no longer live near their families or the towns in which they were raised. Communities are often groups of alienated individuals who live in suburban "ghettos" where there is little communication. Persons are finding it more and more difficult to gain satisfaction from their jobs because of the tension produced by a competitive society. The special feeling that many people once felt for their country has also changed in recent years. Internal political problems, social upheaval, and war have made many people question the values of their society. A society without a purpose often looks for meaning here and now. Drugs offer this type of experience to many individuals who want to "drop out" of this kind of society, rather than stay around and try to change it.

basic terminology

In order to understand any subject, one should first familiarize himself with the basic vocabulary or terminology of that subject. Many persons become confused with drug-related terms because there are no clear-cut definitions of certain words. The terminology discussed in this section is used throughout this chapter; the explanations given are accepted definitions of these terms.

The United Nations has several agencies that are concerned with the international implications of drugs. The Commission on Narcotic Drugs supervises international agreements dealing with narcotics. The Permanent Central Narcotics Board and the Drug Supervisory Body supervise international trade in licit drugs. The World Health Organization (W.H.O.) Expert Committee on Dependence-Producing Drugs decides whether new drugs can cause addiction and should therefore be placed under international control.

DEPENDENCE

Dependence may be defined as a state of psychological and/or physiological dependence on a drug following the periodic or continued use of a drug. There are varying degrees and differing characteristics of dependence, based on the drug that is taken and the length of time that it has been used.

The World Health Organization (W.H.O.) discussed drug dependence in an article entitled, "Drug Dependence: Its Significance and Characteristics." This article appeared in the *Bulletin of the World Health Organization,* Vol. 32, 1965. The statement by W.H.O. was as follows:

"It has become impossible in practice, and is scientifically unsound, to maintain a single definition for all forms of drug addiction and/or habituation. A feature common to these conditions as well as to drug abuse in general is dependence, psychic or physical or both, of the individual on a chemical agent. Therefore, better understanding should be attained by substitution of the term drug dependence of this or that type, according to the agent or class of agents involved. . . . It must be emphasized that drug dependence is a general term that has been selected for its applicability to all types of drug abuse and thus carries no connotation of the degree of risk to public health or need for any or a particular type of drug control."

The W.H.O. makes another important statement that defines psychological drug dependence in the same *Bulletin* article:

"In this situation there is a feeling of satisfaction and a psychic drive that require periodic or continuous administration of the drug to produce the desired effect or to avoid discomfort."

The term dependence is used in place of other terms to describe the state of adaptation to a drug. Such words as addiction or habituation have a "bad" connotation that "dependence" does not have. When one is discussing a drug dependence, your mind should not become clouded with the picture of a "dope fiend" or "dope addict." The adoption of the term dependence allows us to look at the situation the way it really exists. The term dependence applies to all drugs and carries with it no implication of a degree of risk to individual or public health. It is a descriptive term that includes both physical and psychological dependence.

When a person is physically dependent on a drug, his body requires that drug in order to function in what has come to be a "normal" situation for that individual. If the drug is absent for a while, the functioning of the body becomes disrupted until the body is able to readjust to the new situation without that drug. This disruption of functioning results in the *withdrawal syndrome.*

WITHDRAWAL SYNDROME

The withdrawal syndrome is just what its name implies. It focuses on the physical and mental symptoms that result when a drug is withdrawn from an individual. The symptoms of withdrawal depend on the drug from which an individual is withdrawn. Some of the most common symptoms include irritability, anxiety, abdominal discomfort, nausea, convulsions, and delirium tremens. These symptoms will also vary in severity in relation to the type and length of drug dependence. As we get further into our exploration of specific drugs, those withdrawal symptoms that pertain to a drug or group of drugs will be discussed.

TOLERANCE
CROSS-TOLERANCE
AND REVERSE TOLERANCE

Tolerance is a physical reaction of the body to a drug. It is in one sense a survival mechanism that allows the body to be exposed to poisonous substances in large amounts without succumbing to their dangerous or lethal effects. As the cells of the body become accustomed for a particular dosage of a drug, the same amount of that drug cannot produce the desired effect. In order to get that feeling

or effect, the dosage of the drug must be continuously increased. The result is a physical dependence on the drug.

Cross-tolerance is the use of a different drug or drugs to help to relieve the withdrawal symptoms caused by another drug on which an individual is dependent. For example, barbiturates and tranquilizers are often used to help an alcoholic get through the withdrawal period from alcohol. You may then wonder, what could then be done to avoid the withdrawal symptoms that may result from the tranquilizers and barbiturates? The answer is simply that a person does not take enough of these drugs for a long enough period to develop a dependence on them.

Reverse tolerance is the need for less of a substance as time goes on. An alcoholic in the late stages of alcoholism needs less alcohol than when he started drinking.

POTENTIATION
AND SYNERGISM

Drugs that are said to be synergistic work together to produce a much greater effect than if taken alone. Synergistic drugs generally give a similar effect if taken alone; however, when taken together, the effect is so powerful that it may be lethal. For example, do you recall the discussion of a "Mickey Finn" in Chapter 5. This is a drugged alcoholic drink that can knock someone unconscious. The "working together" or synergism of alcohol and barbiturates, for example, produces a total depressant effect that can result in a dangerous condition, coma, or death. The effect of both drugs is much greater than the effect of either barbiturates or alcohol taken separately.

If two drugs are taken together and one strengthens or *potentiates* the action of the other, this is called potentiation. For example, certain drugs are used as local anesthetics in simple surgical procedures. Sometimes another drug is given along with the local anesthetic to aid in keeping the anesthetic in a particular area. A drug that constricts or closes up the blood vessels would have this effect and would *potentiate* the anesthetic.

ANTAGONISTIC DRUGS

Antagonistic drugs are those drugs that have an opposite effect on the body from other drugs. The antagonistic effects are usually temporary but can be valuable in treating overdoses or poisonings. The use of certain tranquilizers in the treatment of an overdose of the drug LSD is one example of how antagonistic drugs work.

drug users, drug misusers, and drug abusers

Just as there were social drinkers, problem drinkers, and alcoholics, there are different types of drug takers. You may be surprised to find out that you most likely are a drug user. A drug user is an individual who takes any type of drugs on a regular basis. A drug misuser is a person that is not responsible in his use of drugs. The drug abuser is the person who self-administers drugs for purposes of achieving a high. These three types of drug takers are discussed in the following section of this chapter.

THE DRUG USER

All of us are probably drug users even though we may not recognize ourselves as such. Alcohol, nicotine, and caffeine are all drugs that many of us take on a daily basis. The prescription pills you get from your pharmacist are also drugs that affect you physically and/or emotionally. These are drugs that are not used with the intention of getting a high and are generally used by the public for legitimate reasons.

Caffeine is one substance that people are constantly surprised to find out is a drug. It fits the definition of a drug in that it does affect the individual both physically and mentally. Caffeine is found in coffee, tea, cocoa, and cola drinks. Coffee was first discovered in Arabia and Turkey and was brought to Europe and eventually to the United States from these countries. Tea was discovered in China and imported at first from that country. The kola nut, from which many cola drinks are derived, came originally from West Africa. Cocoa comes from Mexico, the West Indies, and areas of Central and South America. Chocolate products are made from cocoa. Caffeine can also be found in the Cassina plant and many tribes of American Indians made a caffeine beverage similar to coffee from this plant.

Caffeine has some very specific effects on our bodies. It acts as a stimulant to the central nervous system and produces clearer and more rapid thought processes. It also helps to keep people awake. This aspect of helping people to stay awake makes caffeine a popular drug on the college campus. Pills that are largely made up of concentrated caffeine are frequently popped in all-night study sessions. Caffeine also improves one's appreciation of sensory stimuli and makes some people capable of increased motor activity.

Besides the actions of caffeine on the central nervous system, it also affects the heart rate, heart rhythm, diameter of the blood vessels, circulation, and blood pressure. In some research, caffeine has been linked to the secretion of stomach acids which in excess can cause a certain type of *ulcer* (a lesion or sore in the stomach wall).

Most people do not recognize the drug aspects of caffeine. They usually do not take it to achieve a clear mind or better work but rather because they enjoy drinking coffee. The scientists disagree as to whether one can become dependent on caffeine; however, some researchers have noted withdrawal symptoms at high levels of caffeine consumption. Depression has been found to occur as a withdrawal symptom among heavy coffee drinkers. Some research has indicated that dependence can occur in those who drink more than four or five cups of coffee in a day.

Caffeine can be fatal in extremely large

dosages. It is estimated that a fatal dose of caffeine for a human being would be 10 grams or the amount of caffeine found in 70 to 100 cups of coffee. If you drink coffee, try to answer the question of "why do you drink it?" Did you think of coffee as a drug prior to reading this chapter?

OVER-THE-COUNTER DRUGS

Drugs that are freely sold over the counter (OTC) are also used by many people who often do not understand that these drugs can produce harmful effects. The over-the-counter market is the largest distributor of such drugs as caffeine, nicotine, and alcohol.

Over-the-counter drugs are considered to be generally safe for the public to purchase in the treatment of their own ailments. The over-the-counter drug business is in excess of two and one-half billion dollars a year.

All types of drugs are sold over the counter. Vitamins, laxatives, antacids, pain relievers, cough syrups, and external creams are only a few of the thousands of preparations available in every drug store. The old-fashioned, staid, professional-looking drug store is hard to find these days. Most modern drug stores are basically outlets for packaged drugs that are boldly advertised throughout the store.

One of the most widely used over-the-counter drugs is aspirin. The phrase "widely used" may be a gross understatement considering the fact that Americans are estimated to take more than 40 million aspirin tablets each day. After alcohol, aspirin is the most widely used drug in the world. Aspirin is not a new drug by any means; it was used by the ancient Greeks as far back as 2,400 years ago. Aspirin is sold as a pain reliever and its active ingredient is salicylic acid. Aspirin serves many purposes. It can reduce or block low-level or moderate pain. It

When taken as directed, over-the-counter drugs are relatively harmless, but they can pose a danger if misused.

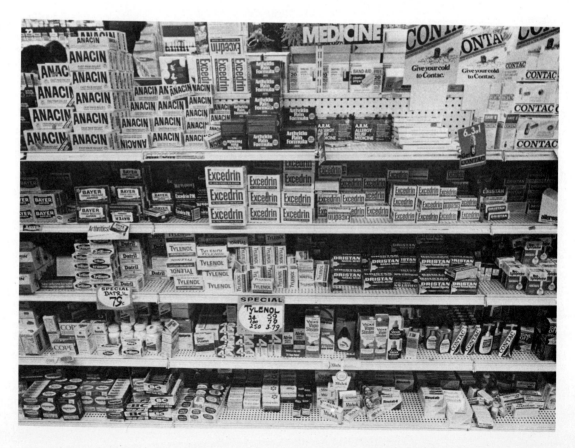

also has the ability to reduce soreness and
inflammation. This is especially valuable in
the treatment of arthritic conditions, especially
rheumatoid arthritis (an inflammation of the
joints). All of you are probably familiar
with the fever-reducing powers of aspirin.
It is a multipurpose drug that has a relatively
low toxic or poisonous level.

There are some problems inherent in taking
too much aspirin. Research has indicated
that excessive dosages may cause bleeding
from the stomach lining. Another serious
condition or even death can result from
an overdose of the substance. Aspirin poisoning causes many deaths each year, especially
among young children in the under-five
age group. "Baby aspirin" is the usual cause
of such deaths. Many children like its taste
and are attracted by its candy color (it is
often orange colored and flavored). Safety
caps and a limit of 36 tablets in a bottle
have helped to ensure child safety.

How frequently do you take aspirin and
for what reason? Have you ever felt better
almost immediately after taking this drug?
This effect may be explained by the way
we have been socialized to accept aspirin
as a "cure-all." From the time we were
children, aspirin has always been the first
remedy prescribed for many discomforts.
Those of you who are in the habit of frequently taking aspirin may "think" you feel
better as soon as you take it. It is a type
of conditioned response. This type of response
occurs with many other drugs. People believe
they are getting a certain effect from a particular drug because they want to believe
it. This interesting aspect of drugs is discussed
later in this chapter.

There has been much controversy concerning
the marketing of over-the-counter drugs,
especially aspirin. Many advertisers make
certain claims for a product that cannot
be proven. One such claim is that a buffered
aspirin is better than a nonbuffered tablet
because it reduces stomach acidity and
speeds up the absorption of the drug. Research

has not shown buffered aspirin to have any
effects that differ from plain aspirin.

PRESCRIPTION DRUGS

Prescription drugs are those that cannot
legally be purchased without a doctor's
prescription. There are a wide variety of
prescription drugs that are taken to relieve
both physical and psychological problems.
Why are certain drugs allowed to be sold
over the counter while others may only be
sold with a prescription? The answer to
this question can be found in the history of
the 1938 Food, Drug and Cosmetic Act.
This act was first introduced to establish
uniform safety laws regarding foods, drugs,
and cosmetics. Many amendments to this
act have been passed over the years but
the problems concerning which drugs should
be labeled as prescription and which should
be sold over the counter has persisted. In
1951, an amendment was passed that clarified
the prescription–nonprescription controversy.
According to this amendment, three groups
of prescription drugs were established. A
prescription drug had to meet these requirements: (1) those drugs that had warnings
on their labels as to their habit-forming
ingredients; (2) those drugs that the Food
and Drug Administration (FDA) had found to
be unsafe because of their poisonous or
toxic effects at high levels; and (3) all new
drugs that had to go through a trial period before they could be sold on the over-
the-counter market.

Many types of drugs are sold by prescription,
particularly those drugs that have psychological effects, the psychoactive drugs. Psychoactive drugs produce a temporary change
in a person's mood, feelings, and behavior.
These drugs include the sedatives, tranquilizers, stimulants, and certain antidepres-
sion drugs. The number of prescriptions
issued each year for these drugs has steadily
increased from 149 million prescriptions in
1964 to 214 million in 1970. These figures
indicate an increase of more than 40 percent
in psychoactive drug prescriptions. It is

interesting to note that the majority of people who take prescribed psychoactive drugs are women. Why do you think that this is the case? Does your own knowledge or experience contradict these findings?

Nicotine and alcohol are not discussed in detail in this chapter because separate chapters are devoted to these drugs. Alcohol was the subject of Chapter 5 and nicotine was discussed in Chapter 6 on Tobacco.

The drugs we may use every day (caffeine, nicotine, and aspirin) and the drugs that are purchased over the counter and by prescription are usually done so without the intention of getting a high. These drugs are taken for relief from a specific physical or emotional problem. This is a legitimate use of drugs. In the next section, the misuse of drugs, frequently for illegitimate reasons, is discussed. The psychoactive drugs are often used in this manner. They are considered as legitimate when used under a doctor's care in the proper dosage. They are misused if taken at one's own discretion and in unsafe dosages.

THE MISUSE OF DRUGS

Drugs are misused in many ways. Some of obvious misuses include excessive cigarette smoking and drinking of alcohol. As was discussed in the alcohol chapter, many people misuse the drug alcohol by taking too much of it and becoming intoxicated. Alcohol can be used legitimately if taken in small amounts that do not adversely affect one's behavior or safety. The same is true with cigarette smoking. If one smokes a few cigarettes to relieve tension or just to have something to do, this may not be a misuse of the drug nicotine. Unfortunately, most smokers are unable to limit their dependence and therefore endanger their health by smoking. This constitutes a misuse of nicotine. This was discussed in detail in Chapter 6

Have you ever taken a medication that someone else has given you? This would be a misuse of a drug. Prescribed drugs should be taken only by the person for

whom they have been prescribed. To take someone else's prescription drug is a misuse that could be very dangerous. People also misuse drugs by either not reading the directions or by not following them. Two teaspoonsful is *not* better than one when you are taking a medication. The dosage is carefully considered by the doctor when he writes his prescription. Dosages are usually based on age, weight, and physical condition and therefore should not be changed by the patient at will. Misusing drugs in this manner can result in uncomfortable side effects and more dangerous complications.

Some people take too much of a ''good thing.'' If they find they are losing a moderate amount of weight on a prescribed diet pill, they may increase the dosage hoping to lose more weight, more quickly. This is a dangerous practice that could seriously affect their physical and emotional health. Never alter a dosage by yourself. If you think the dosage may be incorrect, check immediately with your doctor. Many drugs are potentially harmful, some are deadly—they should be taken responsibly and not be misused.

THE DRUG ABUSERS

Drug abusers may be defined as those individuals who self-administer drugs for purposes of achieving a high or a modification of mood or behavior for any number of complex reasons. Many drugs fit into all the categories discussed. They can be used, misused, or abused depending on the amount taken and the period of time over which they are taken. For example, you could *use* a prescription to help you sleep and if taken properly that would be a legitimate use of the drug. However, you could *misuse* that drug by giving some sleeping pills to a friend or by taking more than the prescribed dosage. If you were to *abuse* the same drug, you could take an overdose and not live to tell about it!

The use, misuse, and abuse of drugs is not a black-and-white, clear-cut matter. It is often difficult to define what actually constitutes misuse or abuse of a drug. It also differs for each individual. What might be considered a misuse of a drug for some people would be an abuse for others. This can be understood in relation to alcohol. Some people cannot tolerate too many drinks and only a few drinks may be a misuse of that drug for that person. Others may be able to drink more heavily without being affected or affecting others. Therefore, a few drinks would not be a misuse of the drug for these people. A person's state of mind also affects whether he is using, misusing, or abusing a drug. A depressed individual will act differently upon taking a drug than if he were elated. Mood has a great deal to do with the way a drug will affect you. If you are in a happy mood, a small amount of alcohol will have a disinhibiting effect. If you are depressed, you may drink more to gain the same effect and you would be misusing or abusing the drug. Have you found this to be true? Do you react differently to a drug depending on your mood or your company? Ask a few of your friends this question. You may not get substantial research findings in this way, but you will have a good indication of how people react to drugs under different conditions.

In the next section of this chapter you will learn about the different types or classifications of the most common drugs. You have probably heard or read about many of these drugs, but you may not be familiar with what they are used for, their physical and psychological effects, and how they are taken.

the classification of common drugs

Drugs may be classified in many ways. Doctors, pharmacists, chemists, and lawyers all have different classification systems for grouping drugs. For example, a doctor will usually classify a drug according to its major medical use; a pharmacist according to the purpose for which it is most frequently sold; a chemist according to its chemical makeup; and a lawyer according to the way it is classified by recent federal drug laws.

In this book, drugs are classified according to their effect on the body, specifically on the central nervous system. According to this classification, our study of drugs will include the narcotic drugs (basically central nervous system depressants), sedative drugs (depressants that have a quieting effect), marijuana (a sedative with some psychoactive or mood-changing qualities), stimulants (drugs that stimulate the central nervous system), hallucinogens (psychoactive drugs that distort time and place), and volatile solvents (mind-altering drugs that are inhaled).

NARCOTIC DRUGS

Narcotic drugs act primarily as a depressant to the central nervous system, but they also act to relieve pain, induce sleep, relieve coughing and diarrhea. Some patients who take narcotic drugs experience a feeling of well-being or euphoria while others experience the opposite effect or dysphoria (a feeling of anxiety, tension, and fear). If taken in excess, narcotics can lead to coma or death from respiratory failure.

Narcotic drugs generally cause a physical dependence in varying degrees. Individuals who do become dependent on these drugs usually develop a *tolerance* for the drug. If you recall an earlier section of this chapter, tolerance was defined as an increasing resistance to the usual effects of the drug.

The pharmacy label accompanying a prescribed narcotic usually bears a warning about its use.

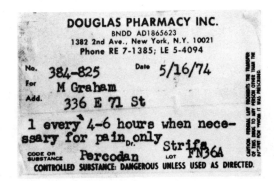

A tolerance also implies that the drug abuser must take more and more of the drug in order to feel well and experience the euphoria that these drugs can produce. If the drug is taken for a medical purpose, at the proper intervals and dosage, dependence will generally not occur. However, if dependence does occur, a lack of the drug will cause a *withdrawal syndrome* (severe even fatal effects due to a lack of the drug).

OPIATES

The opiates are narcotic drugs that are derived from the oriental poppy plant. These red, white, and purple flowers grow best in a very hot and dry climate. They usually grow in India, Turkey, and certain areas of Russia, China, Egypt, and Mexico. The drug opium is the dried juice of the pods or capsules of the poppy plant. Each plant yields a very small amount of juice so many fields of poppy flowers must be planted to get a sufficient opium supply.

In the areas where opium is produced, the field workers cut open the pods of the plant and the white juices come to the surface of the pods. Contact with the oxygen in the air produces a chemical reaction called oxidation, and the white juice turns a reddish-brown color, thickens, and hardens into gumlike, dark-colored balls. This is the natural opium drug. The natural product has a bitter taste and a sweet smell.

Opium has been used for thousands of years. Some persons place its discovery in ancient Egypt around the year 1600 B.C. A document written on papyrus seems to identify opium as a product used to keep children from crying too much. It was also used by the ancient Greeks and Romans, and Homer referred to it as a ''destroyer of grief.'' Opium was thought to be carried to Persia and China by Arab merchants. It reached India in the 1500s and was very popular in that country. India began to grow its own crop of opium poppies and started to export it. Opium was used heavily by the Chinese,

Harvesting opium from the poppy plant.

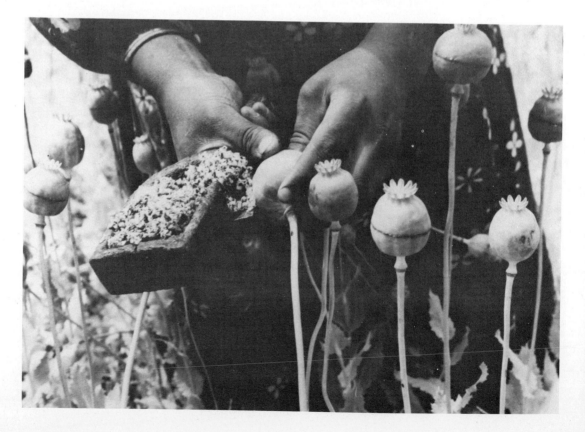

so much so that two "Opium Wars" were fought over it. In an attempt to stop opium use and trade, the Chinese rulers went to war with the British whose trade domination of China was linked to opium smuggling. The British won both wars fought between 1834 and 1858, and the importing of opium became legal.

The legalization of opium led to its widespread use in the United States in the late 1800s. Some people have described the United States during this period as a "dope addict's paradise." Opium was cheaply priced, readily available, and legally sold with or without a prescription. One could buy opium products at grocery stores, drug stores, and even by mail order. There were also numerous patent medicines sold that contained opium. They were sold for all types of problems including teething, coughs, menstrual cramps, and as general pain killers.

Morphine is an opiate drug that is derived from opium. It is produced by chemically refining opium into a product that is about ten times stronger than opium. It is usually found in the form of a cube, capsule, tablet, powder, or solution. It is sold illegally in a capsule called a "cap" or as a powder folded in paper and called "paper" or "package." It is also known on the street as "M," "dreamer," "white stuff," "morpho," "cube," and "monkey." Have you heard any of these names for morphine? Are there other names you have heard that are used for morphine?

Morphine is an excellent pain killer and has a strong tranquilizing or quieting effect on individuals. It alleviates a patient's fear of pain, his anxiety about the pain, as well as lessening the pain itself.

Most morphine that is sold illegally has usually been stolen from hospitals or doctors' offices. It is often obtained by forging stolen prescription forms. Morphine is usually used by drug abusers by injection or taken orally. Different methods of using opiates are explained later in this chapter.

Known as "snow," "stuff," "H," "junk," "horse," "joy powder," and numerous other names, heroin is produced from morphine and is twice as addictive as morphine. It is also 20 to 25 times as strong as morphine and is therefore a very dangerous drug when abused. The danger of dependence on heroin is greater than to other opiates because of the body's tolerance of this drug. Increasingly large doses of the drug are needed within a short period of time in order to get a high.

In its pure state heroin is a grayish-brown powder, but because of its strength it can be diluted many times with milk sugar. This diluting is referred to as "wetting" and as it is diluted the heroin loses its brown color and becomes off-white or white in color. It is odorless and has a very bitter taste. Heroin is usually sold in one-ounce or smaller plastic bags by the wholesalers and is then redistributed by the "pushers" in bags, papers, or capsules.

Codeine is a mild opiate and does not have strong pain relieving or sleep inducing effects. It is widely used in cough preparations as it affects the cough center of the brain. It is derived from morphine or produced directly from opium. It is an odorless white powder that is usually taken in tablet form. Drug abusers will occasionally take codeine if no stronger drug (morphine or heroin) is available. It is not usually abused because it does not produce as strong a high as the other opiate drugs. If one overdoses on codeine, convulsions may occur. On the street codeine is sometimes referred to as "schoolboy." Check your medicine cabinet at home for any cough preparations. Do any of them contain codeine? If so, how does the prescription label read?

ROUTE OF ADMINISTRATION

There are different routes of administration or ways of taking opiate drugs. Beginners usually "snort" or "sniff" the drug. Inhaling the drug results in a very mild "kick" and may also cause an inflammation of the nasal passages. In order to achieve a better high, the drug dose or "fix" is injected into fleshy skin areas. This is called "skin popping."

However, the tolerance to these drugs, especially heroin, builds so rapidly that "skin popping" will not give the desired high after a short period of taking the drug in this way. When the drug abuser begins to inject the drug directly into his veins, he is "mainlining" and a high can be rapidly achieved. Usually three or four "fixes" or more a day are needed to keep the chronic drug abuser from suffering the pain and discomfort of the withdrawal syndrome. This is discussed later in the chapter.

Many drug abusers are not careful about sterilizing their hypodermic needles and other equipment. Infections are often passed from one person to another because of this lack of care. Hepatitis (an infection that affects the liver) is a common disease among chronic drug abusers.

SYNTHETIC NARCOTICS

Synthetic narcotics are made in laboratories from petroleum products or coal tar. They are *not* derived from opium. They are usually taken by mouth. Some of the more easily recognized synthetic opiates include Demerol, methadone, Mepergan, and Nalline. Methadone is frequently given to persons who have been chronically dependent on heroin or morphine. It enables these people to live relatively normal lives without craving other opiate drugs. Methadone is discussed in detail later in this chapter.

Synthetic drugs can also result in dependence. Dependence on Demerol, for example, often occurs in persons involved in the medical profession where the drug is readily available. Withdrawal symptoms result when a person stops taking synthetic drugs.

It is interesting to note that heroin can be synthetically produced. One may wonder why the street sellers are not producing and peddling these products. The answer is in the cost. It is still significantly cheaper to produce opiates from opium than to produce them by synthetic means.

physical and psychological dependence

Physical dependence often referred to as addiction can only occur with the use of certain drugs. These *certain* drugs are all depressants and include alcohol as well as all of the opiates discussed so far in this chapter. One can say that physical dependence has occurred if the drug abuser has built up a tolerance to a drug and if withdrawal symptoms result when the drug is taken away. The reasons why tolerance to certain drugs does occur are still subject to scientific inquiry. However, it is known that after repeated doses of the same drug, the dosage must be increased in order to achieve the same pleasurable effects.

These pleasurable effects often referred to as "a high" are also called a "kick," "bang," or "rush." These terms are often used to describe the feeling a drug abuser experiences after mainlining morphine or heroin. The experience is often described as so pleasurable that many addicts "shoot" the drug just for that purpose. Those who "snort" or "skin-pop" drugs do not feel the "rush" that is associated with mainlining. But these drug users can get just as "hooked" or dependent on the drug as those who "mainline."

When a drug is taken away completely or sharply curtailed in amount, the user suffers from the withdrawal syndrome. This syndrome covers a number of discomforts and more serious physical conditions. The lesser symptoms often include restlessness, tension, irritability, upset stomach, and muscle pain. The more serious conditions may include hallucinations, convulsions, delerium tremens (especially in alcoholics), and delusions.

Have you ever heard of the expression "cold turkey?" It is often used to describe the giving up of a habit in an abrupt manner. Persons who go "cold turkey" on cigarettes suddenly stop smoking. They do not slowly cut down the number of cigarettes they smoke, but give them up all at once. The same expression applies to persons who abuse drugs. However, the expression has more meaning in the case of drugs because it describes a withdrawal symptom—that of goosebumps. The drug abuser who goes "cold turkey" often gets goose flesh or bumps, and his skin looks somewhat like a plucked turkey. This is where the expression is thought to have originated. Have you ever given up a habit by going "cold turkey?" Do you think this is the best way to stop smoking, drinking, or taking drugs?

Psychological dependence is the desire of the user to obtain a drug because he has become accustomed to using it. A person becomes used to a drug or other substance and feels the psychological need for it rather than the physical need. Psychological dependence can develop to any number of things such as coffee, soda, alcohol, cigarettes, and drugs. You probably know people who cannot get through the day without drinking many bottles of soda. They do not physically need to drink it, but it gives them something to do and they think they must continually have it. When people smoke heavily, they feel tense or restless until they light up another cigarette. These are all psychological dependencies. People can develop psychological dependencies on most drugs, including the opiates. People who become psychologically dependent on these drugs feel that they could not function without them. They do not continue to abuse drugs in order to prevent withdrawal symptoms but because they enjoy the high they experience.

DEPRESSANT OR SEDATIVE DRUGS

Drugs that have a depressant effect on the central nervous system are classified in this group. Alcohol is a depressant drug that many people think is a stimulant. However, as was dicussed in Chapter 5, the depressant action of alcohol on the brain results in the symptoms of intoxication. Depressant drugs include alcohol, the narcotic drugs, and

the barbiturates. The barbiturate drugs are drugs used in medicine primarily to induce sleep. These and other depressant drugs are discussed in this section of the chapter.

BARBITURATES

The story behind the name "barbiturates" is unusual and one may only assume that it is true. The story is told that Dr. A. Bayer (of the Bayer Laboratories in Germany, where aspirin was first produced) was doing research with substances combined with urea (a product of urine). The urine for these experiments was supposedly taken from a girl named Barbara and, upon producing the new compound, Dr. Bayer named it *barbiturates* (from Barbara's urates).

Barbiturates act as general depressants and affect all levels of brain function as well as skeletal muscle, smooth muscle, and heart muscle function. They effect judgment, memory, and emotional control, producing effects that are similar to those produced by alcohol. They are most commonly used to induce sleep but can depress the central nervous system so severely that coma or death may result. They are sometimes used as *anticonvulsants* (to prevent convulsions) as in the disease epilepsy. Barbiturates are usually taken by mouth but are sometimes injected. There are frequent side effects from taking barbiturates, including allergic conditions, skin conditions, hangover (similar to that from alcohol), and pain. It is important to note here that both physical and psychological dependence can result from continued use of most barbiturates. Physical dependence implies *tolerance* and the dosage of barbiturates must be continually increased in order to maintain the same effect.

Two of the most commonly prescribed barbiturates are phenobarbital and Seconal. Both are sold only by prescription and are usually prescribed to help patients to sleep. These barbiturates and others are widely used in the United States today. It has been estimated that three to four billion doses of these drugs are prescribed annually in this country. This is the legal consumption of these drugs. It has also been estimated that more than 300 tons of barbiturate drugs are produced each year and about one-half of this amount goes into the illegal market.

Many kinds of barbiturates are taken or "dropped" by drug abusers. These drugs are often designated by their color on the illegal market. Phenobarbital is often sold in yellow capsules and are called "yellow jackets," "yellows," "phennies," or "barbs." Seconal capsules are usually red in color and are known as "redbirds," "red devils," or "pink ladies." Another barbiturate, Amytal, is usually in a blue capsule and is known on the street as "bluebirds," "blue devils," and "blue heavens." When two barbiturates such as Amytal and Seconal are sold in one capsule, it is usually red and blue in color. This capsule is often called a "Christmas tree," "double trouble," or "tooies." The names speak for themselves. Have you heard any other names used to describe barbiturates?

Young people frequently start taking barbiturates at home. They have often been prescribed for their parents and teenagers find them in the medicine cabinet and experiment with them. The effects of abusing barbiturates are similar to those of abusing alcohol. The abuser of barbiturates becomes intoxicated to varying degrees depending on how much of the drug he uses and his tolerance for the drug. If a person is acting as if he were intoxicated but there is no smell of alcohol around him, he is probably using barbiturates. Eventually, barbiturate users will pass out if they take too much of the drug. However, barbiturates are more dangerous than alcohol because all of the drug is absorbed into the body and is rarely vomited up by the user. If barbiturates are abused, they may at first make the drug user feel more relaxed and more sociable. After another dose, he may begin to feel sluggish and tired. If he has taken a large dose of the drug, he will fall into a deep sleep that may be followed by a coma. If medical attention is not promptly received, the person may never come out of the coma and may die in this state.

Many patients take barbiturates in order to commit suicide. It is estimated that about one-fifth of all suicides result from barbiturate poisoning. It is the second most common method of committing suicide (carbon monoxide poisoning is the most used method). Accidental deaths often occur after a person has taken the prescribed dose of the drug and then in his half-awake state reaches out for more pills. If a person has little tolerance for the drug, a small amount could produce deadly effects. Do you or any members of your family take barbiturates by prescription? If so, how does the bottle label read? Where do you or your family keep the drug? Are they aware of its danger?

If you recall from Chapter 5, the taking of alcohol with another depressant drug was discussed. Many people, especially young people, mix alcohol and barbiturates in an attempt to get a "double high." This high is very short-lived as the drug abuser may soon fall into a coma and die from the actions of the two drugs. A combination of barbiturates and alcohol interferes with body functions that help to dispose of these drugs. This causes a toxic or lethal level of the drug to be reached in a relatively short period of time. In addition, the two drugs working together have a *synergistic* effect, resulting in a greater depressant effect than if each drug were taken alone.

METHAQUALONE

This drug is fairly new on the depressant drug scene, but it has received much media coverage in recent times. Known as "heroin for lovers" because of its supposed aphrodisiac (ability to increase sexual desire or powers) effects, this drug has become very popular among young people, especially college students. These aphrodisiac powers have never been proven but a recent survey of Northeastern colleges still finds this drug fast becoming one of the most popular drugs on campus.

Methaqualone is prescribed as a sedative-hypnotic (drug that induces sleep and has a quieting effect). This drug is a central nervous system depressant and is as dangerous, if abused, as barbiturates. If taken with alcohol, it is also as lethal as barbiturates. It has been found that most abusers of this drug started taking it by legal prescription or by getting the drug from someone who had a prescription. At one time the drug did not come under the same strict controls as the narcotic drugs, and many tablets were diverted from pharmaceutical houses to the street. However, methaqualone is now under strict federal drug control. Have you heard of methaqualone? Do you think it is easily obtainable?

TRANQUILIZERS

Tranquilizers are also central nervous system depressants and they are used medically

Are some prescription drugs too easy to get?

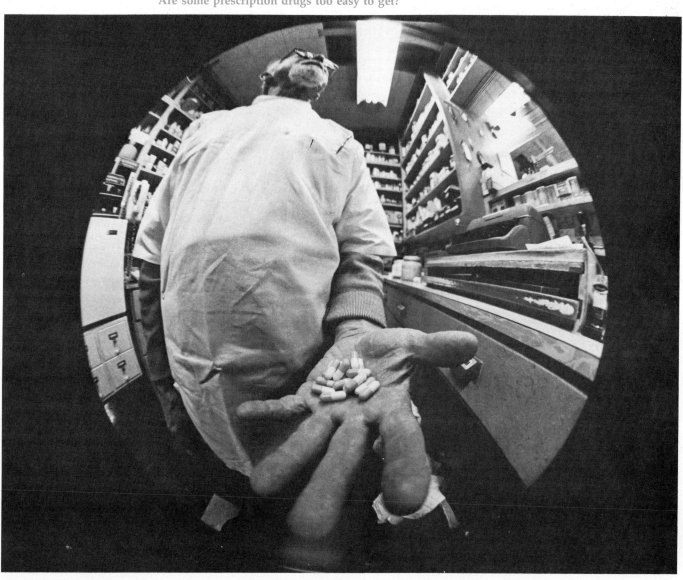

to calm people and relieve highly emotional or nervous states. They are usually grouped as major and minor tranquilizers depending on their strength. The major tranquilizers are used to quiet psychotic (persons who are severely mentally ill) patients. They cannot be used to alleviate everyday tension or nervousness. Their use for this purpose is considered dangerous even at low dosages. However, these drugs are very useful in managing mentally ill patients, especially those who are hospitalized.

Most doctors prescribe the minor tranquilizers for the symptoms of nervousness and tension. Their effects are very similar to the barbiturates except that a dose that is sufficient to reduce nervous symptoms seems to produce less sleepiness than the same dose of a barbiturate. Tranquilizers are widely used for tension and such symptoms of tension as stomach discomfort, fast heart beat, headaches, restlessness, anxiety, and general nervous conditions.

There are many tranquilizers on the market today. Three of the most widely used are *meprobromate* (Miltown and Equanil), *diphenylmenthanes* (Phobex and Atarax), and *chlordiazepoxide* (Librium and Librax). Many of you may recognize some of the names. Some of these drugs (especially Miltown and Librium) have become a part of everyday language. Ask a few friends or relatives if they know what Librium is used for. Were you surprised at their answers?

The minor tranquilizers are not usually abused because they do not produce a high. However, dependence can occur if the dosage of the drug is increased over a long period of time. The dosage prescribed by doctors is safe (if directions are followed) and persons can take prescribed levels of the drug for long periods without becoming physically dependent on the drug. However, psychological dependence may occur if a person begins to feel that he cannot function without his daily dosage of the drug. Physical and psychological dependence on the depressants is discussed in the next section of this chapter.

PHYSICAL AND PSYCHOLOGICAL DEPENDENCE

Physical dependence on barbiturates is similar to physical dependence on alcohol. It slowly builds as the individual increases his tolerance for the drug. Dependence, both physical and psychological, will vary with the dose, length of time one has been taking the drug, and with one's personality. Withdrawal from barbiturates is similar to withdrawal from alcohol. The usual symptoms include delirium tremens, nausea, sweating, and fever. However, heavy barbiturate abusers should never go "cold turkey" as the shock to their bodies often results in death. Withdrawal from barbiturates should take place under close medical supervision.

Psychological dependence on barbiturates is similar to that of alcohol. Barbiturate abusers like the high they get from the drug and feel they would become depressed without it. They often develop a strong psychological need for the drug that may vary in intensity depending on the personality and surroundings of the individual.

Tranquilizer abusers can suffer from physical dependence on the drug if they tend to be dependence-prone. These are individuals who are abusing or have abused other drugs. Such individuals will suffer from withdrawal symptoms that are similar to withdrawal from alcohol or barbiturates. If one has been taking large dosages of tranquilizers, he should not be abruptly withdrawn from the drug. As with the barbiturates, withdrawal should occur under medical supervision.

CANNABIS OR MARIJUANA

Probably more has been written about this drug in recent years than any other drug. No matter how you feel about this drug, you can find someone in a position of authority to back up your opinion. Because of the drug's exposure by the media, you may already be well-acquainted with its effects. This section of the chapter will discuss marijuana in some detail, and you may discover some new facts about the drug.

Marijuana is usually classified as a sedative hypnotic that has some psychoactive qualities. The drug is produced from the Cannabis sativa plant that grows in many varieties throughout the world. The active ingredient of the plant has been indentified as tetrahydrocannabinol (THC). This substance is most highly concentrated in the resin of the plant which is produced by the flowering tops and leaves of the plant.

The term marijuana is probably derived from a Spanish or Portuguese word that means intoxication. Marijuana as it is most commonly known in the United States is a smoking mixture that is composed of the chopped leaves, stems, and flowers of the *Cannabis* plant. Charas or ganja is another form of the drug that is the unadulterated resin obtained from the plant or dried flowers. This form of the drug is much stronger than marijuana and is most often used in India. Hashish usually refers to a powdered form of charas and is stronger than marijuana. Hashish is available in the United States and is often called "hash." There are many street names for marijuana including "pot," "Mary Jane," "tea," "grass," and "weed." Marijuana cigarettes, known as "joints" and "reefers" are the most popular way of smoking the drug. Do you or your friends know any other slang names for marijuana? Is it smoked in any way other than by cigarettes?

What are the effects of marijuana? Is it a dangerous drug? Should penalties for possession of the drug be strengthened or reduced? These are only a few of the questions that are posed each day concerning marijuana. The effects of marijuana are often compared to those of alcohol. It is basically a sociable drug that is smoked with other people to achieve a high. A marijuana high or getting "stoned" is usually stimulating at its onset and is mildly tension relieving. One has a good feeling upon initially smoking marijuana. The latter effects (with continued smoking) usually result in a peaceful, quiet mood. However, periods of uncontrolled laughter may alternate with periods of silence.

Many individuals report that their sensory perception improves and that they experience changes in perception of time and space. Memory may be impaired and the passage of time is frequently overestimated. Most smokers of marijuana report receiving desirable effects from the drug and seem to enjoy pleasant experiences while under its influence.

Are there any long-term effects or adverse conditions resulting from marijuana smoking? This question is difficult to answer as the smokers and the experts all have different opinions. Cases of marijuana-induced psychosis have been reported but they are rare and the condition generally does not occur

Getting "stoned."

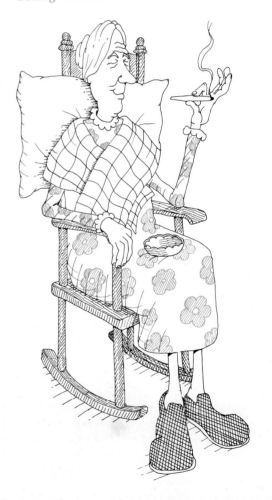

in stable individuals. There has been some research that reports chromosomal damage and birth defects in children born to heavy marijuana users. However, this relationship has not been definitely established. Another side effect sometimes associated with heavy marijuana smoking is a loss of motivation. This effect is difficult to prove scientifically and many so-called "pot-heads" or heavy users of the drug get involved in different life styles that may not stress the goals of the general American society. The following statement from the *Official Report of the National Commission on Marijuana and Drug Abuse* refers to this type of behavioral change. "No evidence exists to date to demonstrate that marijuana use alone caused these behavioral changes either directly or indirectly." It is presently thought that behavioral changes, such as loss of motivation, tend to be short-lived and that marijuana is only one of many contributing factors that may cause these changes. There seem to be no withdrawal symptoms and physical dependence on marijuana has not been established. Psychological dependence, however, tends to be quite strong. Heavy users have demonstrated symptoms of anxiety, restlessness, and insomnia when they abruptly stop using the drug.

Regular marijuana smokers tend to feel a definite psychological need for the drug. They seem to generally enjoy the drug experience and often promote it to their friends. The set and the setting have a great influence on how marijuana will affect the smoker. Different effects are experienced depending on the people and the environment. A happy, noisy crowd will experience marijuana smoking differently than a quiet, unfriendly crowd. Marijuana smokers will often perceive what they want to perceive and will "think" that marijuana is the reason for a certain perception. Frequently marijuana smokers will think they have experienced a change in time, place, or perception because they have heard that this is an effect of the drug.

The legal aspects of marijuana will be briefly discussed here in reference to the Marijuana Tax Act of 1937. The Marijuana Tax Act

attempted to control the use of marijuana by using federal police power and the imposition of penalties on buyers and sellers of the drug. The transfer of marijuana to unapproved or illegal buyers is supposed to be taxed at $100.00 per ounce. Since this transfer is considered illegal by the federal government, the high cost of the tax was designed to publicize dealings in the drug and make the drug difficult to purchase. The Tax Act carries with it maximum sentences of from 10 to 40 years depending on the offense. The Marijuana Tax Act is frequently the subject of debate. Many people think that the penalties are too stiff and should be relaxed. Some states have already adopted laws that lessen the penalties for possession of a small amount of marijuana. Others feel that they are not stiff enough. How do you feel about this law? Should it be changed or repealed?

Research concerning marijuana continues in many areas. You have probably read about some aspect of current research in a popular magazine or newspaper. Two such findings were recently spotted by the author and they provide some interesting information regarding marijuana and your health. Preliminary research at New York's Columbia-Presbyterian Medical Center reported evidence that marijuana smoking may lower the body's resistance to disease by impairing the body's *immunity* (ability to fight off disease or foreign matter). However, this discouraging information has a bright side. In transplant operations it is essential that the body does not reject the new organ. Most rejection takes place because of the body's immune responses toward the "foreign" organ. It is hoped that new drugs may be produced from marijuana that might help prevent transplant rejection. It is also hoped that similar drugs may be developed in the fight against cancer.

In a November 1974 report the Department of Health, Education and Welfare summarized research findings concerning frequent marijuana use. Some of the findings are:

1. Depressed levels of the male sex hormone

testosterone have been found in some men who use marijuana habitually.

2. Marijuana consumed regularly during early pregnancy—while sexual differentiation is occurring—may adversely affect the development of the male fetus.

3. Tests have shown that automobile drivers under the influence of marijuana have slower than normal reaction times and loss of concentration.

This report stressed that although these and other findings are tentative, it is thought that marijuana may be more harmful than was previously thought. The report made no recommendations concerning laws governing the use of marijuana.

Current research being performed at the Long Beach, California, Veteran's Administration Hospital has produced some data that concern marijuana smokers who have angina pectoris or intense chest pains. Persons who smoke "pot" and suffer from this disease tend to show a rapid increase in heart rate and blood pressure. The level of carbon monoxide gas (a toxic gas) in the blood also increased markedly. These researchers feel that their data indicates a potential danger to those known angina patients who smoke marijuana. In your reading, have you come across any new research concerning marijuana? If so, write a brief paragraph describing the findings and discuss it in class.

STIMULANTS

Do you take any stimulants? Your immediate answer to this question is probably "no." However, do you drink cola, coffee, or tea and do you smoke cigarettes? If you answered "yes" to the second question, then you *do* take stimulants. These substances all contain natural stimulants in the form of caffeine and nicotine. Stimulants are substances that speed up the functioning of the body. Caffeine was discussed in an earlier section of this chapter on page 125. You may want to review this section. Nicotine was discussed in detail in Chapter 6.

COCAINE

Cocaine is a natural stimulant drug that is extracted from the leaves of the coca shrub. This plant is native to areas of South America where cocaine has been used for more than 400 years by local inhabitants. These people would chew the leaves of the plant in order to produce the desired effect or high. It is interesting to note that although cocaine is a stimulant drug, it is listed as a narcotic or depressant drug under the federal narcotic drug laws. Cocaine is processed from the coca leaves into an odorless, white, fine crystalline powder and that is why the street name "snow" was given to the drug. Other street or slang names for the drug include "coke," "leaf," "flake," "dynamite," and "joy powder." When cocaine is mixed with heroin, it is called "speed-ball." This combination is sometimes injected by heavy heroin abusers.

Cocaine was first used medically as an anesthetic and as an agent to stop excessive bleeding. It is still used today as a local anesthetic in certain types of surgery. Cocaine taken in moderate doses tends to speed up the heart, dilate the pupils, and increase body temperature. There are many stories told about how cocaine improves one's sexual abilities and how it can make people more daring and brave in the face of danger. However, these stories are purely speculative and hard scientific data has not been found to back them up.

An individual under the influence of the drug becomes very active, talkative, sociable, and feels happy. The high of cocaine does not last long and may be followed rather quickly by a depression. If the amount of cocaine taken is increased, hallucinations may occur and confusion may also result. Some individuals have reported the sensation of feeling that there were bugs crawling under their skin. If the drug is taken in large amounts, a deep sleep, coma, or death may result.

Physical dependence on cocaine has not been established and there are no physical withdrawal symptoms. However, there is evidence of strong psychological dependence

TABLE 7-1 DRUGS: MEDICAL USES, SYMPTOMS PRODUCED, AND DEPENDENCE POTENTIALS

Name	Slang name	Chemical or trade name	Source	Classification	Medical use	How taken
Heroin	H., horse, scat, junk, smack, scag, stuff, Harry	Diacetyl-morphine	Semisynthetic (from morphine)	Narcotic	None in U.S.	Injected or sniffed
Morphine	White stuff, M.	Morphine sulphate	Natural (from opium)	Narcotic	Pain relief	Swallowed or injected
Codeine	Schoolboy	Methylmorphine	Natural (from opium), semi-synthetic (from morphine)	Narcotic	Ease pain and coughing	Swallowed
Methadone	Dolly	Dolophine, Amidone	Synthetic	Narcotic	Pain relief	Swallowed or injected
Cocaine	Corrine, gold dust, coke, Bernice, flake, star dust, snow	Methylester of benzoylecgonine	Natural (from coca, *not* cocao)	Stimulant, local anesthetic	Local anesthesia	Sniffed, injected, or swallowed
Marijuana	Pot, grass, tea, gage, reefers	*Cannabis sativa*	Natural	Relaxant, euphoriant, in high doses hallucinogen	None in U.S.	Smoked, swallowed, or sniffed
Barbiturates	Barbs, blue devils, candy, yellow jackets, phennies, peanuts, blue heavens	Phenobarbital, Nembutal, Seconal, Amytal	Synthetic	Sedative-hypnotic	Sedation, relieve high blood pressure, epilepsy, hyper-thyroidism	Swallowed or injected
Amphetamines	Bennies, Dexies, speed, wakeups, lid proppers, hearts, pep pills	Benzedrine, Dexedrine, Desoxyn, Methedrine	Synthetic	Sympatho-mimetic	Relieve mild depression, con-trol appetite and narcolepsy	Swallowed or injected
LSD	Acid, sugar, big D, cubes, trips	D-lysergic acid diethylamide-25	Semisynthetic (from ergot alkaloids)	Hallucinogen	Experimental study of mental function, alcoholism	Swallowed
Mescaline	Mesc.	3,4,5-trimeth-oxyphenethyl-amine	Natural (from peyote)	Hallucinogen	None	Swallowed
Psilocybin		3-[2-(dimethyl-amino)ethyl]indol-4-ol dehydrogen phosphate ester	Natural (from *Psilocybe mexicana*)	Hallucinogen	None	Swallowed
Methaqualone	Meth, ludes, Quaaludes, soapers	Quaalude, Sopor, Parest, Optimal, Somnafac	Synthetic	Sedative	Sleeping aid	Swallowed

Source: Adapted from *Resource Book for Drug Abuse Education,* Washington, D.C.: U.S. Department of Health, Education and Welfare Public Health Service, National Clearinghouse for Mental Health Information, October 1969.

Usual dose	Duration of effect	Effects sought	Long-term symptoms	Physical dependence potential	Mental dependence potential	Organic damage potential
Varies	4 hours	Euphoria, prevent withdrawal discomfort	Addiction, constipation, loss of appetite	Yes	Yes	No
15 milligrams	6 hours	Euphoria, prevent withdrawal discomfort	Addiction, constipation, loss of appetite	Yes	Yes	No
30 milligrams	4 hours	Euphoria, prevent withdrawal discomfort	Addiction, constipation, loss of appetite	Yes	Yes	No
10 milligrams	4–6 hours	Prevent withdrawal discomfort	Addiction, constipation, loss of appetite	Yes	Yes	No
Varies	Varies, short	Excitation, talkativeness	Depression, convulsions, paranoid delusions	No	Yes	Yes?
1–2 cigarettes	4 hours	Relaxation, increased euphoria, perceptions, sociability	None?	No	Yes?	No?
50–100 milligrams	4 hours	Anxiety reduction, euphoria	Addiction w/ severe withdrawal symptoms, possible convulsions, toxic psychosis	Yes	Yes	Yes
2.5–5 milligrams	4 hours	Alertness, activeness	Loss of appetite, delusions, hallucinations, toxic psychosis	No?	Yes	Yes?
100–500 micrograms	10 hours	Insightful experiences, exhilaration, distortion of senses	May intensify existing psychosis, panic reactions	No	No?	No?
400 micrograms	12 hours	Insightful experiences, exhilaration, distortion of senses	May intensify existing psychosis, panic reactions	No	No?	No?
25 milligrams	6–8 hours	Insightful experiences, exhilaration, distortion of senses	Paranoid delusions?	No	No?	No?
300–600 milligrams	4–6 hours	Relaxation, euphoria	Depression, convulsions	Yes	Yes	Yes

Note: Question marks indicate conflict of opinion.

among heavy users of the drug. Psychological dependence often occurs in people who are somewhat emotionally disturbed and are seeking a way to cope with their problems.

Cocaine is usually "snorted" or sniffed and repeated sniffing can destroy the lining of the nasal passages. Regular users are often called "horners" because of their inflamed and running noses.

Recent statistics have shown a great increase in the number of "coke" users in the past few years. Seizures of illegal cocaine have increased seven times in the past five years. Cocaine use has continued to spread, and a recent survey taken for the Commission of Marijuana and Drug Abuse revealed that in 1972 10.4 percent of all college students have tried cocaine at least once.

Cocaine is sometimes called the "champagne of drugs" because of its high price tag. The street price of cocaine can go as high as $100.00 for a gram of the drug. A heavy user of the drug may snort up to 10 grams a day, so one can easily see that snorting cocaine has become a very expensive habit. Why do you think that the popularity of cocaine has increased in recent years? In your own experience, have you found this to be true?

SYNTHETIC STIMULANTS

Synthetic stimulants are those stimulant drugs that are produced in laboratories. These drugs include the amphetamines, methamphetamines, and the antidepressants. These drugs stimulate the central nervous system and tend to increase the heart and breathing rate, constrict or tighten certain blood vessels, increase blood pressure, dilate or open up the pupils, increase sweating, and cause a dry feeling in the mouth. Most amphetamine users feel happy, more talkative, confident, less tired, and many experience a loss of appetite.

Medically, amphetamines have been prescribed for *narcolepsy,* a disease where the individual may suddenly fall asleep (this may occur many times during the day).

It was also prescribed for troops during World War II to help them stay more active and fight off battle fatigue. Amphetamines have also been used successfully to control *hyperactivity* (overexcitement and increased activity) in children and teenagers. This drug is probably best known for its use in dieting. Many doctors prescribe the drug to control obesity because of its appetite depressant effects. In addition, it tends to speed up body function. These two qualities of the drug make it extremely effective in weight control. However, there are some problems in continued use of these drugs for weight reduction. One problem is that tolerance for amphetamines increases at a rapid rate and heavier and heavier doses are required to gain the same effect. Some individuals who abuse the drug find that they have lost all appetite and some report an inability to swallow. A second problem that often occurs in using amphetamines for weight control is that overeating usually indicates an emotional problem or poor eating habits or both of these conditions. The amphetamines will only provide a temporary "crutch" for the individual and as soon as the drug is withdrawn the old habit or problems will return. Have you ever taken amphetamines for weight control? How did they affect you? Did you lose weight by this means? Generally, do you think that the use of amphetamines is the best way to lose weight?

Amphetamines are frequently prescribed as mood elevators for depressed patients. In recent years antidepressant drugs (discussed later in this chapter) have also been used for this purpose.

You are all probably familiar with some of the street names for amphetamines. "Pep pills," "bennies," "uppers," "dexies," and "wake-ups" are only a few of the names they have been given. Do you know of any others? "Bennies" refer to one type of amphetamine, Benzedrine, and Dexadrine is the accepted name for "dexies." Both of these drugs are medically used for weight control and are abused for the high that they produce.

The "kick" or high that one gets from abusing

a moderate dose of amphetamines results in a "turned-on" or euphoric feeling. Abusers of the drug are usually alert and talkative and many perform impulsive acts that often show a lack of judgment. If the drug is used over a long period of time, sleeplessness and behavior changes may result. Sometimes severe mental illness or *psychosis* occurs where the individual has delusions of superiority or develops suspicious feelings. Hallucinations similar to those of cocaine abusers may also result. Amphetamines can be extremely dangerous when taken by car or truck drivers. If a number of pills is taken at one time by a driver, he may suffer from hallucinations, delusions, or may even "blackout" behind the wheel. In many states it is a felony to drive under the influence of amphetamines. Withdrawals from heavy dosages of amphetamines, called "crashing," often produces a prolonged period of depression, nightmares, restlessness, and an inability to get anything accomplished. Compulsive behavior may also occur where an individual does the same task over and over again. As with cocaine, there is a strong psychological dependence on amphetamines.

METHAMPHETAMINES

Methamphetamines are also synthetic stimulants that affect the central nervous system. They are very similar in structure to the amphetamines, but they give a "better" high to the drug abuser. Methedrine is a well-known methamphetamine that is often called "speed," "meth," "splash," "crystal," or "bombita." Heavy abusers or "speed freaks" take the drug by mouth or frequently inject it either by "skin-popping" or "mainlining." Abusers can stay awake for many days while eating very little food. They later become exhausted or "strung-out." Withdrawal from the drug is often called "crashing" and the heavy user may slip between deep sleep and coma and may resume "mainlining" the drug after a few days. "Mainliners" often develop a paranoia (mental disturbance characterized by fear) that can be dangerous to themselves and others. These individuals tend to become suspicious of others and

are often hostile. This hostility can lead to violence. For this reason many people stay away from "speed freaks" because they cannot be sure of their actions.

Sometimes "speed freaks" will "mainline" a combination of methedrine and barbiturates. They do this to control the effects of "speed" and to help them to fall asleep. However, some "speed" abusers will alternate between methedrine and barbiturates as a personal choice of drug usage. This combination of drugs is extremely dangerous as the user will exhibit highly irrational behavior that is frequently of a violent nature. The methedrine increases the individual's activity and wakefulness while the barbiturates initially produce an intoxicated state similar to drunkenness on alcohol. Users often say: "Barbs make you want to tear up the street, while speed gives you the energy to do it." Do you know anyone that uses one or both of these drugs? If so, how would you describe his behavior?

You have probably read or heard the expressions, "speed kills" and "meth is death." What do you think these expressions mean? Have you had any personal experiences that tend to bear out these expressions?

ANTIDEPRESSANTS

Antidepressants, as the name implies, are drugs that elevate the mood of seriously depressed people. Doctors are presently using antidepressant drugs more frequently than amphetamines to relieve depression. The action of antidepressants in mood elevation is a complex process. It is explained here in simplified terms. An individual's mood is thought to be controlled by varying levels of three hormones within the nervous system. These levels are controlled by an enzyme. This enzyme is able to stop the action and destroy these "mood" hormones within the body. In this way, this enzyme controls the amount of these hormones that are produced and indirectly controls the individual's mood. The antidepressant drugs tend to inhibit the production of this enzyme and bring about an increase of the "mood" hormones. Accumulation of these hormones stimulates the individual and elevates his mood. Marplan, Niamid, and Nordil are a few of the antidepressant drugs that work in this way. Have you known anyone who was severely depressed? If you have, describe his depression symptoms. How do you think severe depression differs from everday depression? Think about this carefully, as it is often very difficult for a "normal" person to imagine the feelings of a severely depressed individual.

HALLUCINOGENS
OR PSYCHEDELICS

Hallucinogenic drugs cause sensory distortions that sometimes induce hallucinations. They tend to produce symptoms that are similar to those exhibited by psychotic individuals. This aspect of these drugs is extremely dangerous as abusers of the drug may become violent and injure themselves or others.

The hallucinogens rose to popularity in the early and mid-1960s. In part under the leadership of Timothy Leary, many young people turned to hallucinogens. "Turn on, tune in, and drop out" was an often repeated phrase of this era. What general meaning does this phrase hold for you? The popularity of these drugs began to wane in the late 1960s for a variety of reasons. One reason was that the so-called "hippie" era of the early and mid-1960s was coming to an end. Hallucinogens and other drugs were considered an integral part of the "hippie movement." Evidence of "bad trips" (dangerous sometimes deadly hallucinogenic experiences) flooded the media. In addition, research appeared that linked the hallucinogen LSD with chromosome damage. Other drugs began to appear that seemed to be somewhat safer and more attractive to drug abusers. In your experience, have you found that the use of hallucinogens has greatly decreased?

In recent years psychiatrists have attempted to use hallucinogens in order to treat patients with severe mental or emotional problems.

Some researchers have experimented on themselves by taking such drugs in order to induce psychotic reactions. Generally speaking, most of the research involving hallucinogens has not produced the expected results and any present research is extremely limited or heavily guarded.

MESCALINE
AND PSILOCYBIN

Mescaline is an hallucinogenic drug that is produced from a natural substance, peyote. Peyote is found in a certain variety of spineless cactus plant that is native to Mexico and certain areas of the southwestern United States. The peyote drug is easily obtainable from the crown of the plant that appears above the ground. It can be eaten or cooked as it is found, but is most commonly dried to produce the peyote or "mescal" button. Indian religious rites often involve the eating of these "buttons."

A person who takes mescaline usually suffers from initial vomiting, cramps, sweating, muscle twitching, and increased pulse rate and blood pressure level. Following these symptoms, the hallucinatory properties of the drug are exhibited. Persons under the influence of the drug report "seeing" beautiful color patterns and hallucinating sounds and sensations. Some have reported "hearing" the colors of a painting or "seeing" music in a variety of colors. Time and space relationships are also distorted (the same effects are noted by LSD users). In order to produce these effects, the drug must be used in high dosages. Although it rarely occurs, a very high dose of the drug may result in death caused by convulsions or respiratory failure.

Psilocybin is another natural hallucinogen that is derived from a variety of mushroom native to Central Mexico. A small amount of the drug will result in a pleasant, tension-reducing experience. At higher doses, the abuser will experience perceptual and body-image distortions. Hallucinations may also occur in some individuals. These hallucinations are similar to those experienced by mescaline users.

LSD (D-LYSERGIC ACID DIETHYLAMIDE-25)

LSD is a powerful synthetic compound that is very potent in small doses. For example, it is said to be 800 times more potent than a similar dosage of mescaline. It is an odorless, tasteless, colorless drug that tends to dilate the pupils, escalate temperature and blood pressure, and increase salivation. Its hallucinatory effects are similar to those of mescaline and psilocybin but are usually stronger. There is sensory distortion or "scrambling" where individuals "hear" color, "see" music, and think that the flames of a fire feel cold to their touch. Upon initially taking the drug, one may feel a tingling and then a numbing sensation of the hands and feet. The LSD abuser may feel that he can think very clearly although an observer would find the individual to be confused or disoriented. Many abusers of the drug (so-called "acid heads") become so disoriented that they try to or succeed in committing suicide. Anxiety and fear are common experiences of the LSD user. A bad experience with the drug is often referred to as a "bad trip" or a "bummer." An overdose of the drug may result in delerium and convulsions. Some people experience "flash-backs" where the hallucinatory effects of the drug may appear from time to time long after drug use was discontinued. This effect is usually caused by the drug and the individual's mental condition prior to taking LSD.

Tolerance to the drug increases at a rapid rate when taken on a daily basis. The same repeated dose of the drug will probably not be effective after four days of usage. Cross-tolerance has been shown between LSD, mescaline, and psilocybin. Physical dependence has not been established for any of these drugs; however, there is a strong psychological dependence. As with other drugs, psychological dependence is very definitely linked to the mental stability or condition of the drug user prior to taking the drug.

STP-DOM

STP and DOM are short-hand for the same synthetic hallucinogen. DOM stands for a compound with a lengthy name, 2, 5-dimethoxy-4-methylamphetamine. The street name "STP" refers to the initials for serenity, tranquility, and peace and the motor oil additive. The effects of STP are similar to those of mescaline and LSD. STP is often substituted for mescaline in illegal transactions. This is a dangerous practice as STP is much more powerful than mescaline and the street dose of the drug is very potent. What have you heard about STP? Do you think it is a frequently used drug on today's college campus?

VOLATILE SOLVENTS— VAPOR SNIFFING

You have probably read something about this subject, but you may not recognize the heading. Does "glue sniffing" sound more familiar? This, too, is a drug abuse because the inhaling of vapors definitely affects both our physical and mental processes.

What substances are sniffed and why do people sniff them? Most people sniff paint thinner, certain glues, hair spray, cleaning fluid, gasoline, and lighter fluid. They sniff them because they contain volatile (gaseous) substances that produce intoxication characterized by sleepiness, dizziness, loss of consciousness, and hallucinations. Many individuals report a light-headed, pleasurable sensation after sniffing these substances.

Many of the symptoms of "sniffing" these products are similar to the early stages of alcohol intoxication. The drug abuser initially acts as if he were drunk and then may become sleepy and fall into a deep sleep or become unconscious.

There are numerous inexpensive products that contain substances that can be sniffed in order to get a high. These products are readily available and most people are not aware of the extensive physical damage that they can cause. These vapors are central nervous system depressants and have an effect on the body that is similar to that of barbiturates and narcotics. The prolonged use of such drugs can result in liver damage, kidney failure, anemia, and death. See if you have any of these products around the house. If so, how do the labels read? Do you think they are adequatley marked?

A number of authorities in the area of drug abuse agree that glue sniffing is physically more harmful than the effects of other drugs. Dr. Samuel Irwin in his book, *Drugs of Abuse: An Introduction to Their Actions and Potential Hazards* ranks the following substances according to their potential physical danger:

1. Glue sniffing.
2. Methamphetamine.
3. Alcohol.
4. Cigarettes.
5. Barbiturates and hypnotics.
6. Heroin and related narcotics.
7. LSD and other hallucinogens.
8. Marijuana.

Of course this does not mean that you are better off if you smoke excessively than if you sniff glue. All of these drugs are potentially harmful; it is a matter of degree of physical harm. Are you surprised at this list? In what order would you have ranked these dangerous substances.

There is an apparent physical dependence to these substances as tolerance rapidly develops. The chronic "sniffer" must continue to increase the amount he inhales in order to induce the euphoric effects of the drug. The word "apparent" was used to describe physical dependence because authorities disagree as to whether these substances are truly addicting. One of the reasons for this disagreement is that there are few withdrawal symptoms associated with solvents. However, there is a strong psychological dependence on these drugs. As with other drugs, psychological dependence is directly related to the emotional stability of the drug abuser.

Synanon was founded in 1958 by Charles E. (Chuck) Dederich. Originally for alcoholics, the organization now is mainly concerned with the rehabilitation of drug addicts. Dederich is still in charge, and his methods of treatment are still in use. Chief among these is the Synanon Game. Each resident of the Synanon community must participate in the Game, which is a form of encounter group. The "players" confront each other directly and express their emotions openly.

treatment for drug addicts

There are many types of treatment available to persons who are dependent on drugs. Most treatment revolves around counseling and group therapy similar to that of A.A. There are private, public, and hospital facilities for the treatment and rehabilitation of drug abusers. There are also therapeutic communities where drug abusers can live together and share their problems in a group experience. Synanon, Odyssey House, and Daytop are a few of these well-known therapeutic communities.

THERAPEUTIC COMMUNITIES

The first of the therapeutic communities was Synanon. The word "synanon" was coined by a drug abuser who had difficulty prounouncing two of the basic words of the group: symposium and seminar. In his efforts to repeat these words, he came up with "synanon." Synanon was established by Chuck Dederich (an ex-alcoholic) in 1958. It grew from a small undertaking to a million dollar enterprise in a short period of time. It has been supported mainly by small donations and private foundations. A drug abuser who enters Synanon must give up his habit completely. He is required to go "cold turkey." If a drug abuser is dangerously ill, medical attention is provided. Synanon provides drug abusers with a place to stay, daily seminars, and small leaderless group therapy sessions. Basic to the Synanon philosophy is "self-help." While A.A. members look to a higher being for strength, Synanon members are told to look to themselves. This philosophy is apparent in the formal Synanon prayer that is read at daily morning meetings:

"Please let me first and always examine myself. Let me be honest and truthful. Let me seek and assume responsibility. Let me have trust and faith in myself and my fellow man. Let me love rather than be loved.

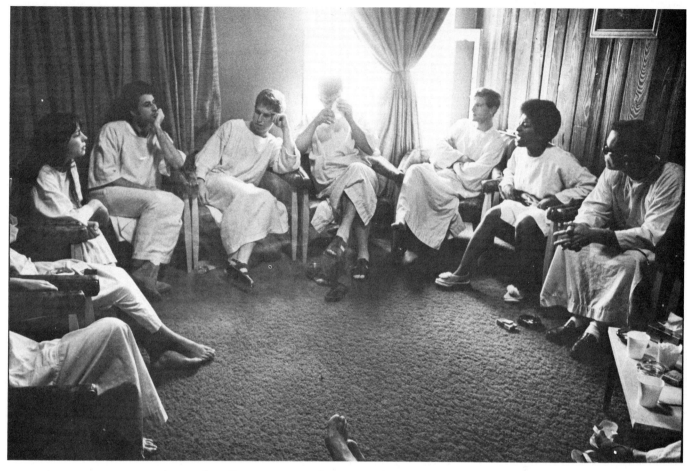

A marathon Synanon group therapy session
that lasted 48 hours. The white gowns remove
distinctions of dress and style among
participants.

Synanon has five
centers in California
and one in Detroit.
The rules are the same
everywhere. Residents
work in offices, shops,
or farms within the
community and are
each paid a salary of
$50 a month. More than
15 percent of the
residents are not
addicts at all; they
joined Synanon
because they liked
its lifestyle.

Let me give rather than receive. Let me
understand rather than be understood."

Synanon and other therapeutic communities
have had their share of problems. A major
problem is zoning laws, where residents
try to keep a therapeutic community out of
their area. Many legal battles have ensued
because of this resistance. Neighborhood
people are fearful of having a drug rehabilitation center in their midst. What are your
feelings concerning this type of situation?

Another problem is the so-called success
rates of these communities. It has been

estimated that Synanon has a one-in-ten
"cure" rate. In other words, only one out
of every ten people who leave Synanon will
remain drug free. Chuck Dederich once
replied to a question of how long it would
take to effect a "cure" at Synanon by saying
"If he's lucky, it will take forever." It is
Dederich's opinion that some addicts can
only remain drug free if they continue to
live at Synanon or other such communities.
If you want to learn more about Synanon
read *Synanon: The Tunnel Back* by Lewis
Yablonsky or *Synanon* by Guy Endore.

Odyssey House is another therapeutic com-

Odyssey House believes that narcotic addicts can get along without drugs of any kind, that they can be successfully treated by psychotherapy and that they have a responsibility to prevent drug addiction in others. The agency was founded in 1966 by 17 former addicts and a psychiatrist, Judianne Densen-Gerber.

Based in New York, Odyssey House also has facilities in several other states. Patients live in. Psychotherapy, education, and vocational training are all provided. At first, new residents do mostly manual work. Later, they are given a share in the running of the community and are trained to recruit other candidates for it.

munity that was started in New York City in 1965 by Dr. Judianne Densen-Gerber. It is based on group therapy techniques and a philosophy of accountability. Each person is held accountable to himself and to the group for his actions. The rehabilitation program is divided into three stages: (1) pretreatment, (2) intensive residential treatment, and (3) posttreatment or reentry. The pretreatment stage is designed to motivate the drug abuser to want the help that a therapeutic community can offer. This stage takes place in the outside community when Odyssey House staff members hold group sessions at Community Involvement Centers. These centers are located in high drug abuse areas. Once motivation is shown by a cooperative attitude and by decreasing one's drug habit, an individual is recommended for admission into the Odyssey House residence. The residents' days are strictly structured, providing little time for leisure activities. Between three and six hours a day are allotted for group meetings. The residents are responsible for house maintenance and necessary clerical work. All of these jobs are a part of the therapy program. The Odyssey House story provides interesting reading in *We Mainline Dreams* by Dr. Judianne Densen-Gerber.

"There is no refuge, finally, from ourselves. Until a person confronts himself in the eyes and hearts of others, he is running. Afraid to be known, he can know neither himself nor any other—he will be alone. Here together a person can at last appear clearly to himself, not as the giant of his dreams, nor the dwarf of his fears, but as a man—part of a whole, with his share in its purpose."

This moving quotation states the basic philosophy of Daytop, a therapeutic community based on the Synanon technique. Read the quotation again, what do you think is basic to the philosophy of Daytop?

METHADONE AND HEROIN MAINTENANCE

Methadone is a synthetic, addictive opiate drug that is used in drug rehabilitation programs as a substitute for heroin. If a heroin abuser is given a daily oral dose of methadone, he can be "maintained" or stabilized. The methadone allows the heroin abuser to satisfy his needs for a drug without taking heroin. (Methadone blocks *only* the effects of heroin; it does not block the effects of other drugs.) In other words, one drug has been substituted for another drug. A person who takes methadone does not experience the high that he received from heroin. However, he does feel well physically and is able to function in society.

There have been volumes written on the pros and cons of methadone maintenance. Many people approve of this method because it helps heroin abusers to lead a "straight" life. They don't have to commit crimes in order to get money for heroin and they can hold jobs and become useful members of society. In addition, the success rates of therapeutic communities have not been overwhelming and methadone does help people to stay "drug" free. People that disapprove of methadone maintenance feel that dependence has only been shifted from one drug to another. They also feel that the drug abuser is never really free of his dependence and must exist from day to day waiting for his next dose of methadone. What are your feelings on this subject? Do you think that methadone should only be used as a last resort?

In England there is a heroin maintenance program. Heroin addicts are given daily doses of the drug in order to keep them from committing crimes. It is thought that the addict who does not have to worry about where his next "fix" is coming from will function better as a member of society than the street addict. What are your feelings about heroin maintenance programs?

149

THINKING IT OVER

1. Explain what is meant by drugs being "people problems." Do you think that this is a healthy way to look at the drug situation?
2. What are some of the reasons why people take drugs? Can you think of any others?
3. What is meant by a "pill society"? Do you think that we live in such a society?
4. Discuss the meaning of the word "dependence." Do you think that "dependence" is a more useful term than "habituation" or "addiction"?
5. Explain what is meant by the "withdrawal syndrome." Have you experienced "withdrawal" from cigarettes? Explain how you felt.
6. Discuss the meaning of the word "tolerance."
7. Explain and give an example of potentiation.
8. Explain the difference between the drug user, drug misuser, and drug abuser. Do you fit into any of these categories?
9. What are over-the-counter drugs? Do you think that the public should be protected from advertising misrepresentation of these products? Briefly discuss your answer.
10. What are the requirements for a drug to be sold by prescription?
11. How are drugs misused? Give some examples. Have you misused drugs, if so, how did you misuse them?
12. What are some of the factors involved in defining whether a drug is being misused or abused?
13. What is a narcotic drug? Discuss the opiate narcotics.
14. What are the effects of barbiturates on drug abusers? What are some of the street names for these drugs?
15. Discuss the many uses of tranquilizer drugs. There have been controversies in connection with the heavy use of tranquilizers in quieting mental patients in institutions. How do you feel about this situation?
16. What type of drug is marijuana? According to what you know and what you have read, do you think marijuana use should be legalized?
17. What is a stimulant drug? Do you take any stimulants?
18. Discuss the drug cocaine. Why do you think more people are using it in the last few years?
19. Why is the name "speed" given to amphetamines? Discuss some of the uses and abuses of the drug.
20. What are the effects of an hallucinogenic drug? Why do you think that so many young people in the 1960s became hallucinogen users?
21. List the major drugs in order of their potential hazards.
22. What is the basic concept behind therapeutic communities for drug abusers? Do you think this is a workable concept? Explain your answer.

KEY WORDS

Amphetamines. Central nervous system stimulants.

Antagonistic drugs. A drug that has an effect on the body opposite from a drug that one is taking.

Antidepressants. Mood elevating drugs.

Barbiturates. Depressant, sleep-inducing drugs that produce intoxicating effects.

Cocaine. A natural stimulant drug extracted from the leaves of the coca shrub.

Cross-tolerance. The use of a different drug or drugs in order to help relieve the withdrawal symptoms caused by the drug on which the individual is dependent.

Dependence. Psychological or physiological need for a drug after periodic or continued use of the substance.

Drug misuser. An individual who is irresponsible in his use of drugs.

Drug abuser. An individual who takes drugs for other than medicinal purposes.

Drug user. An individual who takes any type of drug on a regular basis.

Fix. Slang expression for a dose of a drug.

Flashbacks. The hallucinatory effects of a drug (LSD) that occur long after an individual has stopped using the drug.

Hallucinogens. Drugs that alter mood, behavior, and perception.

Hepatitis. An infection of the liver.

LSD (d-lysergic acid diethylamide-25). A powerful hallucinogenic drug that has physical and psychological effects.

Mainlining. Injecting of a drug directly into the veins.

Mescaline. An hallucinogen derived from peyote.

Methamphetamines. Synthetic stimulants that are similar in structure to the amphetamines.

Methaqualone. A depressant drug that is often abused.

Methedrine. A methamphetamine often called "speed."

Narcotic drugs. Drugs that are central nervous system depressants.

Opiates. Narcotic drugs derived from the opium poppy plant (opium, morphine, heroin, and codeine).

Over-the-counter drugs. Drugs that are sold without prescription.

Peyote. A natural hallucinogenic substance found in a certain type of cactus plant.

Potentiation. When two drugs are taken together and one strengthens the action of the other.

Prescription drugs. Drugs that cannot be purchased without a physician's prescription.

Psychoactive drugs. Drugs that produce a temporary change in mood or behavior.

Reverse-tolerance. The need for less of a substance after an individual has been drug-dependent for a long period of time.

Salicylic acid. The main ingredient in aspirin.

Sedative drugs. Drugs that have quieting or sleep-inducing effects.

Skin popping. Injecting a drug into the fleshy parts of the skin.

Snorting or sniffing. Inhaling of a drug through the nasal passages.

Stimulants. Drugs that stimulate or excite the central nervous system.

Synergism. When two drugs combine together to produce a greater effect than if taken alone.

Synthetic narcotics. Those narcotic drugs that can be produced from chemicals rather than the natural plant ingredients.

Tolerance. The physical reaction of the body to a drug that results in the necessity for an increased dosage to produce the desired effects.

Tranquilizers. Central nervous system depressants that are used to calm individuals and relieve highly emotional states.

Volatile solvents. Substances that are easily vaporized and produce intoxicating effects upon being sniffed.

Withdrawal syndrome. The physical and psychological symptoms that result from the withdrawal of a drug that has been taken over a period of time.

GETTING INVOLVED

Books and Periodicals

Beggs, E.L. *Open House.* New York: Ballentine, 1973. A staff member of Open House, a treatment center located in Marin County, California, discusses suburban addicts, their rehabilitation, their patterns of behavior, and their families.

Brecher, Edward M. *Licit and Illicit Drugs: The Consumers Union Report on Narcotics, Stimulants, Depressants, Inhalants, Hallucinogens, and Marijuana—Including Caffeine, Nicotine and Alcohol.* Boston: Little, Brown, 1972. An authoritative fact book.

Densen-Gerber, Judianne. *We Mainline Dreams: The Odyssey House Story.* New York: Doubleday, 1973. Personal experiences at Odyssey House recounted by one of its founders.

National Institute on Drug Abuse. *Marijuana and Health*. Fourth Report to the United States Congress. Rockville, Md.: Department of Health, Education and Welfare, 1974. About marijuana: the extent of its use by age and locality, its chemistry, its effects on the body, and recent research in this area.

Movies

A Hatful of Rain, with Eva Marie Saint and Don Murray, 1957. Intense, reform-minded movie about drug addiction. Distributed by Films Incorporated.

The Man with the Golden Arm, with Frank Sinatra, 1956. Another pioneer movie about drug addiction. Distributed by United Artists—16 mm.

Monkey on My Back, with Cameron Mitchell, Dianne Foster, 1957. More about the problems of addiction. Distributed by United Artists—16 mm.

PART III
SEXUALITY

8
SEXUAL BEHAVIOR

Are we going through a sexual revolution or evolution? Many think current sexual behavior indicates a drastic change from that of 20 years ago. You may be surprised at what you learn in relation to our "changing" sexual behavior. This chapter explores sexual behavior and attitudes and points out factors that are producing change in our society.

Most of us live by sexual standards that we may not have thoroughly considered or understood. These standards are discussed and their origins are explored. A difficult question for all young persons concerns sexual behavior and decision making. There are no "pat" answers to these questions, but the chapter explores factors that may influence one's decisions and guidelines that one can consider.

The final section of this chapter concerns itself with alternate forms of sexual behavior. The homosexual, transvestite, and transsexual are discussed in relation to their place in present-day society. Prostitution and the social problems that surround it are also explored.

While reading this chapter, think about the following concepts:

■ Sex, although ''governed'' by society, is an individual matter.

■ Life is more humanistic (placing people first) today.

■ There has been an evolution rather than a revolution in sexual behavior.

■ Sexual standards are accepted by each individual in varying degrees.

■ The decision-making process should be stressed in questions relating to sexual behavior.

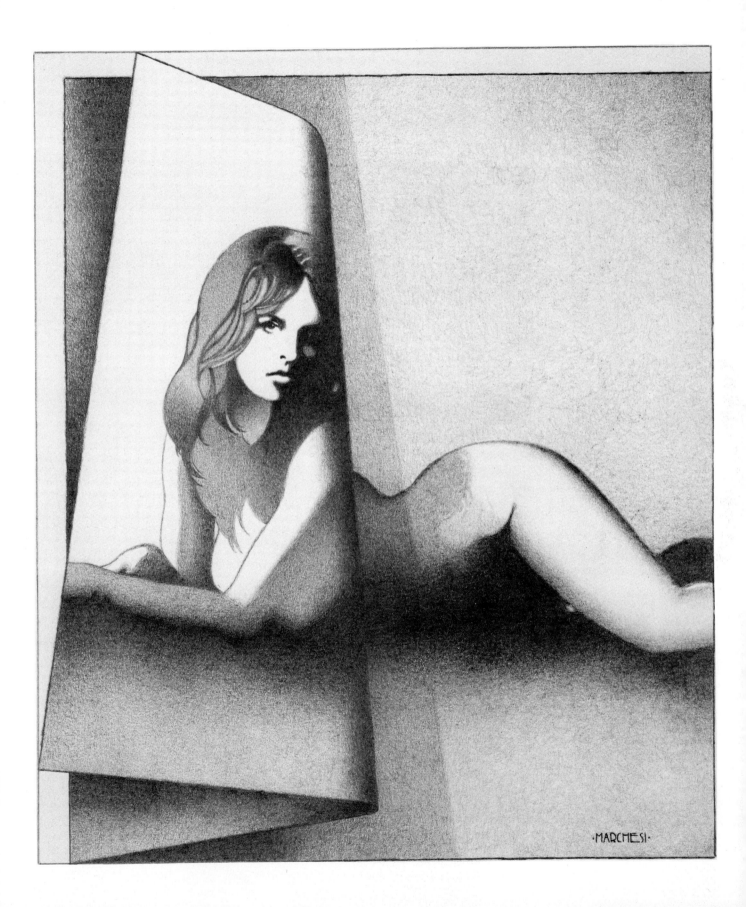

"Sex" and "sexual behavior" are no longer "closeted" terms. They appear with great frequency on radio "talk" shows, television, other forms of media, best-sellers, and movies (even those that are not X-rated). One can say that sexuality has finally been recognized as a basic aspect of human life.

Sex is *not* a synonym for sexual intercourse; the word encompasses a totality of behavior patterns that are primarily concerned with how people relate to and communicate with each other. Although sexual intercourse is frequently the culmination of sexual activity, it is only one form of sexual behavior. Sexual behavior is related to society and how society reviews sexuality at a certain period of time. How would you define "sexual behavior?"

In the next section of this chapter, a few basic terms are discussed in relation to sexual behavior. These terms are used frequently when discussing this topic.

a look at the basics

What was the first word you can remember in a discussion of sexual behavior as a child? If it wasn't *sex,* it was probably morality. The question of defining morality or immorality has been with us for thousands of years. The dictionary defines morality as right or wrong conduct, often implying sexual virtue. Many people today link morality to sexual behavior rather than to values. Morality can only be defined in rather general terms; what is moral in one society or for one individual is not moral for others. In some countries bigamy (having more than one spouse) is both moral and legal, while in other lands it is neither legal nor moral. Morality is often linked to religion. All religions teach the basics of morality and some imply sexual morality in their teachings. Morality is individual; it is what *you* think it is. Your judgment may be influenced by parents, peers, religion, education, and society, but your conception of what is right or wrong (morality) is an individual decision.

Another term frequently used in discussions of sexual behavior is virginity. Technically virginity is the physical condition of a girl or woman who has never experienced sexual intercourse. At one time, virginity was associated with an intact hymen (the connective tissue that closes the external opening of the vagina). Many individuals once thought that the hymen was only broken during first sexual intercourse. However, in most cases the hymen is broken prior to first intercourse. The hymen is often broken through falls, athletic competition, masturbation, and other forms of sexual experimentation or through normal physical activity. Virginity is discussed in further detail in a later section of this chapter.

Promiscuity may be defined as engaging in sexual intercourse on a casual level with many persons. It implies a relationship with many men or women rather than a monogamous or one-to-one relationship. Often promiscuity is labeled as "bad" by persons who do not accept this type of behavior. As with other patterns of sexual behavior, one should not pin a "good" or "bad" label on a practice. What is fine for one person is frequently repugnant to another. If a type of behavior is not harmful to you or your partner, generally speaking it is acceptable. Unacceptable behavior of any type is that which is individually or socially harmful.

Pornography is a word that has come into our everyday vocabulary in recent years. Pornography is sexually arousing (erotic) material presented in such forms as literature, movies, or art. Pornography is difficult to define because one has to be able to recognize what is to be considered erotic. What is erotic to one person may not be to another depending on one's experiences. This has been a major problem in court cases that seek to ban pornograghic films or literature. How is one to decide whether an art form is pornographic? If society decides that something is pornographic do people still have the right to buy it or see it if they so wish? These are some of the social problems that exist concerning sexual behavior and expression. How do you feel about pornography in general? In which ways are an individual's rights threatened by banning certain forms of pornography?

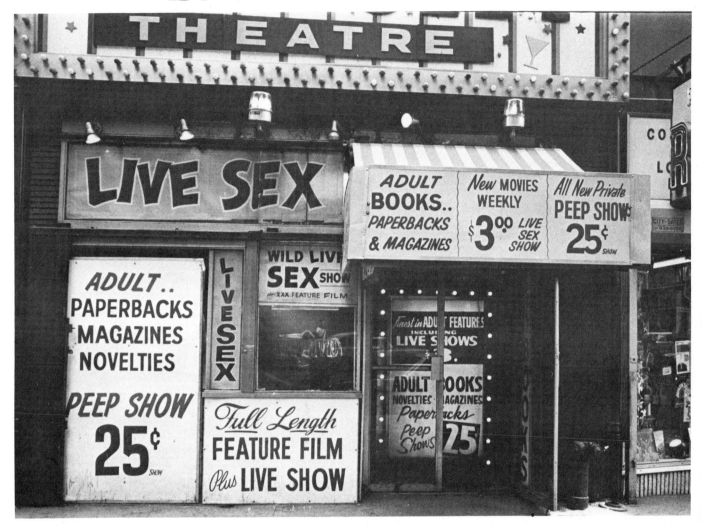

Increasing permissiveness regarding sexually
oriented materials has helped turn pornography into a flourishing business.

All of the words and their meanings discussed
in the previous section have varying definitions among different groups of people.
As was previously mentioned, two persons
could look at the same piece of art and one
will declare it pornographic and the other
will see it as a masterpiece. This applies
to regional groups of people. People from
one area of this country may have an entirely
different definition of a commonly used
sexual term than those from another area.
Sexual behavior is *generally* governed by
society in that there are certain "rules" and
"obligations" accepted by most of society.
However, sexual behavior is an individual
matter and if there are 50 persons in a room,
you are likely to have 50 different opinions
in relation to the meaning of each of the
basic terms previously discussed.

sexual revolution or evolution?

Many articles exclaim that we are going
through a sexual revolution. This implies a
sudden change in sexual behavior in the
past few years. Though sexual activity may
have increased in recent years, one cannot
call this increase a revolution. It was not a
sudden change but a gradual or evolving
change—hence, the word, evolution. What
are some of the reasons for these changes
in our attitudes about sexual behavior?

These reasons are explored in the following section.

A DIFFERENCE IN OUR APPROACH TO LIFE

People are looking at life in a different way. In some ways society is more humanistic today. In a humanistic society, people are concerned with what happens to others and they feel that interpersonal relationships are established for the benefit of both individuals rather than the pleasure of one person. Humanism in sexual behavior is seen in a mutual caring and respect for the partners in the relationship. Partners are more open about their feelings and are doing more of what they want to as individuals rather than simply trying to please the other person. There is no deceit or trickery involved in a humanistic relationship. The feelings of both partners are known to each other and devious behavior is unwarranted.

"The Times They Are a Changing" is the title of a Bob Dylan song that points up a major theme of sexual evolution. A decline of the family in present-day society is often cited as one of the basic reasons why more young people have a different view of sex than did many of their parents or grandparents. Today's family is less structured and domineering than it was in past years. Young people are given responsibility at an earlier age because parents are often away from the home. Many men must commute to their jobs and leave the home early and return quite late. There is less time to spend with children and sometimes a breakdown in communication ensues. More women are working today, providing less adult supervision at home. In the past, many families were "extended." An extended family is one in which the grandparents and frequently other relatives shared the home. When this occurred, young people were exposed to the attitudes of an older generation than their parents. What advantages and disadvantages do you think are offered by the extended family? Today, individual family units are much more the norm and few people live in an extended family situation.

Religion also affects one's attitude concerning sex. Studies have indicated that there is a direct relationship between one's feelings about religion and one's attitudes toward premarital sex, for example. Persons with strong religious beliefs tend to reject premarital intercourse. Many of these individuals have a strong burden of guilt when it comes to sexual feelings. A decline of organized religion in recent years is linked to more permissive sexual attitudes.

Has the media has an effect in bringing about or changing sexual attitudes? How would you answer this question? The answer is "yes" it has. For example, the advertising media is always playing on the role of sexuality in selling their products. Sometimes an advertisement is subtle, but in most cases it is overt. Sex is implied in every conceivable type of "ad." Mouthwashes, toothpaste, hair spray, and even cigarettes are sold using sex appeal as the backdrop. Look for this the next time you watch television or read a magazine. Jot down some of the ideas in a commercial that are sexually oriented.

Besides the use of the media by advertising, other aspects of the media have definitely affected our sexual attitudes. There are documentaries on television that deal with sexual topics, radio talk shows offer sex advice, newspaper columns discuss sex-related questions, and sex is no longer forbidden from our motion picture screens. It was not that long ago that married couples on television had to have twin beds and when movie scenes were on the verge of becoming too erotic, one heard a clap of thunder and the camera panned to a curtain blowing in the wind! Certainly individuals were already changing, but the media made these changes more acceptable to a large segment of the population.

An integral factor in the change of sexual attitudes is the increased self-sufficiency of women in our society. Women today are freer to do what they want with their lives and this freedom extends to sexual attitudes. The guilt-ridden, repressed woman may still exist but certainly to a much lesser

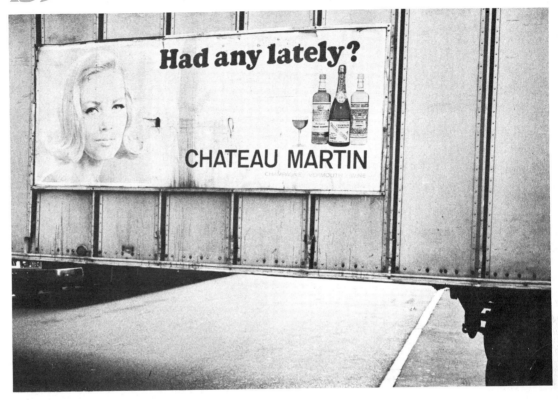

A provocative advertising campaign.

extent than she once did. Women who engage in sexual relationships today are much more open about their feelings and enjoyment of sex. There has been a gradual decline in sexual inhibitions that once prevented women from enjoying sex. Many of today's women view sex as a pleasurable experience that they are as much involved in as their partners. The once accepted attitude that women are passive receivers and men are aggressors in sexual activity is no longer accepted by the contemporary woman.

Sexual attitudes have changed as society has become more secular. Secularism is a belief that morality should be based on the well-being of humanity and not on religious systems. This has become an increasing trend in recent years. Do you find this trend to be true among your friends? Do you think secularism is more dominant among young people than among the older generation? If so, why do you think this has come about?

The "times are certainly a changin' " and with these changes there is a new sexual freedom. The term "freedom" is *not* meant to imply irresponsibility or moral degeneration.

In fact, most recent surveys indicate that most young people are both responsible and humanistic when it comes to sexual behavior. This new freedom removes much of the guilt, shame, inhibition, hypocrisy, dehumanization, and unhealthy fascination with a *normal* aspect of human life—sex. Today's society has a much healthier outlook in relation to all types of sexual behavior than in any time in the recent past.

PREMARITAL SEXUAL ACTIVITY

The most drastic change in attitudes concerning premarital sex occurred in the 1920s. The deprivation of World War I led to a period of intense feelings in all areas. The revaluation in sexual attitudes began in the 1920s and has continued to evolve until the present.

Premarital sexual activity has been increasing

among both men and women in recent years. A recent survey indicates that from 50 to 80 percent of college-age men approve of premarital intercourse. However, only about 65 percent of the individuals had experienced premarital intercourse. In a similar survey of college-age women, more than 70 percent indicated approval of premarital intercourse. However, only about 35 to 50 percent engaged in intercourse prior to marriage. The relationship between premarital sex and love and involvement are discussed in a later section of this chapter.

Our present society is much more open concerning sex than it has ever been before. The increase of premarital sex is only one aspect of this openess. Openess can be seen in the publicity received by such movies as *Deep Throat* and *The Devil in Miss Jones*. Nudity on stage is accepted today as indicated by the record-breaking performance of the Broadway show *Hair*. Family television programs have dealt with the topic of menopause on *All in the Family* and programs such as *Not for Women Only* have spent weeks discussing male and female sexuality. The sexual revolution seems to primarily be in sexual attitudes rather than in sexual behavior. Perhaps, our attitudes have finally caught up with our behavior.

sexual standards

What is meant by a sexual standard? It is a type of behavior that has come to be accepted in varying degrees by society. Many sexual standards are replete with ignorance, superstition, and hypocrisy, and yet they still live on in many segments of society. An example of such a standard is that of masturbation (the self-stimulation of the genitals for purposes of sexual arousal). This practice had been and still is considered by some segments of the population as "dirty," physically and mentally harmful, and capable of preventing an individual from engaging in sex with a partner. Furthermore, with this standard masturbation is tacitly accepted when performed by a boy but totally rejected when performed by a girl. Sexual standards are hard to change. Many individuals who have been educated in these

matters still look to these old standards when it comes to sexual behavior. Why do you think this is so? Do you find yourself resorting to established sexual standards when questions of sexual behavior are raised? Some established sexual standards are discussed in the following sections.

ABSTINENCE

Abstinence forbids intercourse (often termed *coitus*) between men and women prior to marriage. It is a sexual standard that has lost some of its acceptance in recent years. However, many individuals do continue to accept this mode of behavior. Virginity was defined in an earlier section of this chapter. According to our definition virginity can only exist if one has not had sexual intercourse. Therefore, a women whose hymen has been broken by activity other than coitus is still a virgin. It is interesting to note that there are some women who are able to have intercourse and even bear children without rupturing the hymen. This is usually due to either an immature hymen or one that is extremely flexible, allowing penetration of the vagina without being broken.

Many men equate virginity with "purity." They feel very strongly that their wife-to-be should be a virgin. This obsession with virginity has been compared to that of the Kurd society of Mesopotamia. Here virginity in a bride is celebrated by a parade and the bride price is not paid until virginity is proven. Proof of virginity is determined by a marriage cloth which is examined for blood stains (a highly unreliable method of determining virginity).

Many men and women place a premium on virginity and will participate in all forms of sexual behavior except intercourse. This is sometimes referred to as technical virginity. The act of intercourse connotes a certain finality that many individuals are unable to accept. In addition, religious feelings, guilt, and the fear of losing the respect of their partner enters into this decision. The fear of pregnancy is also a strong element in the protection of virginity. What are your feelings

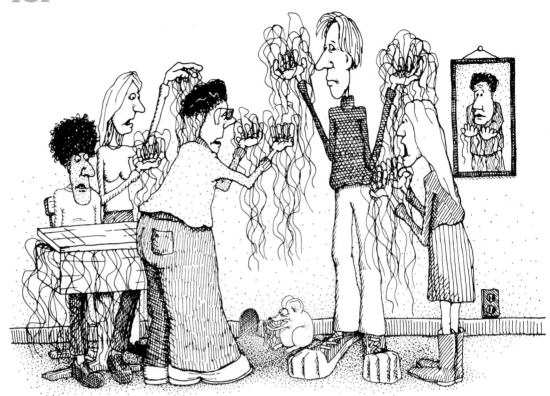

A myth of the 1950's; masturbation caused hair to grow on the palms.

concerning virginity? Do you feel that this sexual standard is less important today than it was when your parents were dating? Why do you think you answered this question the way you did?

DOUBLE STANDARD

The double standard is one of the oldest traditions of Western culture. The accepted meaning of double standard is that men are allowed to engage in premarital intercourse while women are not. The double standard has also been applied to many other aspects of social living in relation to men and women. Can you think of other examples of social rules that apply to one sex and not the other?

There are many problems inherent in a culture that generally accepts the double standard. Women are divided into two groups—the "good" and the "bad." There is no "gray" or in-between. The "good" are those women who are virgins and would be chosen as marriage partners. They are not expected to be interested in sex or derive any enjoyment from it. They are the "mothers"

of the future who are considered by many to be asexual. Difficulty often arises after marriage when these women are unable to approach sex except in a passive, obligatory manner. The men often find it difficult to respond to a "good" woman in a passionate sense. This type of double standard has been referred to as the orthodox standard that describes an extreme view of sexual behavior.

Today's double standard is in transition. There are still many people who accept the orthodox understanding but the majority of people accept a more liberalized viewpoint. There *are* shades of "gray" and women are not usually seen as either "good" or "bad." Premarital intercourse is accepted if the woman is committed to the relationship. Intercourse with involvement is another sexual standard that will be discussed later in this chapter.

The double standard was often taken a step further after marriage. This view of the double standard allows men to have extramarital affairs while women are expected to accept this behavior and not participate in any sexual involvement of their own outside of marriage. This standard has held surprisingly constant over the years, though more and more women in recent times have been engaging in extramarital relations. This double standard is a product of society's view of women rather than of sexuality. Married women were seen as wives and mothers and not as individuals in their own right. In many cases, they were not even considered as sexual beings and therefore a man had the "right" to find sexual fulfillment elsewhere. This standard is also in transition among many segments of the population. Extramarital affairs, if accepted, are usually accepted for both partners. This area of behavior is explored in more detail in Chapter 10.

Although the media may have us believing that the "double standard" is on the way out, the polls do not indicate this trend. An article (May 1974) in *Human Behavior* states "all those new-fangled liberation movements not withstanding, we are still securely hooked into the premise that it's peachy for guys to sow all the wild oats they please, but nice girls don't get sowed upon."

A recent poll conducted by two sociologists, David Berger of Temple University and Morton Wenger from Muhlenberg College, indicated that college students placed a higher value on female virginity than on male virginity. In a recent Gallup poll of college students, 75 percent of all students interviewed approved of premarital intercourse, but 75 percent stated they would prefer to marry a virgin. Although the statistics differ depending on the poll, one can conclude that the double standard is still very much entrenched in American society.

An interesting point concerning sexual behavior and the double standard was revealed in a study conducted by Northwestern University sociologist, Donald Carns. In a survey of approximately 1,800 undergraduates he found that the male students were anxious to discuss their sexual ex-

periences with friends. The women, on the other hand, were less anxious to discuss the subject and if they did at all, it was after careful consideration. Women are fearful of the reaction they might receive when discussing a sexual experience while men are assured of approval.

PERMISSIVENESS WITH AFFECTION

This standard of sexual behavior establishes premarital sexual intercourse as acceptable for both men and women if they are involved in a stable loving relationship. This standard has existed for many years but has come to be more openly accepted in recent times. This type of relationship is nonexploitive. Both partners are totally involved in a sexual relationship because that is what they want. They are committed to the totality of the relationship. This is a humanistic approach to sexual behavior where the person and not the body is valued.

A standard of permissiveness with affection can be seen in the many couples who choose to live with each other without first getting married. Some individuals choose to "try out" marriage in this way. Others have no intention of getting married but do have a committment and affection to their partner. It has been suggested by some marriage counseling authorities that all couples should live together before are they are married. The desired result would be fewer divorces. However, this concept has yet to be proven. Do you feel that people should live together prior to marriage? What would be some of the advantages? Disadvantages? Do you feel that this behavior would be right for you? What might influence your decision?

PERMISSIVENESS WITHOUT AFFECTION

This standard provides for premarital sexual intercourse where there is no affection. Physical attraction is sufficient to justify sexual relations. Many individuals who are promiscuous subscribe to this sexual standard.

However, promiscuous persons may have varying degrees of affection for persons with whom they are sexually involved. Again, behavior necessarily varies with the individuals involved. Affection can be shared with more than one person and be very genuine. Many persons feel that a monogomous relationship is the only "real" relationship but this is not necessarily true for some people.

Generally speaking, surveys have shown that there are relatively few individuals who have sexual relations without affection. The numbers often appear greater than they really are because the media plays up the stories in a sensational manner. Sexual behavior today is remarkably similar to that in your parents' day. Attitudes have changed and sex is more openly spoken about but behavior itself has not significantly changed.

You have no doubt heard or read of "key clubs," "wife-swapping" and similar sexual behavior where permissiveness without affection is the norm. This type of behavior is rarely spontaneous physical attraction. It is usually a well thought out and organized exchange where many individuals are involved through coercion by husbands, wives, or friends. The motivation behind these activities is frequently more involved than a desire for a sexual fling. How do you feel about this type of sexual permissiveness? What do you think motivates an individual to participate in this type of sexual activity?

sexual behavior and the decision-making process

Years ago young people could only date if they were well-chaperoned. They began to date at a later age and families were usually well acquainted with their choice of dating partners. Today young people are dating earlier and chaperones, except at school functions, are nonexistent. This type of courting system forces decisions concerning sexual behavior on young people.

How will young people make these deci-

sions? Many factors have already influenced a young person's life prior to the age of dating. Parental viewpoints, peers, education, religious training, and one's environment all have an effect on how one deals with difficult decisions. Decisions about sexual issues are often tied into how a person decides about other questions such as drinking, smoking, and the taking of drugs. What do you think is the best way to go about making a decision concerning a personal matter? Are decisions made at a young age necessarily final? If not, how would they be likely to change?

Where does sex education begin? The home would be the most likely answer. However, a recent study indicated that *peers not parents* provided initial sex information. In a survey of college students at the Universities of Arizona and Oklahoma, students were asked to recall the sources of information concerning topics such as menstruation, contraception, masturbation, and homosexuality. The most frequently given answer was "friends" followed by answers that ranged in order to include literature, mothers, schools, street language, fathers, ministers, and doctors. Notice how far down the list "fathers" appeared. Why do you think this is so? Can you recall who informed you about sex-related topics?

This study concluded that most children learned about menstruation and reproduction by the age of ten. Most other sexual topics were introduced between the ages of 12 and 15. The study further indicated that many young people thought that the home, school, and church presented sex information in a negative manner. Sex education became "preachy" rather than knowledge imparted to aid an individual in the decision-making process.

Education is a major factor in providing the information and considerations that go into an intelligent decision concerning one's personal behavior. Sex education has become very much a part of most school curriculums in recent years. In most communities sex education begins in the primary grades and continues as a separate program or as part

William Howell Masters (1915–   ) and Virginia Eshelman Johnson (1925–   ) are responsible for the current interest in sex therapy. In their Reproductive Biology Research Foundation in St. Louis, Missouri, Masters and Johnson studied human sexuality and worked out methods of helping couples who are having trouble with their sex lives. Their therapy uses some of the principles of behavioral psychology, such as conditioning. But Dr. Masters and Ms. Johnson (who in private life is Mrs. Masters) are worried that some of the newer so-called sex therapists are not as ethical as they themselves are; and they point out that there is more to sex than just mechanics. For sex to be completely satisfying, the partners must be fully committed to each other.

of the health curriculum in the higher grade levels. What is taught is frequently controlled by local school boards and state-wide curriculums; explicit knowledge of the techniques of sexual intercourse are forbidden in most schools. This came to light in a recent court case that you may have read about in the newspaper. A high school biology teacher (with 24 years of teaching experience) in New York City decided to show an explicit sexual filmstrip to his class. The film depicted various acts of intercourse as well as of <u>sodomy</u> (a variation of sexual behavior that may include sexual intercourse with animals or oral-genital or anal-genital intercourse between humans). The film was not a commercial piece of pornography but a part of a nine-unit sex education program produced for church schools and written by an educator. The teacher felt

that the film answered the "real need" of his students to communicate about realistic aspects of sexuality. Many parents and members of the board of education think that this teacher went too far and are trying to prevent such an incident from occurring in the future. What do you think?

Many persons who seek sex information frequently turn to their doctors. According to an article in *Human Behavior* (July 1974), this may not be the best place to go. Dr. William Masters has been quoted as saying that doctors "know no more and no less about the subject than other college graduates."

Most doctors are limited in their sexual knowledge because of their personalities and training. Their medical courses taught body structure and function but not the fine

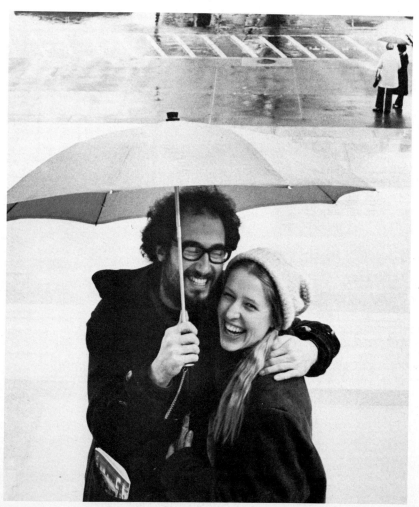

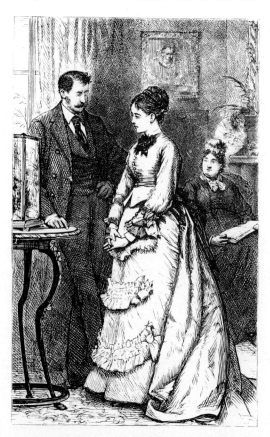

Courting, today and a century ago.

points of human sexual behavior. In addition, few medical students have much time for sexual activity of their own. As recently as 1961, a survey of five Philadelphia medical schools (faculty and senior classes) indicated that half the students believed in the myth concerning masturbation—that it could lead to mental illness. Even more surprising, one-fifth of the faculty held the same belief.

Another report (about five years later) indicated that doctors were not sophisticated in handling problems of a sexual nature. Many of them blushed, giggled, or became hostile when asked questions of this type. Information when given at all was too simplified and did not get to the core of the problem. In this study, it was discovered that more than four-fifths of the doctors interviewed had no training in treating sex or marriage problems. In 1965, a joint committee of the American Medical Association and National Education Association passed a resolution on the need for medical education in the areas of sex and marriage. The Center for the Study of Sex Education in Medicine opened at the University of Pennsylvania. The center serves as a clearinghouse for information, provides curriculum consultation and includes a research center. Recent medical school graduates should be better able to handle sexual questions and problems. Have you ever discussed a sex problem with your doctor? What type of response did you receive?

In general, sex education is not meeting the needs of the majority of people. It can be likened to the three-year-old who asks his mother where he came from. The mother takes the opportunity to tell the boy the entire story of reproduction. When she's finished, the youngster replies, "Mom— you still didn't tell me where I came from— was it New York or New Jersey?" Of course sex education should provide the facts, but it must also discuss behavior questions and provide the foundation for healthy decision making by the individual.

Sex education should teach a student not what to think but how to think. It must provide information on which a young person

can base decisions about an interpersonal relationship. There are no "pat" answers. Each individual must reach his or her own decision based on feelings, knowledge, needs, and the future. Some useful guidelines in helping you to decide what's right for you are discussed in the next few paragraphs.

When determining whether to have premarital sexual intercourse, one must consider what emotions are involved in reaching a decision. Is the decision based on feelings of love and respect or guided by feelings of exploiting one's partner, or using sex as a means to gain status or favor? If you feel that sex is a way of communicating and heightening intense feelings, then your decision would be more rational than if it were based on exploitation.

Many young people enter into a sexual relationship without knowing why they are doing it. Sexual intercourse is an important decision and should be based on careful forethought. The reasons for entering a sexual relationship should be accepted by you and your partner *before* so that you will not be regretful after the fact.

Another consideration is that of *responsibility*. Responsibility covers a great deal of territory. There is the responsibility of preventing conception and venereal disease. But there is a greater responsibility in preventing emotional harm to you and your partner. Individuals who have intercourse are usually very involved with each other from an emotional point of view. If one partner does not share these feelings, should he or she pretend that such an involvement exists?

Sex does not exist by itself—it is one part of life and must be judged on how it fits into the rest of one's life. Readiness for sexual involvement should be based on the ability of an individual to handle life itself on a mature level. One's self-concept is very important to consider. Awareness of self is basic to all life decisions. Do you remember the concept of "I'm OK—you're OK?" How does this concept help one to make decisions concerning sexual behavior?

166

alternate forms of sexual behavior

There are numerous forms of sexual behavior that are termed *alternate* because they are not practiced by the majority of the popula- on. Three of these forms are explored in detail in the following sections of this chapter.

HOMOSEXUALITY

Homosexuality is usually defined as sexual activity between two persons of the same sex. Homosexuality includes members of both sexes; however, the term lesbian is usually used to describe homosexual women. Homosexuality is not a new phenomena. The ancient Greeks accepted homosexual relationships as very natural and on a higher level than heterosexual relationships. Homo- sexuals of either sex may engage in hetero- sexual relationships at some time in their lives. Some homosexuals are married and carry on a "double" life; others either have been married or had intense heterosexual involvements. These individuals are referred to as bisexual.

Who becomes a homosexual? This is a question that psychologists and psychiatrists have been trying to agree about for many years. There are some patterns that seem to lead to homosexuality but none of these have been found to be conclusive. There is evidence that homosexuality may grow out of certain environmental and conditioning patterns. Some homosexuals report that an early homosexual incident accompanied by an environment that did not encourage het- erosexual relationships lead to homosexual behavior. Family histories frequently indicate a strong, possessive mother who has de- veloped an intimate relationship with her son. The young adult feels guilty about having relationships with other women because of his feelings about his mother.

The father is thought to have played a part in homosexual conditioning in some families. Fathers who are too remote or hostile often do not allow for the sex role identification that a young boy needs. Overly masculine fathers who stress manhood and strength often frighten a sensitive young boy. If the child is unable to accept the role his father has established, he may feel unworthy of being a man and may identify more easily with his mother.

Another possibility lies in an hormonal theory of homosexuality. Research has indicated that predominately homosexual individuals tested for male hormones and sperm counts have a lower count for both levels than bisexual or heterosexual males.

The causes of homosexuality have not been definitely established. Family environment may be a contributing cause in some cases but other factors are probably involved. Emo- tional make-up, peer group influence, psycho- logical trauma, and hormone imbalance may all contribute to one's being homosexual.

There are many myths and fallacies that accompany discussions about homosexuals. Homosexuals are people who choose to have a meaningful relationship with a person of their own sex. They are *not* more likely to commit crime, encourage young people to become homosexual, or to dress in strange clothes and affect unusual mannerisms. Some homosexuals may effect atypical behavior but so will *some* heterosexuals.

In recent years, homosexuality has truly come out of the "closet." A "closet" homo- sexual was one who preferred to keep his homosexuality a secret. In most cases, homo- sexuals feel less of a need to remain "closet- ed" at the present time. Homosexuals were frequently discriminated against by individ- uals and employers (this is still true today, but to a lesser degree). In order to make their rights known, homosexuals have formed organizations (sometimes called "gay libera- tion" groups) and have staged sit-ins, peti- tioned, and have tried to have equal rights legislation passed in their states and cities. Much of this legislation has already been approved but there is still much more to be accomplished.

Lesbians in past years had often stayed out of the limelight. But recent changes in social climate have found lesbians to be a strong political group. They are fighting a double

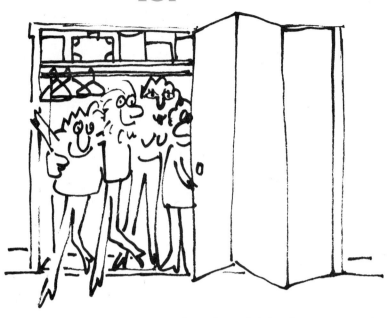

Coming out of the closet.

cause—that of equal rights for women and homosexuals. An interesting book that discusses the "new" lesbianism is *Sappho Was a Right-On Woman* [1] by Sidney Abbot and Barbara Love. The following quotation from the introduction of this book explains the plight of lesbians in today's society:

"We see the Lesbian's life as still filled with complex conflicts which make terrible demands on her. One of those conflicts is a double-bind, a no-win situation, where she can either have external approval and no internal integrity by keeping silent, or can achieve integrity and lose approval by coming out publicly."

What does this quotation mean to you? How have the rights of homosexuals been withheld from them over the years?

TRANSVESTISM

Transvestism refers to a practice of dressing in clothes of the opposite sex. *Transvestites* are individuals who dress in this way. They should not be confused with homosexuals. A recent study of transvestites indicated that less than one-quarter of those interviewed had experienced a homosexual relationship. This percentage is *less* than that of the general public by about 10 percent. Transvestites are usually married and their "dressing-up" is often hidden and occasional.

Why do transvestites "dress up"? They usually do so for erotic or emotional reasons. Dressing in women's clothes provides a sexual gratification that is pleasurable to them. Different transvestites will affect varying patterns of dress. Some will wear only women's undergarments, while others will dress completely as women.

Female impersonators are those individuals who dress as women and appear on the stage in these clothes. They often impersonate a particular female personality and assume her dress and mannerisms. Female impersonators have become increasingly popular in recent years and appear at well-known night spots and occasionally on television talk shows. Barbara Streisand, Marilyn Monroe, and Marlene Dietrich are often impersonated because of their distinct styles and mannerisms. Some female impersonators are homosexual, but many are not. Impersonators often are skilled actors who have worked many years to develop a true-to-life characterization of the individual they are impersonating.

You may have heard the expression, "drag queen." This refers to a homosexual who wears female clothing. To be in "drag" is

[1]From Sidney Abbot and Barbara Love, *Sappho Was A Right-On Woman* (New York: Stein and Day, 1972).

to be in full dress of the other sex and frequently in unusual striking clothes. Some "drag queens" are professional impersonators who make the rounds of gay clubs and parties. These individuals are often witty and comical and display a sense of "camp" (homosexual humor and taste). A fascinating book that takes one into the subculture of the homosexual female impersonator is *Mother Camp* by Esther Newton.

TRANSSEXUALISM

A transsexual is an individual who's anatomy and his or her sex role identification are incompatible. A transsexual knows that he or she is a man or a women and has all the physical characteristics of his or her own sex. However, a male transsexual, for example, feels that he is a woman emotionally and was meant to be a woman physically. He feels that he will not be entirely fulfilled until he has experienced a sex-change operation where he physically becomes a woman. Transsexuals are not satisfied by merely dressing as women because their feelings about their sexuality are more deeply involved in the other sex. Though there are a few female transsexuals, the majority of transsexuals are males who desire to become females.

Sex conversion surgery is not a simple matter. In order to have a sex-conversion operation, an individual must first live as a woman for at least six months. Prior to and during this period, the patient receives female hormones which will help to develop the breast tissue and eliminate a man's beard. Then after recommendation for the operation, an individual goes through lengthy plastic surgery that will reconstruct the external sexual organs so that a female anatomy will be present. Transsexual males are capable of vaginal intercourse following surgery, but they are not capable of giving birth to a child. Female transsexual surgery is much more complicated but it has been accomplished in a few cases.

Some interesting cases of transsexuals have appeared recently. One case involved a male school teacher who had sex-change

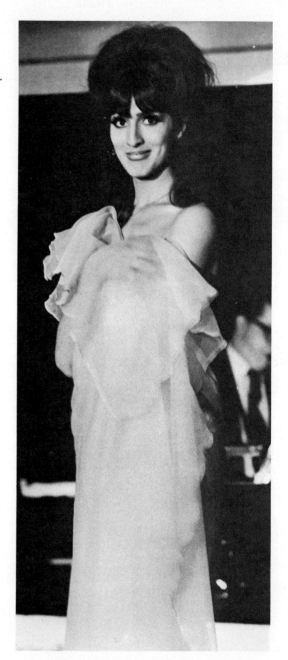

A female impersonator can dress in a deceptively alluring manner that disguises his true sex.

surgery in his 40s. He was and still is married and has children. The story became news when the man—now woman—tried to return to his job as a teacher. He was not allowed to resume his job and has been fighting the case for a number of years. The

Jan Morris (1972–   )
used to be James Hum-
phrey Morris (1926–   ).
James Morris was a
successful writer with
a record of impressive
achievements. He was
an army veteran; he
had scaled Mount Everest.
He was married and had
four children. But since
childhood, Morris had
felt that he was really
meant to be a woman. In
1972 he went to Casa-
blanca for a sex-change
operation and emerged as
Jan Morris. In her book
Conundrum, Morris de-
scribes these events and
also has some unique
things to say about the
differences between a
man's and a woman's
experiences in today's
world.

community feels that he would not be
accepted by his students as a female. The
teacher feels that he is the same person that
he always was, though now he has a new
sexual identity. How do you think a case
of this nature should be resolved?

Another case of transsexualism was recently
documented by a transsexual in the best-
seller, *Conundrum,* by Jan Morris who was
James Humphrey Morris until he underwent
transsexual surgery at the age of 47. James
Morris had been married for over 25 years
and has four children. Now Jan Morris is a
sister-in-law to his wife and an aunt to his
children. His wife of many years speaks of
her present relationship with her former
husband as a "passive friendship"
and accepts the title of sister-in-law. When
asked about her childhood, Jan recalls that
she always wanted to be a girl, even at an
early age. *Conundrum,* the story of how
James became Jan is a first-person report of
great interest and depth. One can learn
much about the feelings of a transsexual by
reading this remarkable account.

prostitution

Although there are many forms of sexual
behavior, none receives more publicity than
prostitution. Prostitution, often called the
"oldest profession," is the participation in
sexual activities for financial reward. Prostitution has been around for a long time and
while the majority of prostitutes are women,
there are some men who engage in this
activity. Male prostitutes may be homosexual
or heterosexual, but most females are
heterosexual.

Who are prostitutes? Many women who are
"dead-ended" become prostitutes. They may
need money to support themselves or an
expensive drug habit. They are frequently
sponsored by an individual who "takes
care of them." This person, the pimp, takes
a portion of the prostitute's money in order
to pay for managing her and arranging for
clients. A high-priced prostitute is referred
to as a "call girl," because her clients usually
phone for appointments.

Prostitution has become a problem in many

large cities. Obviously, dressed prostitutes
often parade the streets looking for clients.
Sometimes clients are mugged and robbed
by accomplices of the prostitute when they
get to a hotel room. Prostitution is illegal
in most states, but the police have a difficult
time keeping these individuals in jail. Most
prostitutes who are picked up by the police
one night are out on the streets the next day.

Many people think that prostitution is a
victimless crime and should be legalized.
In the states where it is legal, there is little
street difficulty relating to prostitution. Legalization of prostitution would reduce criminal
behavior related to pimps, blackmail, and
robbery. It would also greatly reduce the
police effort necessary to control the present
problem. How do you feel about legalizing
prostitution? Discuss some of the advantages
and disadvantages of this type of legislation.

deviant forms
of sexual behavior

The following forms of sexual behavior
deviate from the "norm." Few individuals
exhibit these behavior problems and those
that do usually have deep-seated psychological disturbances.

SADISM AND MASOCHISM

A sadist is an individual who gains pleasure
(in the form of erotic satisfaction) from inflicting physical or psychological pain on others.
Sadism is the form of behavior engaged
in by sadists. Sadism differs from masochism
in that the latter involves sexual gratification
derived from being the recipient of pain.
There are many acts of sadism that are
practiced in varying forms. Biting, whipping,
shackling, and hitting are often used by the
sadist. Psychological sadism may include
name calling, sarcasm, threats, and teasing.

EXHIBITIONISM

An exhibitionist is an individual who derives
sexual pleasure from exposing his sexual
organs to unsuspecting persons. The exhibitionist may come upon women in a subway

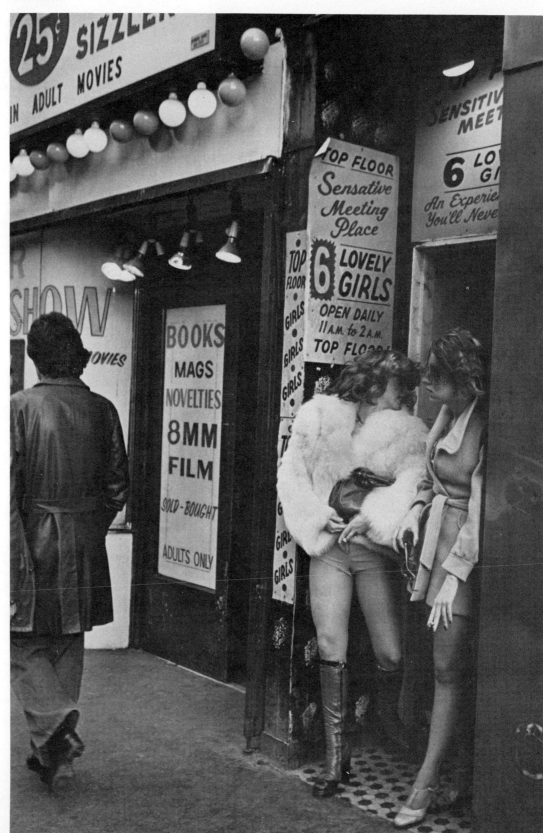

Streetwalkers, New York
City.

or bus station and expose himself and quickly run away. There are some female exhibitionists, but the majority of these people are men.

Most men who exhibit this type of behavior are quiet, passive individuals who in many cases were raised in overly restrictive homes. These individuals are usually not dangerous and are rarely involved in more serious crimes of a sexual nature.

VOYEURISM

You have probably all heard of the expression "peeping Tom." A "peeping Tom" is an individual (usually male) who derives sexual satisfaction from watching other persons who are nude or are engaging in sexual activities. Such a person will look through windows, holes in walls, or use binoculars to see into other people's homes. Voyeurs are often unable to participate successfully in sexual activities. By watching others, they are aroused and yet protected from participating themselves and possibly facing failure.

There are some individuals (often teenagers) who may derive some enjoyment from watching others through binoculars or sometimes at a closer distance. However, if these individuals do this occasionally and not to the exclusion of other forms of sexual activity, then it is not considered to be deviant behavior.

NYMPHOMANIA AND SATYRIASIS

A nymphomaniac is a woman who has an uncontrollable sexual drive. A true nymphomaniac would fulfill her sexual needs no matter what the consequences were to her or society. The male counterpart of a nymphomanic or "nymph" is a satyriac. Satyriasis describes this behavior pattern.

There are very few "true" nymphomaniacs or satyriacs. Many persons use these expressions for anyone whose sexual appetite exceeds their own. Few men understand the "normal" sexual desire of a woman. Some

men use the expression "she's a nymph" to degrade their partner and defend their own sexual capabilities. If both partners in a sexual relationship can openly discuss their feelings and needs, then the use of these terms would be greatly reduced.

The cases of documented nymphomaniacs and satyriacs are few and when discovered, are usually men and women who are overcompensating for sexual deprivation at an earlier age. Some of these individuals may have unexpressed fears of inability to perform sexually or latent homosexuality. Through this overt expression of sexuality, they are protecting themselves from the possible reality of these fears.

THINKING IT OVER

1. Discuss the meaning of the statement: "Sex is not a synonym for sexual intercourse."
2. Explain what is meant by the term "morality." Give an example of this term that was *not* used in the text discussion.
3. Discuss the meaning of the term "promiscuity." Is the text definition different from what you had thought was meant by promiscuity? Explain.
4. What is the meaning of the word "pornography"? Discuss some of the implications for society that are involved with pornography.
5. Explain the difference between a sexual revolution and evolution. Do you think that we are presently experiencing a revolution or evolution of sexual behavior?
6. Discuss two sexual standards and comment on their present acceptance among society in general and among your own peer group.
7. Do you feel that young people are aware of the ramifications of sexual relationship? Explain these ramifications and the reasons for your answer.
8. Discuss your own experiences with sex education. Comment on how sex education (home, school, friends) did or did not prepare you for young adulthood.
9. What guidelines should a young person consider when entering a sexual relationship?

10. Discuss the meaning of the term "homosexuality" and some of the possible
causative factors.
11. How does a transvestite differ from a
transsexual?
12. What is a prostitute? Do you think that
prostitution should be legalized? Explain
your answer.
13. Discuss the deviant forms of sexual behavior mentioned in this chapter. Do
you know of any other deviant patterns
of behavior?

KEY WORDS

Abstinence. A sexual standard that forbids
sexual intercourse prior to marriage.
Bigamy. Having more than one spouse
while the other one is still living.
Bisexual. An individual who enjoys sexual
relations with both sexes.
Coitus. The act of sexual intercourse.
Double standard. The accepted definition
is that men are allowed to engage in
premarital sex while women are not.
Drag queen. A homosexual male who dresses
in unusual feminine attire.
Erotic. That which is sexually arousing.
Exhibitionist. An individual who derives
sexual pleasure from exposing his or her
sexual organs to unsuspecting persons.
Extended family. A family where different
generations of the same family live
together in the same house.
Female impersonators. Men who dress as
women and appear on stage.
Homosexuality. Sexual activity between two
individuals of the same sex.
Humanism. A concern with the feelings
of individuals.
Hymen. The connective tissue that encloses
the external opening of the vagina.
Lesbian. Homosexual women.
Masochism. A deviant form of sexual behavior characterized by receiving erotic
stimulation from pain inflicted by others.
Morality. Conduct that is acceptable or unacceptable; often implying sexual virtue.
Nymphomaniac. A woman who has an
uncontrollable sexual desire.
Orthodox standard. An extreme sexual

standard that implies that certain women
are "good" and marriageable, but asexual.
Pornography. Explicitly erotic material in
the form of films, books, art work, magazines, or records.
Premarital sexual activity. Sexual activity
between persons who are not married.
Promiscuity. Engaging in sexual intercourse
with a variety of partners on a casual
level.
Prostitution. A form of sexual behavior where
individuals seek monetary reward for
sexual activity.
Sadism. A deviant form of sexual behavior
characterized by receiving erotic pleasure
from inflicting physical or psychological
pain.
Satyriac. A man who has an uncontrollable
sexual desire.
Secularism. A belief that morality should be
based on the well-being of humanity
rather than on religious principles.
Sexual behavior. A totality of sexual expression that encompasses the sexual relationship and general communication between
individuals.
Sexual evolution. A gradual change in sexual
behavior and standards.
Sexual revolution. A sudden change in
sexual behavior and standards.
Sexual standard. A pattern of sexual behavior
that is accepted by a large number of
individuals.
Sodomy. Sexual behavior that may include
sexual intercourse with animals or oral-
genital or anal-genital intercourse between
humans.
Technical virginity. Participation in all forms
of sexual behavior except sexual intercourse.
Transsexual. An individual who undergoes
surgery in order to achieve the anatomy
of the opposite sex.
Transvestism. A practice where individuals
dress in clothes of the opposite sex.
Virgin. A girl or woman who has not experienced sexual intercourse.
Voyeur. An individual who derives sexual
pleasure from watching others in the nude
or participating in sexual activity.

173

GETTING INVOLVED

Books and Periodicals

Abbot, Sidney, and Love, Barbara. *Sappho Was a Right-On Woman.* New York: Stein and Day, 1972. Two lesbians tell all about it: the guilt; facing family members; the gay bars; and the role of the women's movement and lesbianism.

Masters, William H., and Johnson, Virginia E. *Human Sexual Response.* Boston: Little, Brown, 1966. The famous scientific study of human sexuality.

_____. *Human Sexual Inadequacy.* Boston: Little, Brown, 1970. The authors describe their methods of treating sexual problems.

_____. *The Pleasure Bond.* Boston: Little, Brown, 1975. A plea for more commitment between sex partners.

Miller, Merle. *On Being Different: What It Means to Be a Homosexual.* New York: Random House, 1971. An autobiographical account by a well-known writer who decided to come out of the closet.

Morris, Jan. *Conundrum.* New York: Harcourt Brace Jovanovich, 1974. Why the author had a transsexual operation; and how being a woman affects one's life.

Seaman, Barbara. *Free and Female.* New York: Coward, McCann, Geoghegan, 1972. Woman's sexual needs and capacities from a feminist point of view.

Movies

Belle de Jour, with Catherine Deneuve, 1968. A society woman has fantasies about being a prostitute. Distributed by Hurlock Cine-World.

Butterfield 8, with Elizabeth Taylor, Laurence Harvey, 1960. The life of a successful call-girl. Distributed by Films Incorporated.

Carnal Knowledge, with Jack Nicholson, Art Garfunkel, Ann Margret, 1971. Two men discover that promiscuity isn't any fun. Distributed by Avco Embassy Pictures.

The Children's Hour, with Audrey Hepburn, Shirley MacLaine, 1962. A mere accusation of lesbianism has disastrous effects. Distributed by United Artists 16.

Everything You Always Wanted to Know about Sex but Were Afraid to Ask, with Woody Allen, 1972. A spoof of transvestism, bestiality, etc. Distributed by United Artists 16.

The Killing of Sister George, with Beryl Reid, Susannah York, 1968. The story of an aging lesbian and her younger lover. Distributed by Films Incorporated.

Midnight Cowboy, with Dustin Hoffman, Jon Voight, 1969. About homosexual hustlers on 42nd Street. Distributed by United Artists 16.

Myra Breckenridge, with Mae West, Raquel Welch, 1970. A totally unbelievable account of a transsexual. Distributed by Films Incorporated.

Rain, with Joan Crawford, Walter Huston, 1932. Somerset Maugham's look at prostitution the way it used to be. Distributed by Budget, Kit Parker, Macmillan, Mogull's, United, Westcoast, and Wholesome.

Sunday, Bloody Sunday, with Glenda Jackson, Peter Finch, Murray Head, 1971. A doctor has to choose between his male lover and his female one. Distributed by United Artists 16.

Records

"The Times They Are A-Changin'," Bob Dylan, *Bob Dylan's Greatest Hits, Vol. 1* album, Columbia. The world is changing—and so are our attitudes about sex.

"Love for Sale," Ella Fitzgerald, *Ella Loves Cole* album, Atlantic. The melancholy feelings of a prostitute.

9
REPRODUCTION

Many of you are probably well-acquainted with the reproductive organs and their functions. However, there are many factors related to reproduction that are misunderstood by people of all ages. This chapter will help to clarify some of these misunderstandings by reviewing the reproductive system and related topics.

Conception, pregnancy, and childbirth are discussed in detail with special attention given to new developments in all of these areas. Do you know that there is a method that can be used prior to birth to determine if a fetus has a genetic disease? Other topics related to pregnancy are also discussed. These topics include the Rh factor, multiple births, and fertility drugs.

All aspects of birth control are explored. The methods and their effectiveness are discussed. In reference to the birth control pills, types of

pills, effectiveness, and potential dangers are discussed in detail. New developments in this area are explained and their present areas of use are explored.

Sterilization procedures for men and women are discussed in great detail. The type of surgery available, its effectiveness, and reversability are considered. In addition, newer methods of birth control are reported including a method of temporary sterilization.

Infertility is a problem that faces many couples. Most people are unaware of the help that is available to couples who have difficulty in conceiving a child. The subject is explored in relation to when and where to seek help.

An issue in the daily headlines is abortion. It is a subject that brings out the strong, often violent, emotions of many individuals. The topic is discussed here from an

objective point of view. You must decide for yourself how you feel about this subject.

While reading this chapter, think about the following concepts:

■ Knowledge concerning reproduction is often incomplete.

■ Menstruation is a natural occurrence and should be accepted as such by men and women.

■ Pregnancy begins at the moment of conception.

■ Pregnancy is a natural state and women need not be treated that differently during this period.

■ Most couples desire to plan their children and there are methods to help them do this.

■ Infertility is as much of a problem to some couples as birth control is to others.

■ The abortion issue, in many cases, has become more emotional than objective.

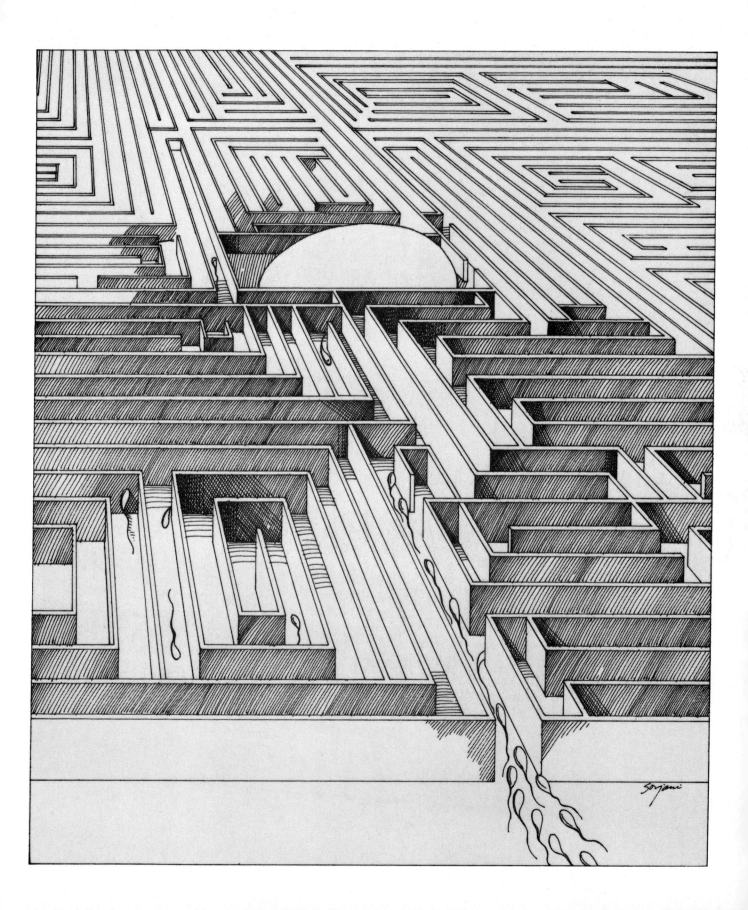

Most individuals think that they are well versed in the anatomy and functioning of the male and female reproductive systems. But much of this knowledge is not based on fact and is frequently accompanied by fallacies. Many persons do not question certain old wive's tales that seem to go along with every aspect of sexual functioning. Where tests of sexual knowledge are given to students of all ages, the wealth of misinformation is astounding. For example, the following is a partial listing of fallacies associated with the *normal* function of menstruation.

1. One should not bathe during menstruation.
2. Athletic activity of all types is dangerous during menstruation.
3. It is dangerous to have intercourse during menstruation.
4. Women are considered "unclean" during this time.
   All of these opinions were given by recent college students!

SIECUS (Sex Information and Educational Council of the U.S., Inc.) was founded in 1964 by Dr. Mary S. Calderone. Its goal is to promote the understanding of human sexuality.

SIECUS believes that everybody has a right to make their own decisions about sex. But this freedom involves responsibilities—to oneself, as well as to others. To decide wisely, one must know all the facts. So the organization provides information about all aspects of sex. If you have a question you would like them to answer, write to SIECUS at Suite 922, 122 East 42 Street, New York, N.Y. 10017.

Misinformation concerning sexual anatomy can be especially harmful when it disrupts sexual functioning. Many individuals do not understand their anatomy or that of their partners and do not fully enjoy sexual intercourse because of this lack of understanding. A recent survey of 1,000 women was conducted to determine the reasons for non-consummation of marriage. Many of the reasons given were based on fear and misunderstanding of the sexual relationship. More than 5 percent of those interviewed reportedly did not consummate their marriage because of the couple's ignorance of where the women's sex organs were located.

Knowledge about the organs of reproduction is essential if other basic areas such as conception, pregnancy, birth, birth control, and venereal disease are to be completely understood. Sex education is far more than the anatomy and physiology of reproduction; it is basic to all areas of sexuality.

male reproductive organs

The reproductive organs of both sexes are often called the genitals. The genitals of the

male include those organs and structures that produce, transport, and deliver the end-product of sperm cells or spermatozoa. The structures involved in this process include the testes, ducts, and accessory structures, and the penis.

THE TESTES

The testes are the paired, primary sex glands of the male. They are endocrine glands which produce substances (hormones) that are released directly into the bloodstream. The male hormones are called androgens, and the two principal androgens are testosterone and androsterone. These hormones are secreted by cells within the testes. Testosterone is primarily responsible for the development of male secondary sexual characteristics. These characteristics include the development of body hair, facial hair (beard), change of voice, skeletal and muscular development of the male sex, and physical and emotional sexual drive. In addition, testosterone maintains the development of these characteristics through adulthood. Testosterone is essential to the development and functioning of all the male sexual organs.

Most "normal" men produce sufficient quantities of testosterone to insure adequate sexual functioning. Men having only one testicle usually have sufficient testosterone production. Many individuals feel that additional testosterone will make them more virile, but this is not true of the "normal" male. However, if hormones are found to be insufficient or out of balance, hormone therapy can be very helpful.

As we continue to discuss the structure and function of the testes, refer to Figure 9-1. The testes are made up of tightly coiled seminiferous tubules. It is within these tubules that the sperm is produced. Production of sperm cells is called spermatogenesis. Spermatogenesis and the production of testosterone occur after puberty and continue throughout life. In between the seminiferous tubules, there are cells that secrete the hormones, testosterone and androsterone. As

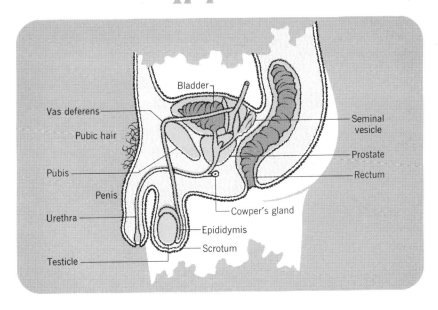

Figure 9-1
Male reproductive organs.

previously mentioned, these are the primary male hormones. The developing sperm move from the seminiferous tubules to the epididymis, which is a tightly coiled connecting tissue. This structure stores the sperm.

The testes are located in a loose pouch of skin found outside of the body. This pouch is called the scrotum. Its location (outside rather than inside) is essential to sperm production. Sperm cannot live at normal body temperature of 98.6°F. The temperature within the scrotum is three to five degrees below body temperature. The scrotal sac has a temperature regulating mechanism of its own. The sac is suspended by the cremaster muscle, which controls the position of the testes in relation to the temperature. If the temperature outside of the body becomes too cold, the cremaster muscle contracts, bringing the scrotal sac close to the body for extra warmth. If the temperature rises, the muscle relaxes, taking the testes away from the heat of the body and allowing them to become cooler.

In some cases, the testes fail to descend into the scrotum. The testes are located in the abdomen of the male child prior to birth. In most cases, the testes descend into the scrotal sac before birth—but not in all cases. In approximately one out of every 50 boys at puberty, the testes have not descended. About one out of 500 male adults will have this problem. In an adult male with undescended testes, there is no sperm production. However, all other sexual functioning is normal. In some cases, testes that have not descended by puberty will begin to and continue to degenerate. If the condition is recognized at an early age, hormone treatment and surgery (in certain cases) will enable the testes to achieve their proper location.

Castration may be defined as the removal of the sex glands (gonads) of either sex. Castration in the male, therefore, is the removal of the testes and in the female the removal of the ovaries. A man can become castrated by injury (often during a war) or surgically because of certain physical conditions. Cancer of the testes or of the prostate gland (a glandular structure that secretes a fluid that is expelled with the sperm) is a major reason for castration.

If castration occurs and if testosterone is not given, a man will gradually experience a weakening of his sex drive and function. A certain amount of feminization may also take place. However, men who have been castrated and receive hormone therapy will be able to function in a relatively normal manner. The greatest problem of castration, especially for men, is usually psychological. Because of his appearance and feelings about himself, he is bound to go through a very difficult emotional period—that may last throughout his life.

VAS DEFERENS

The vas deferens is a small tube that takes the mature sperm from the epididymis where it had been stored. The vas deferens are lined with tiny hairs called cilia, which help to move the sperm through the vas deferens to the base of the urinary bladder. Here, the vas deferens meet with the seminal vesicles, which will be discussed in the following section. The vas deferens is the tube that is severed when a man undergoes a vasectomy. This operation for male sterilization is discussed later in this chapter.

Accessory organs. The seminal vesicle mentioned briefly before is a gland located near the base of the urinary bladder. Its primary function is to produce an alkaline secretion that joins with the sperm (from the vas deferens) to increase the sperm's mobility. Some sperm is also stored in the seminal vesicle. The sperm and the seminal vesicle fluid drain into a common ejaculatory duct. This duct passes through the prostate gland, a gland that surrounds the neck of the urethra. The urethra is the tube that conveys urine from the bladder, through the penis, to the outside. In the male, the urethra also conducts the semen (sperm and the secretions of the seminal vesicles and the prostate gland) through the penis to the outside. The prostate gland secretes an alkaline solution that further aids in sperm mobility.

The Cowper's glands are tiny pea-shaped glands located just below the prostate. Like the prostate, they secrete an alkaline fluid that drains into the urethra prior to ejaculation. Ejaculation is the sudden expulsion of semen through the urethra of the penis during sexual intercourse.

THE PENIS

The penis is the organ by which sexual intercourse is performed. In its unexcited state,

it is flaccid or soft. It is made of spongy erectile tissue that is capable of dilating with increased blood flow. This results in the organ becoming stiff and large. The penis will increase in both size and diameter from the flaccid state to the erect state. This erect state or erection is caused by sexual excitement and culminates in the height of sexual stimulation called the orgasm. During orgasm, the semen is released into the vagina. However, ejaculation can occur at other times than during sexual excitement. Such nonsexual stimulation as a full bladder or tight clothes can also cause ejaculation.

Ejaculation can also occur during nocturnal emissions, commonly known as "wet dreams." These dreams may occur throughout life but are usually more frequent among men in their teens or early twenties. They do not begin to occur until puberty when the secretion of sperm begins. "Wet dreams" are usually the result of an erotic dream. They occur because of the psychological stimulation of the sexual process. Ejaculation may also occur through masturbation or self-stimulation with or without erotic thoughts, books, or pictures.

The tip or head of the penis is covered by a hood-like, retractable membrane called the prepuce. The prepuce is often referred to as the foreskin. This membrane surrounds the glans penis, which is the highly sensitive head of the penis. The prepuce or foreskin is often removed soon after birth in an operation called a circumcision. At one time, circumcision was limited to certain religious denominations (it is a religious rite among Jewish people), but it has since become an accepted medical practice for most newborn males. The reasons for circumcision are basically hygienic. The secretions of the penis form a substance called smegma. It is a white sticky substance that collects under an uncircumcised foreskin and causes an unpleasant odor and can also be a source of irritation and bacterial growth.

Research has shown that an accumulation of smegma may be a contributing factor in cancer of the penis. However, this research has not been definitely proven and statistics

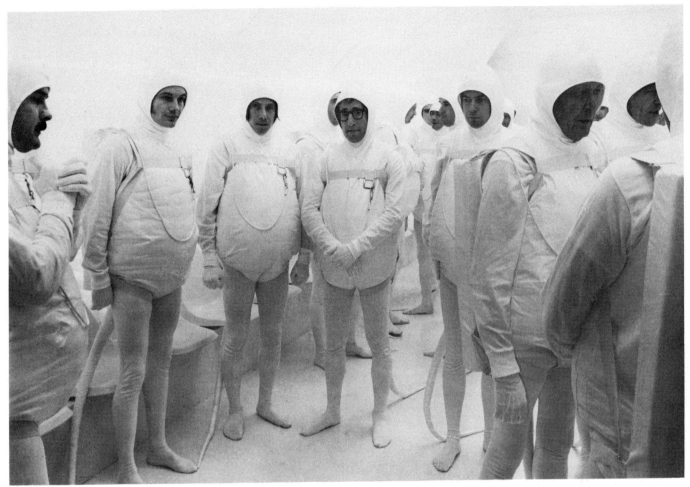

Woody Allen and his fellow sperm awaiting
signal to blast off in a scene from *Everything
You Always Wanted to Know About Sex But
Were Afraid to Ask.*

indicate that there is no greater incidence
of penile cancer among uncircumcised men.
There has also been some research data that
supports a theory that uncircumcised men
may predispose their sexual partners to cervical cancer. Again, this research is still in
its early stages.

As previously mentioned, the urethra conveys
both urine and semen; however, not at the
same time. A muscle at the neck of the
bladder prevents ejaculation and urination
from occurring simultaneously.

EJACULATION

At the height of sexual excitement (orgasm),

the male will ejaculate. Ejaculation is accompanied by a highly pleasurable feeling similar
to the feeling a woman receives from climax
or orgasm. The strength of the act of ejaculation will differ according to the individual.
Some men tend to ejaculate with great force
while others have a more mild ejaculation.
Strength of ejaculation has no relation to the
size of the penis or pleasure of orgasm.

During the act of ejaculation, the sperm is
discharged from the penis through the urethra.
The sperm has mixed with secretions from
the seminal vesicles and prostate and is in
the ejaculatory duct, which is located at the
meeting of the seminal vesicles and urethra.

The average ejaculate (substance ejaculated) contains between 250,000,000 and 500,000,000 sperm. Sperm counts will vary with each individual. The sperm count, however, will decrease if frequency of ejaculation increases. Less sperm is able to be produced and stored if ejaculation is very frequent. This becomes an important factor in conception (the fertilization of an egg by a sperm) and is discussed later in this chapter.

You may have heard of the term "premature ejaculation." This term is often associated with a sexual problem that many men experience. Premature ejaculation may be defined as ejaculation soon after entering the vagina. It becomes a problem because most women need more time than men to achieve sexual satisfaction through orgasm. Statistics indicate that ejaculation occurs before a woman reaches orgasm in about 50 percent of all acts of intercourse. Premature ejaculation has always been a problem but has become more openly talked about in recent years. In the past, most women would not have felt "right" in discussing this matter with their sexual partners.

The problem has come to be openly discussed on television and in magazines primarily because of the work of Masters and Johnson and their research into sexual malfunctions. The reasons for the problem are numerous. Some frequently given reasons include: (1) hostility between the sexual partners; (2) neurosis; and (3) stressful conditions during a young man's initial sexual experiences. Much work has been done in this area and sexual therapists report great success in quickly controlling the problem in a majority of cases.

female reproductive organs

The female reproductive organs or genitals involve the ovaries, Fallopian tubes, uterus, and vagina. In addition, the female has external genitalia. In this section, the structure and function of the female reproductive organs are discussed.

Ovaries. The ovaries (paired organs) are located deep in the female pelvis. One ovary is located on each side of the body. Each ovary is about the size of a small egg and has similar functions to the testes of the male. The ovaries produce the ovarian hormones, estrogen and progesterone. One major function of these hormones is the preparation and maintenance of the uterus or womb for possible implantation of a fertilized egg. However, estrogen and progesterone also function in the development of the female genitalia and female sexual characteristics, including breast development and general maintenance of physical and emotional health.

The ovaries also function in the development and release of ova or eggs. The release of ova is tied to the menstrual cycle which is under the direct influence of the female hormones. This aspect of the female reproductive system is discussed in a later section of this chapter.

Each ovary consists of a number of tiny cavities called follicles. These follicles contain an ovum in some stage of development. Some ovum have not yet begun to grow while others are maturing and still others are mature enough to be released. At birth a female has all of the ova that she will ever have. The number of ova is estimated at between 200,000 and 400,000. However, this number will decrease to about 10,000 at the time a girl reaches puberty. The release of ovum does not start until the menstrual cycle begins at the approximate age of 13. In a lifetime of ovulation (about 35 to 40 years), the average woman discharges only 400 to 500 mature ova. The remaining follicles and ova will deteriorate.

FALLOPIAN TUBES

The Fallopian tubes are tiny tubes that carry the ovum to the uterus (where the fertilized ovum will develop). The Fallopian tube (see Figure 9-2) flares out into fingerlike structures called *fimbria* that catch the ovum upon its release from the ovary. The tubes are lined with *cilia* that move the ovum toward the uterus. The ovum is usually fertilized in the Fallopian tube and then the fertilized egg attaches itself to the wall of the uterus where development begins. However, if the ovum is not fertilized, it passes through the tube and is expelled with the lining of the uterus during menstruation.

You may be familiar with the term "tubal pregnancy." This simply means that the fertilized egg has implanted in the Fallopian tube rather than in the uterus. This occurs very rarely and most such implantations usually terminate by themselves in a few days. Occasionally, development continues and this can become a dangerous situation. However, it is usually discovered because of the pain and discomfort felt by the woman. Surgery is usually required to remove the developing embryo.

UTERUS OR WOMB

The uterus is a pear-shaped organ where the fertilized egg is received and nourished until development is complete and birth occurs. The organ is thick and muscular and is located slightly below the Fallopian tubes.

The muscular makeup of the uterus allows for great expansion during pregnancy. The uterus is wider at the top than at the bottom, and the bottom or neck of the uterus is called the cervix. The cervix opens into the vagina. About a third to one-half inch of the cervix extends into the vagina. It is here that the sperm passes from the vagina into the cervix of the uterus. During pregnancy, the cervix is often blocked by a mucous plug, which closes off the uterus from the vagina and prevents infection and possible damage to the developing ovum.

VAGINA

The vagina is a muscular, elastic passage. It receives the erect penis during intercourse and is also the birth canal. It is able to dilate significantly to allow for intercourse and birth.

The *hymen* (refer to Chapter 8 for additional information) is the membrane that partially closes off the entrance to the vagina from the outside. The membrane does not usually close off the vagina entrance completely because menstrual flow must pass through

Figure 9-2
Female reproductive organs. (*a*) Side view; (*b*) front view.

(a)

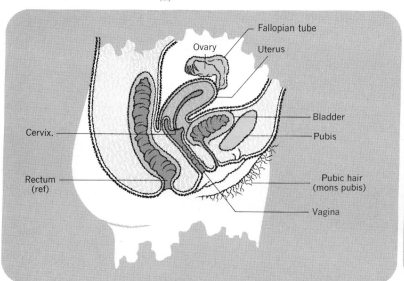

Side view

(b)

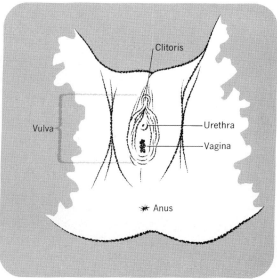

Front view

the vagina. In most cases, the hymen has been partially ruptured prior to first intercourse. However, some women may have a completely intact hymen prior to intercourse. At one time, the *myth* of an intact hymen was considered a sign of virginity. However, in most cases, this myth is no longer accepted.

If a woman feels that her hymen is intact and may cause pain during intercourse, she can consult her physician or gynecologist (a doctor who specializes in the treatment of the female reproductive system) for advice and treatment. If the gynecologist finds a thick membrane, he may advise dilation or minor surgery to correct the situation. This type of surgery is usually performed in the doctor's office under a local anesthetic.

EXTERNAL FEMALE GENITALIA

The external genitalia of the female is often collectively referred to as the vulva. The vulva consists of the clitoris, the labia minora and labia majora, mons veneris, vestibule, and the urethra. Each of these structures and their function are discussed in the following sections.

The *clitoris* is located in the upper folds of the *labia minora* (small lips) and *labia majora* (large lips). Consult Figure 9-2 for location of the structures. The clitoris is highly sensitive and has a *glans* similar in function to that of the head or *glans* of the penis. The clitoris is composed of erectile tissue that, like the penis, is capable of becoming filled with blood and increase in size. This usually occurs during sexual stimulation. It is clitoral stimulation that is an important element in causing female orgasm. However, research has shown that orgasm can occur even if the clitoris is not present. The entire vulval area is sexually responsive and can produce orgasms.

The *labia majora* are folds of skin that are covered by pubic hair on the outside and contain sweat glands on the inner sides.

The *labia minora* are smaller folds of skin that are located inside of the *labia majora*. They enclose the *clitoris* and richly sup-

plied with blood vessels and nerve endings. The *labia minora* are highly sensitive structures.

The *mons veneris* is the fatty tissue that covers the pubic bone and has pubic hair growing on it. This area is very sensitive to erotic stimulation.

The *vestibule* is the area that is enclosed by the labia minora. It is called by this name because within this area is found the openings to the urethra and vagina. This is a highly erogenous (responsive to sexual stimulation) area. The Bartholin's glands are located on either side of the vaginal opening. They function in the secreting of a lubricating fluid which may be helpful in penetration by the penis during intercourse. However, the amount of secretion is very small and some researchers do not think that it can aid penetration.

The *urethra* in the female, unlike the male, has no function in sex or reproduction. Its function is to transport urine out of the body during excretion.

the menstrual cycle and ovulation

The menstrual cycle is an on-going process that lasts from menarche (the onset of menstruation during puberty) to menopause or climacteric (the cessation of menstruation). The menstrual cycle is interrupted only by pregnancy. During the years that a woman menstruates, she is able to become pregnant and bear a child. However, when menstruation stops, the ability to bear children also stops.

The term "cycle" is used in discussing menstruation because certain events occur at a given time each month throughout the years a woman menstruates. The normal range for the length of the menstrual cycle is between 21 and 35 days. However, cycles do vary greatly and individuals tend to have different cycles.

The menstrual cycle (see Figure 9-3) is controlled by hormones secreted by the ovaries (estrogen and progesterone) and pituitary gland hormones. The pituitary gland is located at the base of the brain and secretes many hormones. Two of these hormones are gonadotropic (reproductive organ stimulators), the follicle stimulating hormone (FSH) and the lutenizing hormone (LH).

The blood hormone levels determine the events of the cycle. In the early part of the cycle, an egg matures in the ovary and the lining of the uterus (endometrium) begins to thicken in preparation to receive a fertilized ovum. Following menstruation, the cycle begins all over again. Approximately 12 to 14 days later, the mature ovum is released from the ovary and the lining of the uterus is thick and engorged with blood. The release of the ovum from the ovary is called ovulation. It occurs 12 to 14 days *before* the menstrual cycle begins. If the ovum is fertilized in the Fallopian tube, it will implant itself in the endometrium and begin to grow. However, if the egg is not fertilized, it will degenerate and be expelled with the thick uterine lining. This expulsion of blood and fluid usually lasts from three to seven days and is called menstruation.

These are the basic events that occur each month in preparation for the implantation of a fertilized ovum. There are many physical

Figure 9-3
The menstrual cycle. Solid arrows indicate the production of follicle stimulating hormones; dashed arrows indicate the production of luteinizing hormones, which causes the ruptured follicle to transform itself into corpus luteum and brings about the production of progesterone.

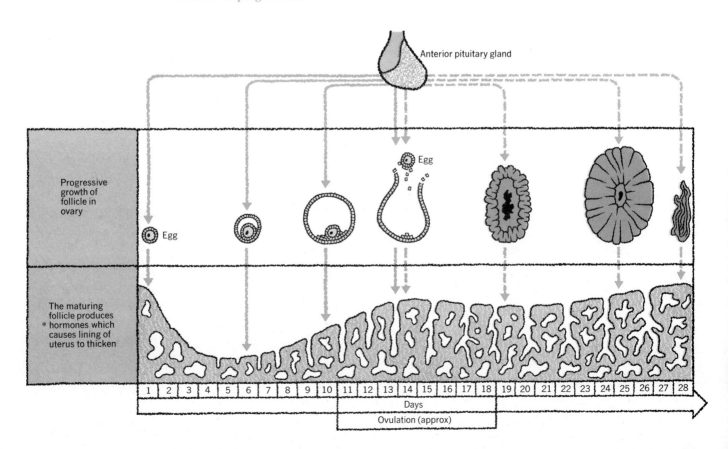

and psychological factors involved in the monthly cycle. Some women experience what is called "premenstrual tension." This term covers a variety of physical and emotional disturbances. Some women feel very irritable; others feel moody or depressed. Headaches, stomach distention, fatigue, nervousness, increase of size and tenderness of the breasts, and general body discomfort are all recognized symptoms that women feel prior to menstruation. Some women are able to feel "ovulation beginning" within them. This occurrence in the middle of the cycle is often distinguished by a sharp pain in the lower abdomen. The pain is called the mittleschmerz.

In the beginning of this chapter, some of the myths that accompany menstruation were discussed. However, in recent years most individuals realize that menstruation is a very normal function of the female body and one's life is altered very slightly by its occurrence. Most women do not experience significant premenstrual or menstrual discomfort and are able to function quite normally.

Attitudes have changed concerning menstruation. When a well-known actress can do a television commercial for a sanitary napkin, then we can see how attitudes have changed in just a few years. It is not a "dark secret" or "curse" that cannot be discussed. "Those days of the month" are rarely alluded to by the modern woman who wants to enjoy all of the days of the month.

It is interesting to note that research indicates that girls are menstruating earlier than did previous generations. The age of *menarche* (the onset of menstruation) has steadily declined in industrialized countries. While the average age of menarche in the United States in 1905 was about 14½ years, it is now about 12½ years of age. The reasons for this change are not entirely known. However, one can assume that improved nutrition may have played an important role. What does earlier menstruation mean to a young girl? Many individuals feel that earlier menstruation indicates a physical maturity but not an emotional maturity. A twelve-year-

old may be physically mature but is she able to handle the responsibility that goes with it?

Do you think there is a conflict between early menstruation and the emotional capabilities of a young girl? Can these conflicts be resolved?

The responsibility of pregnancy, for both the male and the female, is obviously not something to be taken lightly. Becoming a mother or father is a relatively easy task; becoming a parent is a far more complex responsibility.

Do you agree with the above statement that differentiates between the responsibility involved in becoming a mother or father and becoming a parent?

conception, pregnancy, and birth

The beginning of a new life occurs as soon as conception (the fertilization of the ovum by the sperm) takes place. Pregnancy (the state of having a developing life within one's body) also occurs at the time of conception. Birth is the time when the developed infant is expelled or taken from the uterus. These three areas are discussed in the following sections of this chapter.

CONCEPTION

After the sperm are ejaculated into the vagina, they swim up the uterus and into the Fallopian tubes. If there is an egg present in the tube (usually in the farthest one-third), conception may take place.

Many sperm cells will surround the egg; however, only one will penetrate the egg and fertilize it. An enzyme (a substance that initates or speeds up a chemical reaction) produced by the sperm cells helps to break down a protective coating around the egg so that one sperm may enter the egg cell.

The sex of the child is determined at the moment of conception. Both the sperm and egg have 23 chromosomes, one of which is a sex chromosome. The egg cell carries an X chromosome and the sperm cell carries

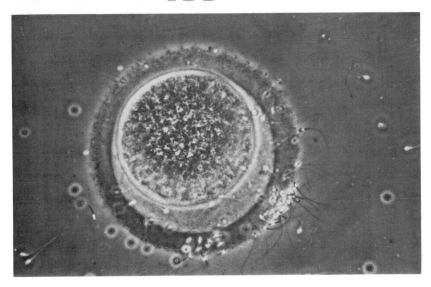

Human egg and sperm at fertilization.

either an X or a Y chromosome. Therefore, the father is the determiner of the sex of the child. If a sperm carrying an X chromosome enters the egg, then there is a XX configuration or a girl child. If the sperm carries a Y chromosome, then the resulting configuration is XY or a boy child. The sex of the child cannot be altered following conception.

Many articles have been written about determining the sex of a child prior to birth. Most of these articles present scientifically unproven information. However, some research has indicated that the time of conception may influence the sex of the child. Dr. Landrum B. Shettles, a research scientist in the area of human conception and development, supports a theory of sex determination that is based on the vitality of the "male" or Y-sperm as compared to the "female" or X-sperm. The Y-sperm are shaped differently than the X-sperm and they tend to swim more rapidly. However, they lose their vitality more quickly than the X-sperm. Female sperm travel more slowly but are stronger and can live longer than the Y-sperm.

Applying these facts to sex determination, Dr. Shettles supports that a couple that desires a female child should have intercourse three or four days prior to ovulation. By so doing, the "male" sperm would tend to die out, leaving a majority of the stronger "female" or X-sperm to fertilize the egg. An acid

douche (vinegar and water) is also recommended prior to intercourse because "male" sperm have greater difficulty surviving in an acid climate.

If a couple desires a male child, then intercourse should take place immediately after ovulation. This would allow a faster swimming "male" or Y-sperm to penetrate the egg. An alkaline douche (baking soda and water) is suggested to counteract the acid environment of the vagina.

This information is not accepted by all researchers and, of course, there are no guarantees. Individuals who wish to find out more about this topic can consult their physician or gynecologist and read some of the research articles written by Dr. Shettles and his co-workers. The time of ovulation is essential to these methods and a doctor can help a woman to determine when ovulation occurs.

An interesting theory concerning sex determination is based on parental stress. This theory proposes that the parent who is under the *least* stress at the time of conception will tend to produce a child of his or her own sex. This theory was tested by studying children born out of rape. One may assume that a woman who is raped would be under greater stress than her attacker. In a study of ten rape-caused births, nine of the children were boys. This is an interesting theory, but at this point it is still a theory.

Can a child's sex be determined following conception? The answer is "yes." Through a method called amniocentesis, a small amount of amniotic fluid is withdrawn by a needle from the pregnant woman. The fluid that is collected will contain some of the cells of the child and will indicate chromosomal makeup—XX or XY configuration. Amniocentesis is performed when serious genetic disease is a possibility. By studying the chromosomes of the developing child, certain diseases can be ruled out or be positively identified. Although sex may be determined by this procedure, amniocentesis is *never* used solely for this purpose. If a couple feels that they may have a genetic problem, they should seek an appointment with a genetic counseling service.

Once the fertilized egg (now called an embryo) has traveled down the tube, it will usually implant in the thick, spongy lining of the uterus. This is the beginning of embryonic development.

PREGNANCY

Pregnancy begins at the moment of conception. However, the signs and symptoms of pregnancy do not usually occur for a few weeks, or even a month or two later. Symptoms of pregnancy frequently include "morning sickness." This is a nauseous feeling usually occurring upon awaking in the morning, but in some cases it may persist for the entire day. The breasts may also become fuller and there may be a darker coloration of the pigmented area of breast. Fatigue and increased urination are also early symptoms of pregnancy. The most apparent symptoms of pregnancy is the cessation of the menstrual cycle. If a menstrual period is missed, then pregnancy might very well be the reason. *Of course,* there are numerous other conditions that would effect the cessation of menstruation. A doctor should be consulted if one or two regular menstrual periods are missed.

Pregnancy tests are very helpful in determining pregnancy after a certain period of time has elapsed. A hormone from a woman's urine can be used to determine pregnancy and this test is highly accurate if taken about two weeks after a menstrual period is missed. This would mean that a woman was approximately four weeks pregnant at the time of the test. Another type of pregnancy test that has been used in the past has come under recent criticism. This test provides for the oral administration of the hormone progesterone. If a woman were pregnant, nothing would occur upon taking the hormone. However, if she were not pregnant, then menstruation would begin. Recent findings indicate that a number of women who were pregnant at the time they took the pills gave birth to a greater than normal number of children with birth defects. This research is still in the preliminary stages of investigation.

As soon as a woman thinks that she is pregnant, she should go for a checkup. A hospital clinic, family doctor, or gynecologist will provide the necessary care to produce a healthy child and mother. Many women feel that prenatal care (medical attention prior to the birth of a child) is unnecessary. This is a very dangerous viewpoint for both mother and child. Each person is different and care must be specifically suited to each pregnant woman. Medical care will provide for counseling in reference to diet, weight gain, vitamins, special medications, and problems of a physical and a psychological nature. Prenatal care is essential for all pregnant women; it is as important to the woman expecting her fourth child as it is to the women expecting her first child!

Adequate diet and exercise is essential for the pregnant woman. Her caloric intake should be just slightly higher than her normal diet. Many women gain excessive weight during pregnancy which is both dangerous to the health of the mother and child and also very difficult to take off following the birth of the child. Some women take the opposite approach and literally starve themselves because they fear excessive weight gain. This is an extremely dangerous procedure. Recent studies have indicated that weight gain should be between 18 and 25 pounds. Many physicians thought that less weight gain than this was appropriate. However, low birth weight children have been born to mothers who have gained only a small amount of weight during pregnancy.

The average pregnancy or period of gestation is about 280 days. In order to determine the approximate date of delivery, the physician adds seven days to the beginning of the last menstrual period and counts back three months. The date arrived at is the approximate date of birth.

As the embryo begins to develop in the uterus, the amniotic sac (bag of waters) is also developing. It is this sac filled with amniotic fluid that will protect the developing embryo. The fluid-filled bag helps to equalize the pressure around the embryo and prevents injury from sharp jolts or pushing. The fluid environment also allows function of movement for the embryo.

The placenta is the rich lining of the uterine wall that provides a medium of exchange for oxygen and nourishment between the mother and developing embryo. The mother's blood and the blood of the child *never* mix. They have two separate circulatory systems, and nourishment and the removal of waste is accomplished by diffusion and absorption between the blood vessels.

The umbilical cord forms at about the fifth week of pregnancy, and it suspends the embryo within the amniotic fluid. The cord connects the mother to the embryo and provides the blood vessels where the exchange of nourishment and waste products occurs.

Some substances can pass through the placenta, although it does provide a barrier to many dangerous substances. It has been determined that certain drugs can pass through the placenta and affect the developing life. One of the most tragic examples of this placental breakthrough was seen in the case of the drug thalidomide. Thalidomide was used in parts of Europe as a mild sedative. However, the drug was linked to serious birth defects in infants born to mothers who had taken the drug. The drug was subsequently removed from the market, but it was too late for the many young victims of the drug. Children born to heroin-addicted mothers are also addicted to the drug and must go through a painful withdrawal period immediately following birth. Alcohol and cigarette smoking are also linked to some problems in the newborn child. German measles and syphilis (a venereal disease) can also pass through the placenta and be injurious to the developing child.

Following implantation in the uterine wall, the fertilized ovum is called an embryo. Embryonic development results in the differentiation of three cellular layers: The ectoderm, the mesoderm, and the endoderm. The nervous system, sense organs, mouth cavity, and skin are derived from the *ectoderm*. The muscular, skeletal, circulatory, excretory, and reproductive systems are derived from the *mesoderm*. The digestive and respiratory systems arise from the *endoderm*.

Following the eighth week of development, the embryo is referred to as a fetus. At this time, most of the early development of the body systems has taken place and the fetus continues to grow from about one inch in length to a birth length of about 20 inches. Fetal development continues for the next seven months until it is time for the baby to be born.

By the time the fetus is three months in development, it resembles a miniature person. It is fairly well formed and weighs less than an ounce (see Figure 9-4). In the last four months, the fetus will have attained about 90 percent of its birth weight. Fifty percent of this weight is put on in the final two months of pregnancy.

The term "test-tube babies" has been making headlines in recent times. At a July 1974 meeting of the British Medical Association, Dr. Douglas Bevis of Leeds University declared that three children had been born to women whose ova had been fertilized in the laboratory and then implanted into their

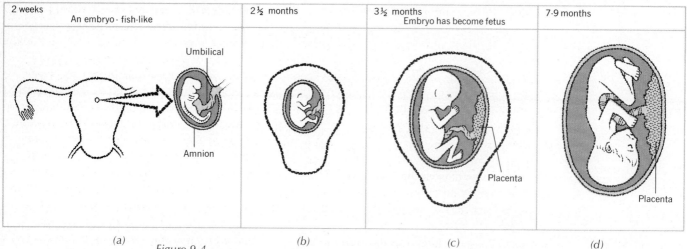

| 2 weeks | 2½ months | 3½ months | 7-9 months |
| An embryo - fish-like | | Embryo has become fetus | |

(a)   (b)   (c)   (d)

Figure 9-4
Fetal development (*a*) 2 weeks, an embryo,
fishlike in appearance; (*b*) 2½ months; (*c*) 3½
months, embryo has become a fetus; (*d*) 7-9
months.

wombs. These children would then be the *first* babies ever conceived in this manner. A test-tube baby is conceived by taking an ova from a woman and mixing it in a culture with her husband's sperm. Eggs that are fertilized are allowed to grow and divide as they would in the uterus. The ovum is then reimplanted in the uterus to continue its growth. Earlier experiments of this type met with no success. The fertilized ovum was usually flushed away during the next menstrual period.

Many individual are protesting this type of research because they feel that humans are exerting too great an influence in the creation of life. Research like this is thought to be a forerunner of complete genetic control of future offspring. Research scientists, however, discount this point of view and feel they have made great strides in helping couples to have children who otherwise could not. How do you feel about this type of research? Some individuals also protest this research because of the potential damage to the fertilized egg while it is being grown outside of the uterus. Do you think that this is a valid objection to research of this nature?

The research described here differs from artificial insemination. Artificial insemination is the implanting of a husband's or donor's sperm into a woman where normal fertilization and embryonic development will take place. Conception takes place in the same manner as it would through intercourse. There is no growth of the fertilized ovum outside of the body.

In recent times, artificial insemination has been taken one step further. Sperm has been frozen and stored for possible future insertion via artificial insemination. This is a costly procedure, and there are only a few locations throughout the country where this is done. There are a number of reasons why some men will do this. Some men with extraordinary talents want their sperm preserved for possible future fatherhood. Other men who are terminally ill may want to preserve their sperm for possible implantation at a date after their death. Men having a sterilization procedure may also want to preserve their sperm. Some individuals who are planning a sex change operation may want to preserve their ability to father a child. Because of the few available frozen sperm banks and the high cost, such a procedure is usually out of the range of most people. How do you generally react to the freezing and storing of sperm for future use? What problems do you see in the utilization of frozen sperm?

BIRTH

Childbirth is the process by which the child is expelled into the outside world. This process is often called parturition, and it usually occurs some time during the ninth month of pregnancy. Many women are better prepared today for childbirth than they were in the past. Prenatal care and classes in birth and child care (often given at a local hospital) teach the pregnant woman what to expect and what is expected of her during preliminary and later stages of birth. Some hospitals allow the father to be with the expectant mother during the early stages of birth. Other hospitals allow the father into the delivery room (if he has completed a course of training) to help the expectant mother in certain exercises and methods of relaxation. The author has a close friend who not only participated in the birth of his son but took home movies of the event.

One method of childbirth that is gaining in popularity is that of natural, or "pain-free" childbirth. This technique is also known as the Lamaze method after the French physician Fernand Lamaze (1890–1957). With the Lamaze method the pregnant woman is taught exercises that will both relax her and relieve pain during childbirth. Fathers who have attended classes in this method can be very helpful in all stages of childbirth. Most women who participate in Lamaze childbirth do not require any medication and are fully awake during the delivery of the child.

About one month prior to birth, the fetus usually assumes the head-down position in preparation for birth. The uterus will usually "drop" or descend into the lower pubic area about 12 days prior to birth. One can usually see and feel that the fetus is lower in the body at this time. This is one sign of approaching birth.

You have probably heard the term "labor" used to describe the process of birth. The term is really quite appropriate in that labor involves a great amount of work by the mother. Early signs of labor may include uterine contractions that vary in strength and duration. There may also be a "bloody show" which is a blood-stained discharge from the vagina.

Frequently, the amniotic sac will rupture. This is often called "breaking the water." Fluid flows from the vagina and in most cases this is a fairly positive sign of labor. However, occasionally the bag of water may break prior to the onset of labor. In some women, the amniotic sac must be broken by the physician after the woman is in labor. This is a fast and painless procedure. A doctor will usually ask a woman to go to the hospital when any of the above signs have occurred and if the uterine contractions are fairly strong and occurring at regular intervals.

The process of labor is usually divided into three distinct stages. The first stage of labor

Figure 9-5
Childbirth.

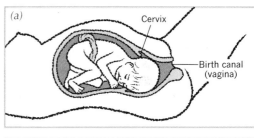
(a) Cervix / Birth canal (vagina)

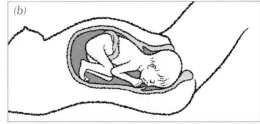
(b)

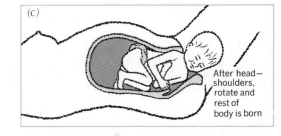
(c) After head—shoulders, rotate and rest of body is born

serves to dilate the *cervix,* or neck of the uterus, so that the child's head can pass into the vagina. This is the longest stage of labor. The length of the first stage varies greatly but, for the average first birth, it is usually from 16 to 20 hours in duration. If a woman is giving birth to a second or third child, the number of hours is reduced to between 6 and 10 hours—often less.

The second stage of labor is the birth of the child (see Figure 9-5). This stage may be as short as ten minutes or may last a few hours (especially if it is a first birth). It is during this stage that certain types of anesthesia are used to relieve pain. The physician will ask the mother's cooperation in "bearing down." This technique helps to gently push the child out of the vaginal canal.

During the final moments of the second stage of labor, the physician may have to perform an episiotomy. This procedure involves a small incision to make the vaginal opening wider for the child's head to pass through to the outside. The incision prevents tears in the vaginal tissue and facilitates the passage of the baby's head.

Most children are born in the headfirst position, but there may be cases of breech birth where the child's buttocks is presented first. The physician may be able to turn the child into the headfirst position. Occasionally, a child presents an arm, shoulders, or hand first. The physician will try to alter the baby's position. If he cannot, a Caesarean section may have to be performed. This is a surgical procedure where the baby is delivered

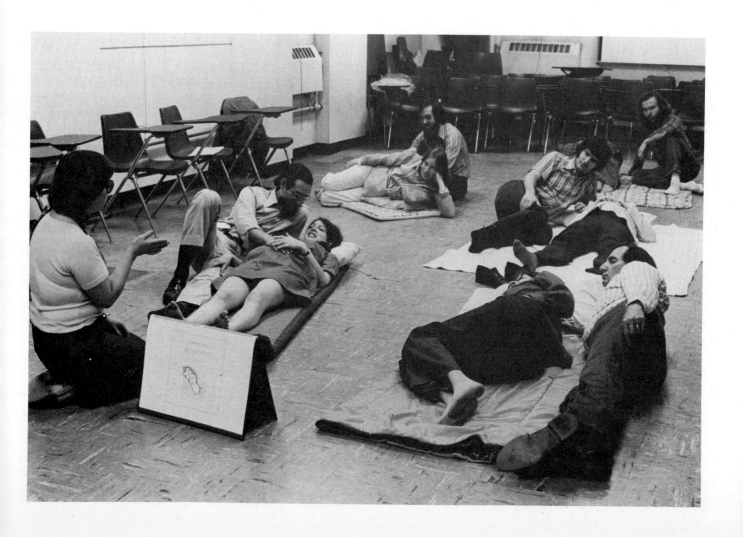

These days more and
more husbands are
helping their wives
through pregnancy and
childbirth by partici-
pating in prenatal classes
and assisting their
wives during delivery.

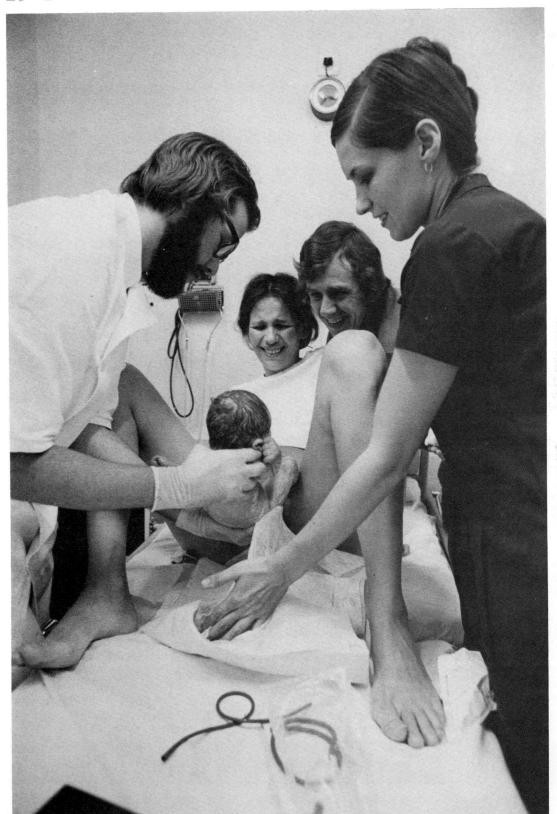

through an incision in the abdominal and uterine wall. Caesarean sections are routinely performed in hospitals for a variety of reasons.

The final or third stage of labor is the expulsion of the placenta. This usually occurs without any aid of the physician within 10 or 15 minutes after the birth of the child. This material, commonly called afterbirth, is accompanied by bleeding which will continue for a number of weeks after delivery.

Once the baby is born, the physician will tie and sever the umbilical cord. Most babies will cry following birth without any help, but sometimes the doctor will slap the child to start him breathing on his own. A few drops of an antibiotic drug will be put in the baby's eyes to guard against gonorrhea infection. The child is then bathed and given to his or her mother to hold for the first time. This completes the cycle that started many months ago—a new life has come into the world.

A new concept of welcoming the newborn into the world is the LeBoyer method. Rather than glaring lights and the sterile conditions of the delivery room, Dr. LeBoyer is concerned with providing soft lighting, subtle sounds, gentle touching, and warmth for the newborn so that the transition from the womb is not as harsh as is presently experienced by newborns under conventional procedures.

some points to ponder

There are some factors associated with pregnancy and birth that you may have heard about, but they may not be too familiar to you. In this section, we will discuss some of the more interesting topics concerned with the reproductive process.

POSTPARTUM DEPRESSION

Most people would imagine that the birth of a child should bring unprecedented happiness. However, many women experience a period of "blues," technically referred to as postpartum depression. The "blues" tends to last for a few days following delivery but may last for weeks or even months. This type of depression is characterized by crying, unwillingness to see or touch the baby, a desire to be left alone, and a fear of caring for the infant. Sometimes depression will result in a desire to sleep excessively and an inability to function at normal household tasks. Depression of this type is usually due to hormonal and emotional instability. The hormones will usually level off by themselves, while emotional problems, if not understood, will cause a deepening depression.

What are some of these emotional problems? The tension and excitement built up during pregnancy comes to a climax at the time of birth. During pregnancy most women receive a great amount of attention, but after the child is born this attention is suddenly turned to the baby. In addition, the woman may not feel capable of caring for the infant, especially if she is unfamiliar with baby care. Babies are a tremendous responsibility and involve almost around-the-clock care. This is a frightening reality to many women. A woman who feels "blue" should try to find out exactly why she is depressed. She should talk openly to her physician and husband. Sometimes just knowing that one's husband or some other close relative is there to help is sufficient to aid in fighting depression. Do you think there are any preventive steps a woman can take in avoiding a postpartum depression *before* it develops?

A recent study taken among new parents highlighted some interesting factors associated with adjustment to parenthood. The study included 511 couples who had had a child from 6 to 56 weeks before the study. The study concluded that there is a slight or moderate degree of crisis associated with the entry of the first child into the family. This feeling was more evident among the new mothers than among the fathers. The woman's problems seemed to center around fatigue, nervousness, loss of figure, and personal appearance in general. The man's

problems were usually associated with financial worries, in-law interference, and a
heavier work load. Lower levels of crisis
were found among those couples who reported a happy marriage. In general, the
study indicated that the gratifications of
parenthood were greater than the crises
brought about by a new baby. How do you
think you will react to parenthood? If you
are already a parent, reflect about your
reactions during that first year of being a
mother or father.

RH FACTOR

The Rh factor is a blood protein. If an indi-
dividual has this factor, then he is Rh positive.
More than 85 percent of the American population is positive for this blood protein. If
the substance is not present in the blood,
then an individual is known to be negative
for this factor or Rh negative. If blood from
an Rh positive individual is given to an Rh
negative individual, the result can be the
formation of a substance that would be
antagonistic to any later transfusions of Rh
positive blood.

What does all of this have to do with childbirth? If a husband and wife have different
Rh factors, then the child could be harmed.
If an Rh positive father and an Rh negative
mother conceive an Rh positive child, some
of the Rh positive blood cells from the child
may enter the mother's bloodstream. If this
occurs, an anti-Rh substance may be formed
by the mother to fight off the positive red
blood cells from the baby. In a first pregnancy, the child is usually not harmed.
However, subsequent pregnancies may be
affected because the mother has built up
these anti-Rh substances that could destroy
many of the developing child's red blood
cells. If the condition is very serious, a child
could be born anemic, jaundiced, or be dead
upon birth. Children who are born alive but
very ill have a complete blood exchange
performed shortly after birth.

There is less chance today than ever before
that a child will die because of the Rh factor.
This is due to a substance called Rho-gam,
which was introduced a few years ago. If a
woman with an Rh factor problem is innocu-
lated with Rho-gam within 72 hours after
the delivery of her child, then subsequent
children will not be affected by the anti-Rh
substance. The Rho-gam is able to break
down this substance and, in this way, prevent
future Rh problems.

MULTIPLE BIRTHS

If you think one baby is enough, have you
ever thought that you may have twins, triplets, or even quadruplets? Twins are the
most common of multiple births, occurring
about once in every 80 births. There are two
types of twins: fraternal and identical. Fraternal twins are conceived from two individual
eggs. They are as alike as brothers and
sisters. Fraternal twins may be of both sexes
or the same sex. Identical twins occur when
a single egg cell is fertilized and then splits
to result in the formation of two identical
individuals. The twins are always of the
same sex and look very much alike. However, environment will affect their psychological traits and personality.

Triplets are less common than twins and
occur approximately once in every 6,400
births. Triplets may be either identical or
fraternal. The most famous of all multiple
births was that of the Dionne quintuplets,
who were identical in that they all split from
one fertilized egg. However, the greater the
number of children born at one time, the less
chance that all will survive.

A recent factor in the increase of multiple
births is the fertility drugs. These drugs are
given to women who have had difficulty in
conceiving a child. In many cases, the fertility drugs have resulted in numerous ova
being discharged and simultaneously fertilized. Many women are willing to take the
risk of multiple birth in order to have a child
of their own. How would you feel if you
were faced with a similar decision?

It might be interesting to read about a family
that experienced a multiple birth. There are
numerous articles written about these families.

Planned Parenthood Federation of America, Inc., was founded by Margaret Sanger in 1917 —when family planning was taboo and it was illegal to provide contraceptive information or services. But times have changed; now Planned Parenthood operates 700 clinics for contraception, pregnancy testing, voluntary sterilization, abortion, and infertility therapy. Planned Parenthood—World Population is the national headquarters of this movement. It is also the American representative to the International Planned Parenthood Federation. In this capacity, it provides family planning information and services to the less developed areas of the world.

A variety of birth control devices: IUD's, pills, contraceptive foam, condom, diaphragm and jelly.

It is fascinating to see how parents handle four or five infants and how they react to the publicity involved. A recent article in *Redbook* (November 1974) discusses the Anderson quintuplets (born without the "aid" of fertility drugs). These quintuplets joined two brothers, aged four and three, at the time of their birth. The story provides for very interesting reading and an understanding of what it must be like to care for five babies at the same time!

birth control

We have discussed the reproductive process from conception to birth. An essential factor of reproduction is the ability to control conception, if one wishes to do so. There have been great strides in this area and in this section we consider some of the methods thare are available if one does not wish to conceive a child.

In order for pregnancy to take place, there must first be normal sperm production and transportation, normal male and female reproductive systems, and effective and appropriate coital technique. If any of these factors are disrupted, then pregnancy may not take place. Infertility (the inability to conceive a child) is discussed in a later section of this chapter.

Most couples desire to plan their children for a variety of reasons. If too many children are born too close together, both the parents and children may have a difficult time. Financial considerations are also an important influence on how many children to have and when to have them. Fortunately, there are many methods available to help a couple plan their families. Some of these products and techniques are less effective than others (see Figure 9-6). In our discussion, the least effective methods will be discussed first.

One method that in reality should not be considered as a method of birth control at

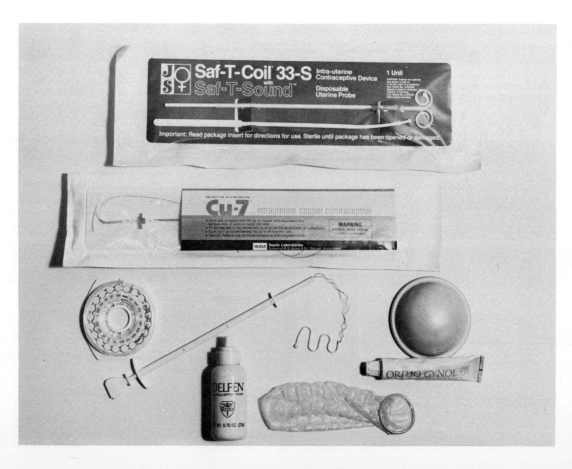

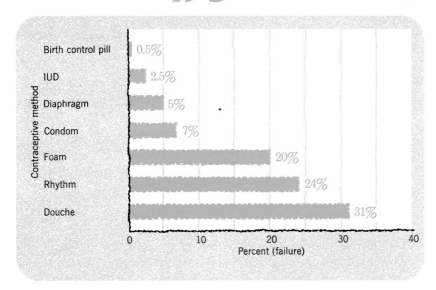

Figure 9-6

Effectiveness of various contraceptive methods.

Alan Frank Guttmacher (1898–1974) was the president of the Planned Parenthood Federation of America for a dozen years. After his death, the organization renamed its research division in his honor. Dr. Guttmacher believed that every child should come into the world "gleefully wanted and loved" by its parents. He wrote many books on the subject; the last was *Pregnancy, Birth, and Family Planning.*

all is the douche. The douche is the flushing of the vaginal tract with a cleansing or spermicidal solution. It is mentioned in this section because many people still think it is an effective method of birth control. Douching may be used, if desired, for cleansing, but it is an ineffective method of birth control.

COITUS INTERRUPTUS

Many individuals choose to rely on coitus interruptus as a method of birth control. With this method the penis is withdrawn from the vagina before ejaculation occurs. This, too, is not a very effective method of birth control. It is very difficult for the man to withdraw before ejaculation, and the pre-ejaculatory fluid might contain some sperm. In addition, this is an unsatisfactory way for a couple to have sexual relations. There is a great amount of stress put on both partners if this is the only method of birth control being used.

RHYTHM

The rhythm method has been in use for many years and is the only method of birth control sanctioned by the Roman Catholic Church. Rhythm involves abstinence from sexual

intercourse except during a certain period of time called the "safe" period. However, this "safe" period is only safe if a woman knows exactly when she ovulates. Ovulation can be determined by taking the first day of the menstrual period and counting *back* 14 days. This should give the *approximate* time of ovulation. In order to "practice rhythm," a woman would have to abstain from intercourse a few days before, during, and a few days after ovulation takes place. The difficulty with the calendar method of determining ovulation is that very few women (less than 30 percent) have regular menstrual cycles. Ovulation can also be determined by taking one's temperature. There is usually a slight temperature dip at ovulation and then a slight rise. However, many women show no temperature fluctuation and other factors could affect temperature change. There is an additional problem intrinsic in the use of the rhythm method. Ovulation may occur spontaneously at other times of the month, and it is thought that sexual excitement might also trigger ovulation. For all of these reasons, rhythm is certainly not the most effective method of birth control.

It is interesting to note that women who are breast feeding often think that they cannot become pregnant until their menstrual cycle returns. While breast feeding will prolong the cycle, it is possible to conceive prior to the first period following birth. This holds true for women who are not breast feeding as well. Many women are surprised to find the are pregnant again, and they have never had a postpartum period. Birth control methods must be utilized or abstinence followed until the first menstrual period arrives and a woman's regular cyclic pattern begins again.

CREAMS, JELLIES, and FOAMS

Vaginal creams, spermicides, jellies, and foams are readily available on the market without a physician's prescription. However, these products used as a sole means of birth control are not totally effective. They must be inserted into the vagina about ten minutes before ejaculation occurs and should be reapplied if intercourse is repeated. The foam products have the best effectiveness as compared to the other products. All of these products, however, are quite effective when used with the condom.

CONDOMS

The *condom* or "rubber" is usually made of a thin rubber substance or from the intestine of a sheep. It is also called a prophylactic and is often referred to as a "safe." But how safe are "safes?" If used properly, they are quite effective and can prevent venereal disease as well as pregnancy. The only problems in using a condom is breakage during intercourse or the possibility of it slipping off during the sexual act. If a man wants to be sure that a condom is safe, he should blow air into it before using it. In this way, he will be able to see if there are any holes in it. When putting it on, a space should be left at the tip to catch the semen. After intercourse, he should hold the condom while withdrawing from his partner. This will prevent the possible spillage of semen into the vagina. Condoms are readily available without a prescription and are quite effective in birth control. However, many women and men do not like to use condoms because lovemaking must be disturbed in order to put

it on and sexual intercourse becomes less spontaneous with its use.

The methods that were previously discussed do not require a doctor's prescription. The methods we are about to discuss do require such a prescription. If these methods are not used under a doctor's direction, they may not be effective as birth control techniques.

DIAPHRAGMS

The diaphragm is a thin rubber cup that is stretched over a metal ring and fitted into the cervix of the vagina. Its placement in the cervix blocks the sperm from entering the uterus. It should be used with a contraceptive cream or jelly to enhance its effectiveness. A diaphragm must be fitted by a physician to be sure of the correct size and placement. The physician will teach a woman how to use it. The diaphragm does not in any way interfere with the enjoyment of the sexual act by the woman or her partner. The diaphragm may be put in place many hours prior to intercourse (this aids in sexual spontaneity) and it can be worn for as long as 24 hours after intercourse. It should not be removed until about five to six hours following sexual relations. This allows for the spermicidal cream to destroy all of the

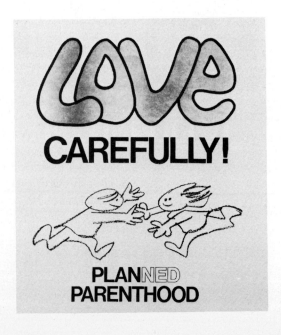

sperm. The fit of the diaphragm should be checked periodically by one's physician to insure proper protection.

IUDs

The IUD or intrauterine device is a medically prescribed contraceptive device. It must be inserted by a physician and remains in the uterus permanently except during checkups or when a woman desires to become pregnant. If a woman wishes to become pregnant, the device is removed and repositioned after childbirth. Most IUD devices are made of a plastic material and they are placed in the uterus. It is thought that the device somehow prevents the fertilized egg from implanting in the wall of the uterus. It does work, but exactly how it works is not known. A thread that is attached to the IUD is present in the vagina. The woman can easily check the presence of the thread, and it is her assurance that the IUD is still in place.

There are many types of IUDs on the market. They are available in "loop" form, "T" form, and in other shapes. They are all highly effective as birth control devices but do have some side effects that cause certain women difficulty. Some women expel the IUDs from the womb, sometimes without being aware that the IUD is no longer in position. Some women report heavy bleeding, uterine cramps, infection, and general discomfort. The more recent developments in the "loop" IUDs have reduced many of these side effects. IUDs have grown in popularity and are used by more than two million women in the United States. It is inexpensive, lasts for a very long time, and does not have to be removed after each act of intercourse.

IUDs are not usually recommended for women who have never been pregnant. There is greater pain upon insertion of the device in these women and they are more likely to spontaneously expel the device than are women who have been pregnant.

BIRTH CONTROL PILLS

The birth control pill or oral contraceptive contains synthetic sex hormones (estrogen and progesterone) that are taken in such a manner that they prevent ovulation. The early research on the pill was conducted by Drs. John Rock and Gregory Pincus in the early 1950s. The pills were used in widespread well-controlled studies in Puerto Rico and Haiti in the mid-1950s.

How does the pill work? Taken daily as prescribed, the pill raises both the estrogen and progesterone levels in the bloodstream. A high level of these hormones prevent the eggs from maturing and ovulation from taking place.

There are two types of pills that are currently being used. One type is the combined pill where a combination of estrogen and progesterone are taken daily for 20 days, beginning on the fifth day after the menstrual period. It is preferable that the pills are taken at the same time each day. Menstruation will begin between two and five days following the last pill. The pills should then be resumed on the fifth day of the menstrual period (in most cases the period will have stopped about the time the pills are to be resumed).

Sometimes the menstrual period does not occur. In this case, the physician will usually advise a patient to start taking the pill again seven days after the last pill was taken. A woman should always consult her physician if there is any problem associated with the birth control pill.

The other type of pill is the sequential pill. In this method, the first 15 pills usually contain estrogen and the other five pills contain both estrogen and progesterone. There is some concern that the use of the sequential pill is related to the incidence of cervical cancer. Some sequential pills include 21 hormonal pills and seven placebos (inert substances). The inert pills are included so that the woman takes one pill for every day of the menstrual cycle. In this way, she does not have to stop and start taking the pills again.

There has been much concern about the potentially harmful effects of long-term usage of the pill. There has been research that indicates that the pill does statistically increase the risk of thromboembolic disease. This is a disease where blood clots form and can result in death. There have been reports that three out of every 100,000 women may die of thromboembolic disorders. While this may be true, few people realize that many more women die of complications due to pregnancy, childbirth, and the postpartum period. At present, most endocrinologists (physicians who specialize in hormonal disorders) and gynecologists feel that the pill is safe and, if taken properly, is 100 percent effective in preventing conception.

Other lesser side effects have been associated with the use of the pill. Nausea, weight gain, bloated appearance, fatigue, headaches, bleeding between periods, and anxiety have all been associated with the use of the pill. Most of the symptoms will disappear in the first few months after usage has begun. If symptoms persist, one should consult with her physician. Many doctors will try a different pill or will suggest that a woman stop taking the pills for a while.

What about the advantages of the pill? The most important advantage, of course, is its effectiveness. Related to this advantage is an improved sex life reported by most couples where the woman uses the pill. Intercourse is more frequent because most couples feel secure that they cannot conceive a child if they are using this method. There is also a high degree of spontaneity in sex in that there are no diaphragms that must be worn or condoms that have to be put on while the couple is making love. There is also no conclusive evidence of any type of cancer being related to the use of the pill, with the exception of some recent concern about the sequential pill.

Women who use the pill should see their doctor at least once a year for an internal examination and a pap smear for cervical cancer. At this time, the doctor can discuss any problems that might be related to taking the pill. The prescription for the pill is usually given for six months or a year and an examination is necessary prior to renewing the prescription.

Birth control pills are relatively inexpensive (about $25 a year) and rely heavily on a woman's memory to be sure that one is taken each of the required days. Pills are often used for reasons other than birth control. They are very effective in regulating the menstrual cycle.

Birth control pills should not be used by nursing mothers because they tend to suppress milk production. Some research also indicates that the hormones from the pill may adversely affect a male infant.

The mini-pill is one method of birth control that is currently under consideration. This pill contains no estrogen and little progesterone. It works on the premise of making the mucuous of the cervix extremely thick and sticky. This would prevent the sperm from entering the cervix. However, there has been a great amount of breakthrough bleeding and other complications associated with this pill.

The so-called "morning-after pill" is already in limited use. The drug is called by this name because if taken following intercourse it will not allow the fertilized egg to implant in the uterus. It must be taken following fertilization but prior to implantation (within a 4 or 5 day span). This drug is called diethylstilbestrol or DES, and it is very powerful and may have some side effects. It should not be fully administered because of its potential danger. However, it may be used in cases of rape, incest, or in cases where individuals should not have children for physical or emotional reasons. Much research remains before this drug can be used in a routine manner.

STERILIZATION

Sterilization procedures are methods that in most cases permanently prevent the ability to impregnate (in the case of a man) or to conceive (in the case of a woman). It is currently estimated that more than six million Americans have voluntarily had sterilization operations. According to a 1970 study of national fertility, one-sixth of all married couples in this country who were using contraceptive methods in that year had been sterilized. Sterilization in 1970 was the most popular form of contraceptive among women between the ages of 30 and 44. Since 1970, sterilization procedures have been performed at about 1,000,000 per year.

Why are so many people turning to this permanent method of birth control? The reasons will vary according to the couple, but many people are not satisfied with the alternative methods of birth control. Many women who have been taking the pill for a long time feel that they do not want to risk potential or unknown harm that may result from continued use. Others have had complications with the IUD and still others feel that methods such as rhythm, condoms, and diaphragms are ineffective, awkward, and uncomfortable to use. There have been numerous unwanted pregnancies due to the use of these forms of contraception. In some cases, the method may have been used incorrectly but, if a pregnancy results, the method is still ineffective. It has been estimated

that one-third of couples who practiced some type of birth control conceived a child within five years. The ineffectiveness of existing birth control methods is one of the major reasons why couples seek a form of sterilization.

Another reason for an increase in sterilization is the perfection of the operation for both sexes. It is a relatively simple and painless procedure that can be accomplished in a short time. The female operation may require a longer period of recovery than the male procedure but is also a quick and relatively painless technique. Both male and female sterilization surgery are discussed in the following paragraphs.

The sterilization procedure for males is known as a vasectomy. It is a simple procedure that involves the cutting of the *vas deferens* (see Fig. 9-7). This operation prevents the sperm from traveling up the *vas deferens* from the testes where the sperm is produced (refer to earlier part of this chapter where the male reproductive system is discussed). A vasectomy, therefore, prevents the sperm from mixing with the other seminal

Figure 9-7
Vasectomy.

Figure 9-8
Tubal ligation.

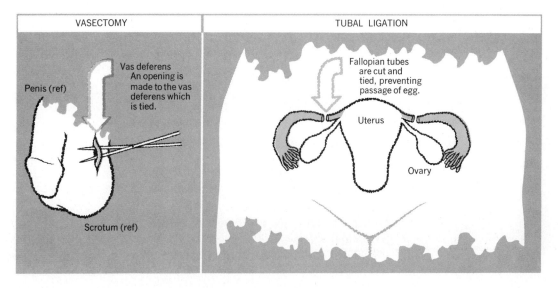

fluids. Sperm is still formed in the testes, but it is not able to travel out of the body. The sperm that is formed is attacked by the individual's antibodies and are carried away by the white blood cells. The operation is usually performed by a urologist and can be performed on an out-patient basis under local anesthesia. Does the operation affect sexual response? The answer is unequivocally "no!" The other fluids are still produced upon ejaculation and the amount of ejaculate is of little difference than before the surgery. Sexual response is the same as it was prior to the vasectomy. In some cases, it is better because the individual no longer needs to be concerned about the possibility of an unwanted pregnancy. Some men may have psychological problems concerned with a feeling of reduced manhood. However, in most cases, mature men decide on the operation and they realize that the ability to impregnate a woman has little to do with virility.

The advantages of a vasectomy are numerous. It is a very effective method of birth control, having a failure rate of far less than one percent. It is an inexpensive procedure when looked at over a long-term basis and involves no use of additional birth control methods. The operation is quick (about 20 minutes), safe, and relatively painless.

The disadvantages include the fact that there is an initial cost of between $50 and $250 and the surgery does not provide immediate protection. Other forms of birth control must be utilized until the sperm count is zero. This usually necessitates about 12 ejaculations. There may be slight pain and bleeding, and there is a possibility of infection. In a very small percentage of cases, some men may have granulomas or swellings that are caused by the seepage of the sperm from the severed vas deferens. They are treatable and additional problems are rare. The operation can be reversed in about 50 to 80 percent of all cases. However, reversal surgery is more complicated and expensive and there is *no* guarantee that fertility can be restored. It is all-important that a couple know that in most cases sterilization proce-

dures are permanent. For this reason, couples should carefully consider their age, marital stability, age of their children, and the possibility that at a later date they might want to consider starting a family or adding to an existing family.

The sterilization operation for women is known as tubal ligation. Tubal ligation involves the tying, cutting, or cauterizing the Fallopian tubes (see Figure 9-8). Cauterization is a technique where heat is applied to the tubes to make the sides of the tube come together, prohibiting the passage of the egg. Tubal ligations are performed in different ways, the end result being the same—the egg cannot reach the sperm and become fertilized. A woman who has had such surgery will menstruate as she did prior to the procedure. Sexual response is the same or better and nothing except for the interrupted journey of the egg has changed.

In one method of tubal ligation, a major surgical procedure, the tubes are cut and a small section of the tube is removed. The ends of the tube are tied so they are unable to rejoin. This method successfully prevents the ova from meeting the sperm. This is an expensive operation (about $350 to $400) and involves a 4 to 5 day hospital stay. Following this type of surgery, a woman may need from three to four weeks of postoperative recovery. It is very difficult, often impossible, to rejoin the tubes once they have been severed.

A newer sterilization procedure for women is known as laparoscopic sterilization. This is often called "Band-Aid surgery" because Band-Aids are sufficient to cover the small incisions that result from this type of surgery. This surgery is performed by making a small incision in the navel and another about one inch below the navel. The laparoscope (a lens that transfers light but not heat) allows the surgeon to look into the depths of the abdomen. The laparoscope is inserted through the incision in the navel allowing the doctor to see the uterus, ovaries, and Fallopian tubes. Through the other incision, a forceps is inserted that is used to cauterize the tubes. This type of surgery takes a few minutes. When completed, the incisions are stitched and Band-Aids are placed over the incisions. This operation can be done vaginally, but the uterus has to be in a certain position for the surgery to be accomplished in this manner.

The advantages of this operation are numerous. It is very effective, quick, relatively painless, and usually requires an overnight stay in the hospital. In some hospitals, it is being performed on an out-patient basis. It is also immediately effective. The disadvantages include the expense, which may be about $500. It may involve some complications, although they are very rare (around 1 percent). These complications may include pain, discomfort, bleeding, infection, irregular heartbeat or electrical skin burns. Once performed, the operation cannot be reversed.

A form of sterilization that is reversible has recently been developed. In this operation, removable clips are placed on the Fallopian tubes in order to prevent the meeting of the sperm and egg. When a woman desires to become pregnant, the clips can be removed. It is minor surgery and requires little aftercare. This operation may be offered on an out-patient basis. The greatest advantage of this procedure is its reversibility.

Are there any psychological problems involved in male or female sterilization procedures? Few long-term studies have been conducted. In one study, the psychological problems of a group of couples where the husband had a vasectomy was compared to another group where the wife took the birth control pill. Initially, the couples where the husband had a vasectomy reported greater psychological problems than the other couples. Two years later, however, the problems of the vasectomized couples were less numerous and intense. Four years later, there seemed to be *no* difference in reported difficulties. Both groups of couples tended to rate their marriages the same, frequency of intercourse the same, and about the same number of men from each group reported problems with impotency, premature ejaculation, and sex drive. The study concluded that

the couples where the man had a vasectomy may have initially been under greater stress. Once the couple could cope with their psychological feelings, stress became less apparent in the relationship. The study, however, did confirm that men who had a vasectomy showed an increase in what was called "masculine-confirming" behavior.

Many physicians will try to discourage young couples, single people, and couples without children from having this type of surgery. Do you feel that this should be done or that individuals should be able to make their own decisions concerning the desire to have or to not have children?

NEW METHODS OF BIRTH CONTROL

Can we look forward to better and safer methods of birth control in the near future? There is presently much research being done in this field with some methods already in the testing stages. New research is looking into male as well as female birth control techniques. Research continues in order to perfect a male birth control pill. One that was developed a few years ago resulted in a reduction of sex drive, inability to have an erection, and disorders when used with alcohol. Other research presently includes a male pill that will incapacitate the sperm's ability to penetrate the egg. Research along these lines is still in its very early stages.

New methods in female contraceptive technique include the mini-pill (which was discussed earlier) and an implant beneath the skin that works in a similar way to the mini-pill. These implants would contain progesterone, and they would slowly release the hormone over an established period of time (could vary from a month, to a year, or many years). The capsule would be removed if the woman desired to become pregnant.

Another method is the progesterone-coated vaginal ring that would fit like a diaphragm. This ring would release sufficient progesterone to suppress ovulation. The ring would be removed monthly to allow for menstruation.

An injection of a drug called *Depo Provera*

is also being studied. This drug could be injected once every three months to prevent ovulation. There are some side effects including no real menstrual period, irregular bleeding, and a delay in ovulation (for many months) following the taking of the drug. This drug is presently being used on a limited basis.

One development that might be an important method of birth control in the future is the prostaglandins. These substances are hormone-like and are found in semen. They are able to cause uterine contractions and have potential use in inducing a menstrual period if the woman has already conceived. Some people refer to this technique as a "mini-abortion." It might be used in the form of an injection or vaginal suppository and would be taken if a woman thought she were pregnant or had definite proof of pregnancy. In its present stage of development, however, there are too many serious side effects to allow for its use as a birth control technique.

infertility

Most of this chapter has been concerned with reproduction and how to prevent conception. However, there are many thousands of people who found that they are infertile or unable to have a child. Infertility is usually due to a dysfunction of the male or female reproductive organs or of the organs of both sexes. Studies indicate that between 10 and 15 percent of the population is infertile. In about 40 percent of these cases, the dysfunction appears in the male.

If a couple is in good health and of childbearing age, they should wait at least a year before seeking a reason for infertility. After a year or more has passed, the man and woman should be checked for general reasons why conception has not occurred. In many cases, a male's sperm count is too low. If this is the case, treatment may be a possibility. The initial examination of a woman would include the reproductive organs, presence of infection, and whether her menstrual cycle was regular. If these

conditions are found to be normal, then a series of diagnostic tests are conducted to determine possible causes of infertility.

Common causes of infertility in the female include absence of ovulation, ovarian cysts, blocked Fallopian tubes, and internal physical problems. Most of these conditions may be treated by medication, surgery, and other forms of therapy. It may take some time to determine the cause, but in many cases new methods of treatment for infertility have resulted in a subsequent pregnancy.

abortion

There are three types of abortion. Spontaneous abortion is often called miscarriage and occurs when the fetus is unintentionally expelled from the uterus. This usually occurs within the first few weeks or months of a pregnancy. Reasons for miscarriage vary and may result from an abnormal fetus or an external blow or other injury. Therapeutic abortion is an intentional removal of the fetus by various legal techniques. A criminal abortion is one performed illegally, often by persons unqualified to perform this technique.

ABORTION PROCEDURES

There are a number of legally accepted abortion procedures performed in United States hospitals today. One method, dilation and curretage (D and C), is usually done prior to the twelfth week of pregnancy. This procedure is done under anesthesia and the patient's cervix is stretched and dilated. Following dilation, the uterus is scraped with an instrument called a curette. The embryo is removed from the uterus in this way.

Another method that is used in early pregnancy is vacuum aspiration. The embryo is sucked out of the uterus through a vacuum pump. It is a quick, efficient method of abortion that is being used in many hospitals and clinics.

A third method that is usually performed if a pregnancy has gone beyond three months is the saline (salt) solution method. The fetus is "salted" out by the injection of a certain amount and strength of a salt solution into the amniotic sac. A spontaneous abortion will usually follow in less than 24 hours.

THE ABORTION ISSUE

Abortion is certainly a dominant issue in today's society. The news is often crowded with pro- and anti-abortion stories. Groups representing both sides are active and vociferous in presenting their views pertaining to abortion. Bumper stickers are often used in campaigns. One popular slogan of the anti-abortion movement is "Adoption not abortion!" The major proponents of abortion are women's groups, especially those groups concerned with women's liberation. The major opponents of abortion are the Roman Catholic Church and other religious denominational groups.

The women's movement has been very active in speaking out for the right of a woman to have the final decision on what to do with her own body. They feel strongly that a woman who is not allowed to have an abortion is being denied her civil rights. Such proponents of abortion feel that if a woman does not wish to bear a child, then she has every legal right to abort that child. Women's organizations and other groups who are in favor of abortion have abortion counseling clinics, women's centers, and hot-line information available to those who need help concerning abortion.

The major opponent of abortion is the Roman Catholic Church. The present church attitude is more than 100 years old. In 1869, Pope Pius the XI decreed that all abortion regardless of circumstances was prohibited. This decree had not been true throughout the history of the church; at other times, abortion had been allowed in the early weeks of pregnancy. However, today the church regards abortion as murder and, therefore, will not condone it under any circumstances. Such groups as the *Right-to-Life* support anti-abortion legislation and have a large number of followers. How do you feel about the abortion issue?

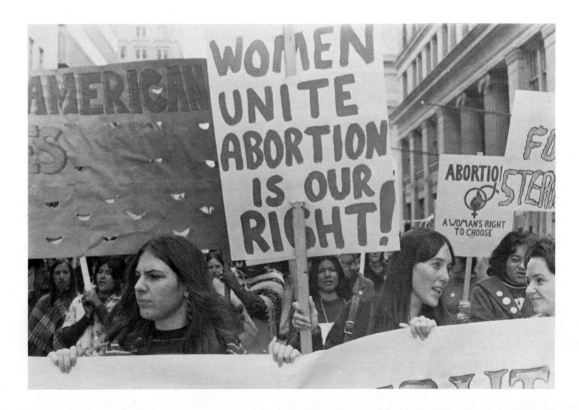

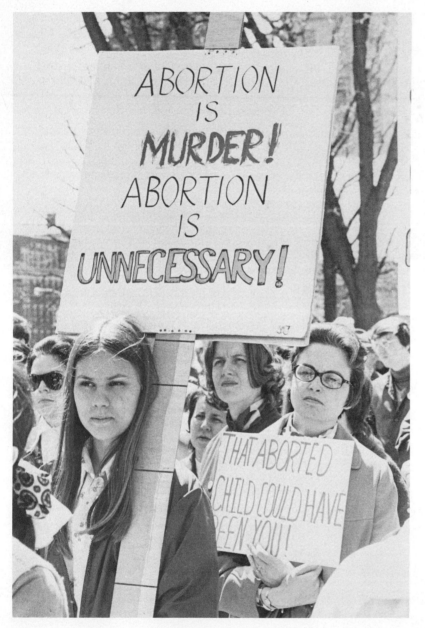

ABORTION AND THE LAW

The present law in relation to abortion was decided in January 1973. The U. S. Supreme Court ruled seven to two that states cannot pass legislation prohibiting abortion. In a later decision, the Supreme Court said that states cannot limit abortion legislation to medical or therapeutic reasons. Women, therefore, have the right to abortion for any reason, medical or personal. However, many groups including the Right-to-Life movement are trying to overturn the original Supreme Court decision.

It has been estimated that more than a million abortions have been performed in a recent year, many of them illegal. Illegal abortion is one of the major reasons why there has been support for abortion legislation reform.

The Right to Life Committee, founded in 1967, is an anti-abortion organization whose members believe that the unborn child, like other human beings, has a moral right to live. In many communities, the committee sponsors a Birthline/Hotline—a telephone consultation service where troubled pregnant women can find out about all the the alternatives to abortion.

Many women have died at the hands of unskilled abortionists.

Presently, legislation that would make abortion legal is pending in many states. But the fight goes on. While new legislation is pending, existing legislation is under fire. The legislatures of states where abortion is presently legal are under strong pressure to return to previous abortion laws. What are the laws regarding abortion in your state? Is there any legislation pending in relation to abortion reform or repeal?

THINKING IT OVER

1. Why is it important to understand the structure and function of the reproductive organs of both sexes?
2. Explain the term ejaculation. Can ejaculation occur at times when there is no sexual stimulation? What is meant by a "wet dream?"
3. Why is circumcision performed on most newborn boys?
4. Discuss the definition and some of the reasons for premature ejaculation.
5. Does the urethra in the male and female serve the same function? Explain your answer.
6. Briefly describe the functioning of the menstrual cycle.
7. How is the sex of a child determined? Are there any methods that can be used to determine the sex of a child prior to conception?
8. What is meant by the term amniocentesis? How is this technique used to help both the parents and future child?
9. Why is prenatal care essential for all pregnant women?
10. Can any substances pass through the placenta and harm the fetus? Explain your answer.
11. Is a "test-tube baby" the same as a child that results from artificial insemination? Explain your answer.
12. What is the Lamaze method of childbirth? How does it differ from more traditional methods?
13. Explain the three stages of labor and what happens at each stage.
14. Why do you think that many women suffer from postpartum depression?
15. What methods of birth control are available without a prescription? Discuss those methods that are available only with a prescription.
16. Discuss the common methods of sterilization for both men and women. What implications does the increase of sterilization surgery have for society in general?
17. What is infertility? What should people do if they have this problem?
18. Discuss the three types of abortions that may occur. How do you feel about the abortion issue? Do you feel that you have been influenced by any individual or group? Explain your answer.

KEY WORDS

Abortion. The therapeutic or crminal removal of an embryo or fetus from the womb.

Amniocentesis. A technique of withdrawing amniotic fluid from a pregnant woman and analyzing the cells to determine possible genetic disorders.

Amniotic fluid. The fluid that is within the amniotic sac.

Amniotic sac. The fluid-filled sac in which the fetus develops.

Androgens. Male sex hormones.

Androsterone. Male sex hormone secreted by the testes.

Artificial insemination. The fertilization of an ovum by inseminating a woman with her husband's or a donor's sperm.

Birth control pills. Hormones that prevent ovulation.

Breech birth. When a part of the body other than the head is presented first at birth.

Caesarian section. An abdominal incision to deliver the baby when it cannot be born vaginally.

Castration. The removal of the sex glands of either sex.

Cowper's glands. Pea-shaped glands located below the prostate and secreting an alkaline fluid that is used with the semen.

Cervix. The neck of the uterus.

Circumcision. A surgical procedure where the foreskin of the penis is removed.

Climacteric. The cessation of menstruation.

Clitoris. The highly sensitive structure that responds to sexual stimulation.

Coitus interruptus. The withdrawal of the penis during intercourse prior to ejaculation.

Conception. The fertilization of the ovum by the sperm.

Condom. A sheath that fits over the penis and catches the semen.

Cremaster muscle. The muscle that regulates the position of the scrotal sac.

Diaphragm. A rubber cup that catches the semen and keeps it from entering the cervix.

Douche. Flushing of the vaginal tract.

Ectoderm. An embryonic cellular layer from which the nervous system, sense organs, mouth cavity, and skin are derived.

Ejaculation. The sudden expulsion of semen through the urethra during sexual stimulation.

Ejaculatory duct. A duct that passes through the prostate gland and carries the sperm and other fluids.

Endocrine glands. Glands that produce hormones and release them directly into the bloodstream.

Endocrinologist. Physician who specializes in hormonal disorders.

Endoderm. An embryonic cellular layer from which the digestive and respiratory systems arise.

Endometrium. The lining of the uterus that is prepared monthly to receive a fertilized egg.

Epididymis. A structure within the testes that stores the sperm.

Episiotomy. An incision made between the vaginal opening and the rectum in order to create a wider passage for the child's head at birth.

Erection. The dilated penis increased in size and stiffness by increased blood flow.

Estrogen. Ovarian hormone.

Fallopian tubes. The tubes that carry the ovum to the uterus, where conception usually takes place.

Fetus. The embryo after the eighth week of development.

Follicles. Tiny cavities of the ovary where the ova develop.

Foreskin. The prepuce that covers the head of the penis.

Fraternal twins. Twins conceived from two ova.

Genitals. The male and female reproductive organs.

Glans penis. Highly sensitive head of the penis.

Identical twins. Twins conceived when one ovum splits.

Infertility. The inability to conceive a child.

IUD (Intrauterine device). A device inserted in the uterus that prevents the fertilized egg from implanting.

Lamaze method. A method of childbirth where the woman is trained to relax through exercise and deliver a child without the aid of drugs.

Laparoscope. A light lens that allows a physician to see the Fallopian tubes (used in tubal ligation).

Menarche. The onset of menstruation.

Mesoderm. An embryonic cellular layer from which the muscular, skeletal, circulatory, excretory, and reproductive systems arise.

Miscarriage: Spontaneous, natural expulsion of the embryo or fetus from the womb.

Orgasm. The height of male or female sexual stimulation.

Ovaries. The female sex organs that produce the ova.

Ovulation. The release of an egg from the ovary.

Parturition. The process of childbirth.

Penis. The male organ of copulation or intercourse.

Placenta. The rich lining of the uterine wall.

Postpartum depression. ''Blues'' or depression following the birth of a child.

Prenatal care. Health care of the mother prior to birth.

Prepuce. The retractable membrane that covers the head of the penis.

Progesterone. Ovarian hormone.

Prostate gland. A gland surrounding the urethra in the male and secreting a thin, milky fluid that makes up part of the semen.

Rh factor. A blood protein that one may or may not have.

Rho-gam. A substance injected into Rh-negative mothers (after the birth of an Rh-positive child) to avoid problems in subsequent pregnancies.

Rhythm. The abstinence from sexual relations except during "safe" periods.

Scrotum. Loose pouch of skin outside of the body that contains the testes.

Semen. The secretions of the seminal vesicles, prostate glands, and sperm.

Seminal vesicles. Two pouches located on either side of the prostate which produce an alkaline secretion.

Seminiferous tubules. Coiled tubules within the testes where the sperm is produced.

Smegma. The secretions from the penis.

Sperm cells. The male germ cell that is capable of fertilizing the ovum.

Spermatogenesis. The production of sperm.

Spermatozoa. The sperm cells of the male.

Sterilization. A procedure where conception permanently (in most cases) is prevented.

Test-tube babies. An ovum fertilized and grown to a certain stage of development outside of the mother's body.

Testosterone. Male sex hormone secreted by the testes.

Testes. The paired sex glands of the male that produce sperm cells.

Thalidomide. A sedative drug used in Europe that caused many birth defects.

Thromboembolic disease. Disease where blood clots may form.

Tubal ligation. Female sterilization where the Fallopian tubes are cut or tied.

Umbilical cord. The cord that attaches the fetus to the placenta of the mother and provides a medium for exchange of food and waste products.

Urethra. The duct that carries both the urine and the sperm but not at the same time.

Urologist. A physician who specializes in disorders of the urinary tract of both sexes and the reproductive system of men.

Uterus. The pear-shaped organ where the fetus develops.

Vagina. The muscular, elastic organ that is the birth canal and receives the penis during intercourse.

Vas deferens. The small tubes that carry the sperm from the epididymis to the seminal vesicles and urethra.

Vasectomy. Male sterilization where the vas deferens are cut.

"Wet dreams". Ejaculation usually stimulated by erotic dreams.

GETTING INVOLVED

Books and Periodicals

Boston Women's Health Book Collective. *Our Bodies, Ourselves.* New York: Simon & Schuster, 1972. A guide to help women understand their own bodies.

Fisher, Florence. *The Search for Anna Fisher.* New York: Fawcett, 1974. An adoptee's search for her real parents.

Guttmacher, Alan F. *Pregnancy, Birth, and Family Planning.* New York: New American Library, 1973. "A guide for expectant parents in the 1970s."

_____. *Understanding Sex: A Young Person's Guide.* New York: New American Library, 1970. The family-planning advocate discusses sex.

Nilsson, A. Lenart; Ingelman-Sundberg, Axel; and Wirsen, Claes. *A Child Is Born: The Drama of Life before Birth.* New York: Delta, 1967. The stages of fetal development in words and pictures.

Movies

Each Child Loved, with Candice Bergen, 1971. Documentary about illegal and legal abortion. Distributed by Planned Parenthood Federation of America, Inc.

Records

"Having My Baby," Paul Anka. On *Paul Anka* album, United Artists. The joys of parenthood from a male (chauvinist?) point of view.

10 MARRIAGE AND THE FAMILY

What are the traditional roles of family members? Have they changed in recent years? In this chapter, the present-day roles of mothers, fathers, and children are explored. Changes in the family structure, including the breakdown of the extended family, are also discussed. The different types of "mixed marriage" that exist today are presented and explored.

Are people finding alternatives to the traditional framework of marriage and the family? The answer is a resounding "yes." More and more couples are sharing household duties so that women can return to work if they so desire. The "open marriage" concept is discussed and the way it applies to the individual as well as the marriage is explored. Other alternatives such as the childless marriage, adoption, foster care, communal living, living together, trial marriage, and homosexual marriage are also explored.

How does it feel to be single in a "married society"? This question and the problems that pertain to single persons are discussed. Divorce and the reform of certain state divorce laws are also considered. Can something be done to save a marriage prior to divorce? Some of the alternatives are presented and marriage and sex counseling techniques are discussed. It is hoped that this chapter will present some of the options that are available to individuals regardless of their marital status.

While reading this chapter, think about the following concepts:

■ Traditional roles of family members are breaking down.

■ There are alternatives to traditional marriage and family life.

■ It is important that individuals do not lose their identity in marriage.

■ Attitudes toward sex and living together without marriage are changing.

■ The single person is more accepted today than ever before.

■ Happiness is dependent on your self-concept — not your marital status.

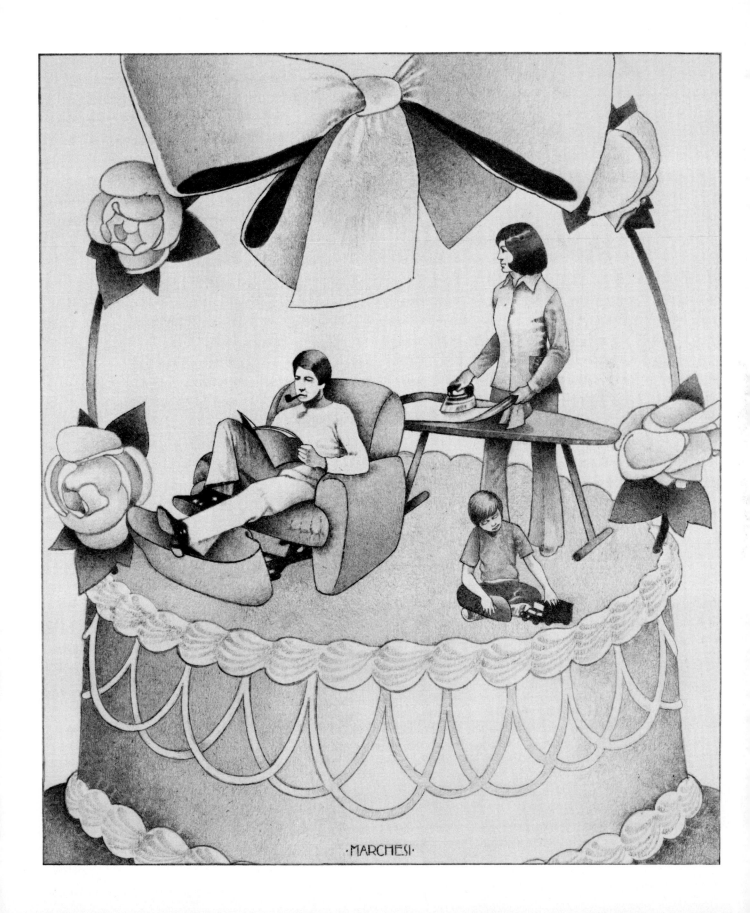

·MARCHESI·

Marriage and the family in the traditional sense is very much a topic of discussion today. Are more and more young people choosing to live together while their married parents are "splitting" in the divorce courts in record numbers? Both of these questions can be answered in the affirmative. Yes, more couples are living together without being married than previously reported. The United States Census accounted for 34,000 such couples in 1960 and 286,000 in 1970. However, these figures may not be completely accurate because many couples who were living together in 1960 probably did not report their status. Divorces continue to increase, but more than two and one-half million marriages were performed in 1973. It is estimated that about 910,000 divorces were obtained in that same year.

The statistics give only one side of a complicated story. What are some of the reasons for these statistics? An examination of traditional roles of family members and how they have changed to meet the needs of a contemporary society will shed some light on the "why" behind these statistics.

a historical and sociological look at marriage and the family

The monogamous marriage is one of the oldest traditions of the human race. Monogamy is the practice of having only one husband or wife at a time. While there are today, and have been in the past, many cultures that are polygamous (more than one wife or husband), monogamy has and continues to dominate the majority of societies. Why did a family structure based on monogamy achieve the role it holds in present-day society? Is it a more successful way for families to exist than bigamy, polygamy, or perhaps no marriage bonds at all? This chapter will *attempt* to answer some of these questions. The word *attempt* is used purposely as marriage in the traditional sense is under a great amount of pressure in these times. Many individuals are predicting an end to

the so-called traditional family unit. Some of these views are also explored later in this chapter.

The generally accepted view of monogamous marriage usually gave the following reasons for the marriage covenant:

1. The procreation of children.
2. To stop sin and avoid promiscuous sexual relations.
3. To develop society and provide help and comfort to each of the marriage partners.

These reasons are often set forth in the marriage services of most religions and they have dominated the traditional view of marriage for many cultures. The word "love" is often not an essential component of the service. In traditional marriage, love was the "icing on the cake." Many young people were not given a chance to "fall in love" but were introduced to their marriage partners a few days (and in some cases a few hours) before the wedding. All of you have probably heard your parents or grandparents discussing such arranged marriages. Do you think that marriages are still arranged today? Do you know of any that have been arranged? How do you feel about such "arrangements"?

Since the 1950s young people have been brought up to have romantic expectations about marriage. They have been "brainwashed" by romantic ideals of movie-star weddings, motion pictures that made us feel that bells would ring when we met our future mates, television commercials that exploited the myth of the forever happy marriage, and romantic novels that overlooked many of the day-to-day problems that appear in marriage. This romantic ideal is one of the major reasons why some couples are very disappointed in marriage. Marriage is a union of two people, and people have problems, faults, emotions, and feelings. One must approach marriage with this in mind and work at making it a better relationship. Margaret Mead, the well-known anthropologist, in a magazine article (*Life*, August 23, 1968) stated that, "We ask too

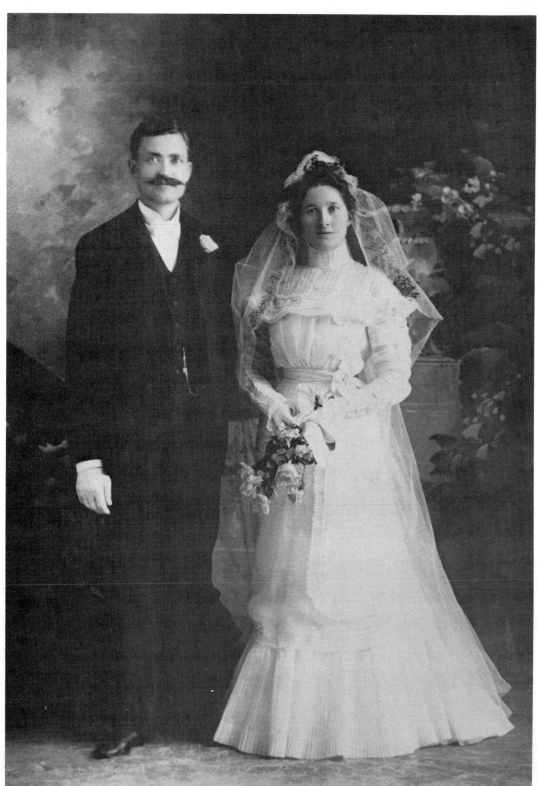

. . . to love, honor, and obey . . .

much of marriage and not getting it we despair too quickly and break it off.''

There are many reasons for the change in the accepted role of marriage and the family. Some of these reasons are based on changes in the traditional roles of family members and in family structure. These changes and their effects on marriage and the family are explored in the following sections of this chapter.

TRADITIONAL ROLES OF FAMILY MEMBERS

The traditional role of the father was to be head of the household. He was usually the sole support of the family and made most of the important decisions. A family dominated by the father is known as patriarchal family.

The traditional mother was seen as the homemaker and child bearer. She was most often dominated by her husband and was limited to the home for most of her activities. The role of the children was to obey their parents, grow up, and become mothers and fathers themselves further carrying on the traditional values.

How have these traditional roles changed? The father's role has changed with the times. The father of the past usually worked at home or close to home. He was constantly around to supervise and dominate his family. The present-day father is usually employed away from home (often many miles away) and he may rarely see his family except for weekends. Men who commute long distances often take buses and trains at early hours and return late at night. If they have small children who are in bed early, they may never see their children. These men are not around to make household decisions or be strong disciplinarians in the home. Many children view their fathers as people who make money but with little emotional attachment. Fathers are often related to great responsibility without enough time for fun and joy. Surely there are countless fathers who take time to spend with their families, but many fathers seem too engrossed in

making a living to have much time left for their families.

What about the mother's role? Has it changed dramatically from the traditional role? There are many women who consider their major role as that of homemaker and childbearer, and they are very content to do so. These women may not be traditional in that they are very involved in outside activities and make important household decisions. However, the woman's movement has educated many women to understand that one can have more than one role—it is a matter of choice. Many women have chosen to return to work after their children have gone off to school. Others have elected to return to work soon after having a child. Children are either cared for by hired nurses, family members, or day-care centers or nurseries. In some cases, men have chosen to stay home to care for the children while the woman goes to work. In an ideal situation, both men and women are able to work and share the responsibilities of caring for home and children. This concept is explored further in a later section of this chapter that considers the alternatives to the traditional framework of marriage and family. In general, today's mother is a more involved person who is not solely tied to caring for the home and children.

The children of today have been strongly influenced by the mass media, and they have had to adjust to rapid changes in society. Children are encouraged to be more independent than they were in the past. Many children grow up faster than they did in the past because they are less protected and have greater responsibility. They are encouraged to form their own opinions and make many of their own decisions. Increasing numbers of children are being brought up in homes where there is only one parent. This is a difficult situation where children often carry some financial responsibility as well as responsibility for younger brothers and sisters. Children are aware of the options open to them and can think in nontraditional ways. They do not see marriage as the necessarily ''right'' answer for them. They may

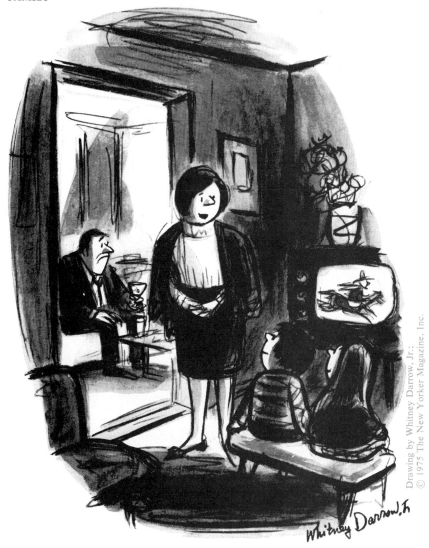

*"Come on, kids. Daddy's going to tell us about
the sort of day he had."*

choose to remain single, live with someone, or live in a group such as a commune. All of these options will be discussed in greater detail later in this chapter.

CHANGES IN FAMILY STRUCTURE

The extended family (refer to Chapter 8) is breaking down for many reasons. Children usually move away from their homes when they seek a job or go to college. Many communities cannot support all of the young people who are born there. In addition,

many young people are adventurous and choose to seek their fortunes elsewhere. Parents, sisters, brothers, and other family members are left behind. Older parents are frequently left living alone in homes that were once filled with children. Married and single children often find themselves in communities where they do not know anyone. This is especially difficult for a young woman with small children. If she is at home, her isolation is compounded by having no friends.

At one time parents, children, grandparents,

and other family members lived in the same household or nearby. Family members could depend on each other to help them financially or with child care. Today's young families are usually "loners," sometimes by choice. Many young people choose to start their life in a new place and "escape" from family ties. Studies have shown such young persons to feel isolated and in a sense "lost."

They have no one to call upon for advice in making important decisions. Children of these couples do not benefit from the experience of having grandparents, aunts, and uncles around them. In many cases, there are few close family ties. In many families cousins do not know each other. How do you feel about the breakdown of the extended family? What are the advantages and disadvantages of close family ties?

"The Times They Are a Changin'" is certainly true as reflected by changes in the traditional roles, redefinition of marriage by many persons, and the breakdown of the extended family. The times continue to change as shown by the increase and greater acceptance of intermarriage. This aspect

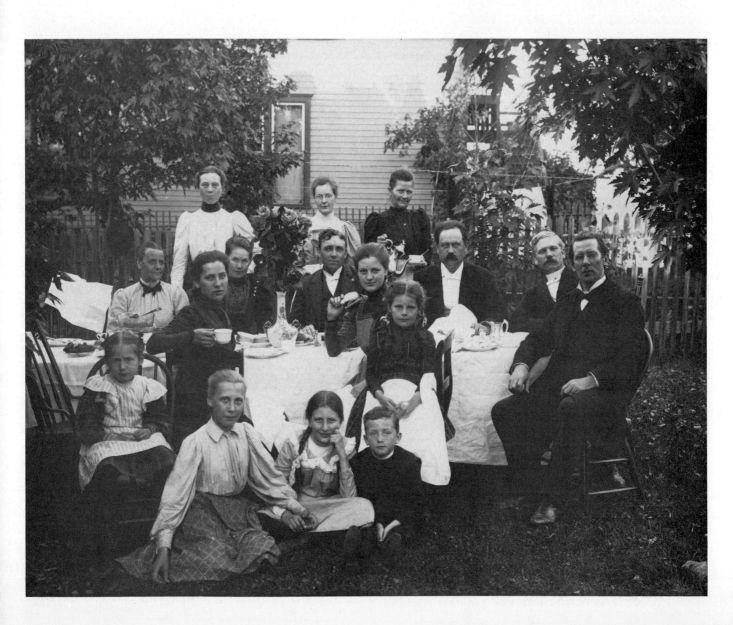

of marriage is discussed in the following section.

"MIXED MARRIAGE"

Mixed marriage or intermarriage encompasses a variety of possible marital relationships. Intermarriage may be defined as the marriage of individuals who have different religious, racial, or ethnic backgrounds. If the background of either person differs in any one of these ways, the couple is intermarried.

Interreligious or interfaith marriage is between two people of different religions. They are occurring with greater frequency in the United States today and have found increased acceptance among individuals of both generations. The younger generation has a tendency to be less influenced by organized religion than in the past. The older generation may not voice total approval but, in a large percentage of cases, they accept the choices of their children.

Interethnic marriages are marriages between persons of different ethnic backgrounds but the same religious background, (for example,

Only a few generations ago the extended family was the most common type but the demands of today's more mobile lifestyle have changed this pattern. Older parents now frequently live alone.

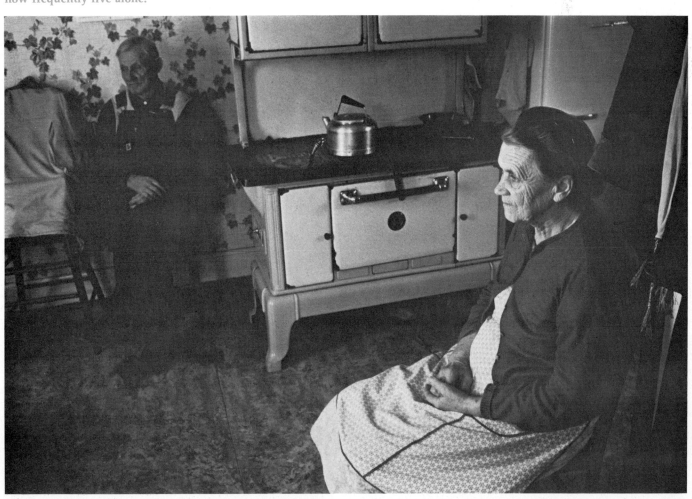

the marriage of an Irish Catholic and an Italian Catholic). These marriages occur with greater frequency than do interfaith marriages. At one time, this type of marriage was looked down upon by the older generation, but this is no longer as true as it once was. Individuals do not tend to live in the ethnic ghettos that were their homes in the early and mid-1900s. Persons arriving in the United States during this period usually settled in an area where they had family or friends. In this way children of the same ethnic background stayed together and frequently married each other. Today, because most people live in urban or rual areas that are mixed, children are exposed to all types of social relationships and are more open to "mixed marriage."

Interracial marriages exist when two people of different races marry even though they may both be of the same religion. Interracial marriage may be between a variety of "people combinations" such as a Caucasian (white) person and an Oriental. There are any number of interracial combinations but most Americans are exposed to black–white marriages and white–Oriental marriages. Both have increased in recent years. There has been an obvious increase in white–Oriental marriage because of the United States' partic-

ipation in both the Korean and Vietnam wars. Many American servicemen have brought back Oriental wives. Many servicemen have also chosen to remain with their wives in Korea and Vietnam.

Black–white marriages are increasing but are still not totally accepted by many people. One could say that "we have come a long way, baby" but probably not far enough. In a recent television program four black–white couples discussed some of the difficulties they have in finding suitable places to live and in bringing up their children. Many of these couples found that they felt most accepted in university environments. Perhaps, as the numbers of such couples increase, they will become acceptable to more people as was the case in other types of "mixed marriages." How do you feel about "mixed marriage?" How have your feelings been influenced by a particular person or incident?

Another type of marriage that is often thought of as "mixed" is the interclass marriage. This type of marriage is between people of different socioeconomic groups. This, too, was once frowned upon and bitterly contested by parents—especially the parents in the higher socioeconomic group. This, again, is no longer as true as it once was. In

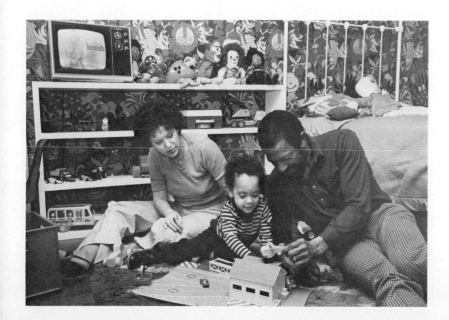

The number of interracial marriages has increased; has this been accompanied by increasing acceptance?

the 40s and 50s, college was often restricted to the middle and upper classes, and certain schools were the domain of the social elite. Today and for the past 10 or 15 years, college doors have opened for everyone. Increased financial aid and open enrollment programs have made all colleges accessible to students from a variety of socioeconomic backgrounds. These students meet each other and are usually unaware of class or financial position. Many persons might object to including interclass marriages in a section discussing "mixed marriage." Class is no longer the barrier it once was. Do you think that interclass marriages are "mixed marriages" in the true sense of the term?

LEGAL ASPECTS OF MARRIAGE

When individuals enter upon a marriage, they rarely consider the legal partnership that they are agreeing to. A marriage license is issued and, if all goes well, neither party will be involved in finding out about what they have signed. Marriage is indeed a legal partnership that is covered by different laws in each state. If a couple decides to divorce, they may be surprised at the extent to which these laws will govern their separation. There are many considerations, such as child custody, out-of-state or country divorces, alimony payments, contesting the divorce, grounds for divorce, and numerous other legal aspects. The newest of which is the no-fault divorce which is being hailed by many as a revolution in its own right. This and other legal aspects of divorce will be discussed later in this chapter.

It is, however, important to understand that a marriage is not only a commitment between two people but also a commitment to the laws of that state regarding marriage, subsequent children, and how that marriage will be nullified if the couple so desires. It would, of course, be possible for a couple to separate without a legal separation or divorce; however, neither person could legally remarry without first obtaining these papers.

There have been many suggested alternatives to traditional marriage and the legal involvement of this relationship. Many individuals express the feeling that it is love, not legal terminology, that should bind them. They feel that if they wish to leave each other, it is a personal decision that the state has no right to infringe upon. How do you feel about such viewpoints? Do you think that marriage should only be between the two individuals that are involved in the relationship?

alternatives to the traditional framework of marriage and family life

What are some of the alternatives to traditional patterns of marriage? One noticeable change in many households is the sharing of everyday duties by all family members. This has come about for two major reasons. Women make up a greater proportion of the work force than ever before, and they do not have the time to perform all of the functions they did when they were home. The woman's movement has encouraged women to expect more from other members of the family and has likewise encouraged family members to participate in every-day duties. A woman now is able to look at herself as an individual in her own right who must look for fulfillment. Sometimes that fulfillment is in the home and sometimes it must be sought outside of the family. Many men once found it difficult to accept the fact that their wives were working. They felt they were not manly if a woman had to help support the family or go to work for any other reason. Although this is still true, especially among certain ethnic groups, the "working wife" is becoming more acceptable.

The traditional views of male and female roles are also breaking down. Such phrases as "man's job" and "woman's place" are being used less and less these days. When they are used, it is usually not long before someone picks up on it and labels the saying as sexist. Sexist is a relatively new term made popular by the woman's movement. It means

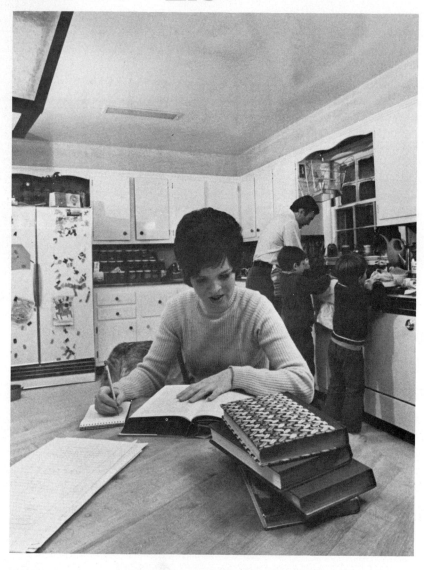

Homework and home-making: an interchange of roles.

that one is categorizing things into traditional male or female roles. For example, if one refers to a telephone operator as a female, he or she is implying that only females work in this capacity because they traditionally did so. However, if one thinks this is true, try calling information—you may be quite surprised at the voice at the other end of the phone! Can you think of any examples of the word "sexist?"

NEGOTIATION IN MARRIAGE

The breakdown of traditional male and female roles is not an easy transition in many families.

For a variety of personal and social reasons, many individuals resist altering their roles. If both partners in the family are equally resistant, then the relationship will usually proceed quite well. For example, if a woman enjoys her home and children and does not want any help from her family, then she may be content with the traditional mother role. If her husband is also content with his traditional role, then the relationship will remain essentially unchanged. However, if one partner is discontent with his or her role, then pressures are put on the other partner to change. This is where *negotiation* can play an important role.

219

A new type of therapy called behavior modification is looking into marriage negotiation. Behavior modification, as the term implies, is the changing of one's behavior to achieve certain goals. An "I'll scratch your back, if you scratch mine" type of technique is being utilized in marriage negotiation therapy.

A couple seeking help will go to a trained behavioral therapist and discuss all of the problem areas of their marriage. Values are assigned to each of the areas. These values depend on the occurrence of certain situations (too often or not enough). For example, if a couple were disagreeing about sharing duties, then one duty would be assigned to each person. If one did not perform his or her duty, then the other would refuse to do his or her part. For example, the husband might agree to wash the bathtub if the wife agreed to cook a meal. If one reneged, then the other would also refuse to do his or her job. Punishment and rewards can be added if they fit into the situation. If a woman wants to converse more with her husband, then a conversation may be a reward for a particular duty that she accomplished. The principle behind this type of therapy is to teach couples to try to derive pleasure from their relationship by not becoming discontent about problems that can be solved. Each party should try harder to please the other party. How do you think negotiation of this type would work in a marriage? Would you be willing to experiment with it?

MARRIAGE CONTRACTS

One step beyond this type of planned negotiation is the marriage contract. A marriage contract is a document that is drawn up between two people and includes such items as money, property, valuables, children, responsibilities, and other possible sources of conflict in the marriage. The contract allows for frank and open disclosure of problems that are likely to creep up after the marriage ceremony. Writing such a contract requires the two parties to think about some of the areas of marriage that most persons

never think about before the marriage. Differences are clarified, negotiated, and agreed upon on paper and a sounder relationship can result from this action. Of course, once married, there will be other considerations that may have not occurred to the couple prior to marriage. However, these aspects can be discussed and added to the contract; such a contract is open-ended and is really a forum for discussing and solving problem areas. How would a marriage contract of this type be helpful? Which types of situations should be explored in a marriage contract?

Some individuals are "performing" their marriage contracts at the wedding ceremony. In recent years, more couples are writing their own marriage vows which often include "contractual" obligations. These vows express how they plan to relate to each other in their marriage. Have you heard couples reciting vows that they have written at their wedding? Would you like to do this at your wedding?

"OPEN MARRIAGE"

The concept of open marriage became popular in the book by the same name. Open Marriage was written by two anthropologists, George O'Neill and Nena O'Neill. The concept of open marriage is essentially that a husband and wife should try not to lose their individual identities. This means that each partner in a marriage should have his or her own life that is apart from the marriage itself. Men and women should be able to have their own friends, not only friends of the couple. Classes or social functions could be attended by one member of the marriage without the other partner coming along all of the time.

O'Neill and O'Neill list the basic guidelines for an "open marriage" as:

living for now and realistic expectations
privacy
open and honest communication
flexibility in roles

George O'Neill and Nena O'Neill are a husband-and-wife team of anthropologists. They are interested in the problems of modern living. Their studies of today's marriage led them to an interesting conclusion: that marriage is most satisfying when both partners remain independent. In a good marriage, the husband and wife each feel free to pursue their separate interests.

open companionship
equality
trust

These are guidelines that may seem appropriate to any marriage but few people do implement them in their relationships. The concept of *Open Marriage* is primarily based on a consideration of each partner's needs, both individual and mutual.

How do sex and love fit into the "open marriage" concept? The O'Neills feel that sex, love, affection, care, concern, and responsibility are an expression of an individual's identity—they are his or hers alone to give and share with another person. None of these qualities of the relationship should be owned, demanded, or controlled by another person.

In an open marriage where both partners are secure in their own identities and trust each other, outside sexual relationships can exist and will not harm the marriage. The term fidelity does not have to be interpreted as sexual faithfulness to each other. The love relationship of the married couple can expand to include other people. The open marriage concept implies that outside relationships tend to augment rather than diminish the marriage. Sex outside of marriage is not recommended by the O'Neills but is given as an option that may work for some couples. The marriage is indeed "open" with many possibilities, including extramarital sex, that might be explored. Do you feel that the "open marriages" concept can work? Do you see any potential problems in this type of relationship?

The "open marriage" concept is more difficult to implement when there are children in the family. The O'Neills feel that motherhood should be optional and should be disentangled from the wife's role. In general, the book emphasizes that both parties of a marriage should work outside of the home, as domestic life tends toward mediocrity. How do you feel about this? Do you think that an "open marriage" concept could be instituted in a home with children? What might be some of the problem areas?

GROUP MARRIAGE

Group marriage may be defined as a "marriage" between three or more people. *Marriage* is in quotes above because this type of arrangement does not constitute a legal marriage. In a book titled *Group Marriage,* Larry and Joan Constantine explore the relationship of more than 100 such groups. Group marriage is a radically new approach to the traditional family. In such a marriage, each member of the relationship is responsible to and cares about the other members. If, for example, there are two men and one woman, there should be no jealousy between the men. All individuals share the responsibility for household chores, and, if there are children, they are brought up by three or four parents rather than two.

The classic definition of group marriage included two couples rather than odd numbers of people. In the traditional sense, these two couples would live together, work together, and have sexual relations with each other. A contemporary view of group marriage allows for there to be more members of one sex than another. If, for example, there are three men and one woman, then very likely the men are also sexually involved with each other as well as with the woman. If another marriage partner is desired by one of the members, then all of them would have to vote on whether or not to accept the new member.

In the Constantine's study of group marriage, they found that more such marriages existed in urban than in rural areas. The majority of these individuals were college graduates, many with advanced degrees, representing a variety of occupations. Among those studied were college students, professors, sales personnel, farmers, mechanics, psychologists, social workers, nurses, and doctors. There was also a minister and a student of religion. The median income for these families was about $10,000 per year. The usual number of people included in a group marriage was four. Most frequently these individuals were already formally married prior to forming a group marriage with another married couple. Triads, or three-member marriages, were the

ALTERNATIVES TO THE
TRADITIONAL
FRAMEWORK OF
MARRIAGE AND FAMILY
LIFE

221

next most common type of group. Large groups (five or six people) are rare but do exist. The Constantines had heard of eight- and twelve-member groups but were unable to locate them.

The terms co-wife and co-husband as well as multilateral marriage are used by the Constantines to explain this relationship. The marriage is multilateral in that it has many sides, few of which are exclusive to the entire group. A co-wife and co-husband are usually deeply attached to all group members. In some larger groups (four or more persons), some individuals may be more involved with some members than with others. The larger the group, the more difficult it is to keep all of the involvements on the same level. Do you think that group marriage is a workable concept? What type of group has the greatest chance for survival? Do you feel that you might be interested in becoming a part of such a group?

THE CHILDLESS MARRIAGE

One alternative to the traditional family is electing to have a marriage without children. The fact that more and more people are choosing to do this and their decision together with the liberalization of abortion laws has produced a noticeable decline in births in the last few years. The July 13, 1974, issue of *Business Week* reported that the total number of babies born in the United States in 1973 dropped to 3.1 million, the lowest level since World War II. This compares with 4.2 to 4.3 million births in the years from 1956 to 1962. The birth rate per family is now 1.9 rather than the 2.1 children needed to replace the parents. The number allows for the women who do not have children. This, however, is not zero population growth, which implies that as many persons are born as those who die. Therefore, the population would not increase at all. Today there are still more persons being born than there are persons dying. It will take a number of years, if births stay at a low level, before ZPG can be achieved. This is discussed in greater detail in Chapter 20.

Deciding to remain childless is often a difficult question for people to resolve. Many young people are brought up with the idea that someday they will have children. Many individuals who marry never think that they do have an option not to have children. There may be pressures on young people from parents and friends. Well-meaning individuals often produce feelings of guilt in couples who remain childless after a few years of marriage. They are called selfish, immature, irresponsible, and the women are looked upon as being unfulfilled. The couple is often told that they are "missing one of the great joys of life." These individuals are relating their own feelings to the childless couple, frequently because they would like a grandchild, nephew, or friend who is also at home with a child.

In a recent study by J. E. Veevers, a Canadian sociologist, 52 urban, middle-class women were interviewed concerning their choice to remain childless. All of the women had been married for at least five years. Two-thirds of these women had not made a definite decision but kept postponing childbearing until it was not brought up again. Another third discussed the possibility of adopting, in order to avoid confrontation. The final group had decided prior to marriage that there would be no children and signed an informal contract with their husbands attesting to this decision.

There are many couples who, upon marriage, are not quite sure what their position will be concerning children. There are groups that have been formed to educate people about the alternatives of childlessness. They want people to know all the ramifications of parenthood and to find out for themselves whether they would or would not make good parents. "Parenting" is much more than the biological ability to bear a child. One such group, the National Organization for Non-Parenthood, has provided much information concerning how to counter remarks about being childless, what to consider when deciding about whether or not to have children, and how to enjoy childlessness. This group is not against children; they want people to consider the possible alternative. Do you

National Organization for Non-parenthood (NON), founded in 1972, hopes to change our culture's attitudes about having children. It wants to make childlessness a socially approved option. In this way, NON hopes to help ease population pressures on the individual, the community, and the environment.

think that most young people consider the possibilities of *not* having children prior to marriage? If you answered "no," why do you think this is so?

ADOPTION AND FOSTER CARE

Another alternative to traditional family life is the adoption or foster care of children. Persons who are unable to have their own biological children or who do not desire to have children for a variety of reasons may choose to adopt a child. There are many private and public institutions that can help a couple who wish to adopt. However, in recent years, since abortion reform, there have been fewer babies available than in the past. This has been especially true in the case of Caucasian infants. Many persons who wish to adopt have had to pay large sums of money (often illegally) in order to adopt a child. It is always best to go through a legitimate agency where both the parents and the child are protected.

Some persons have looked to adopt children from other countries. There were a great number of parentless children left in Vietnamese orphanages following the war. There are agencies in the United States that specialize in bringing these children into American adoptive homes.

The large number of children who have handicaps, belong to minority groups, or who are older are difficult to place. These children are very much in need of adoptive homes and are frequently overlooked. The healthy Caucasian infant is easy to place, but what about all of the other children who desperately need homes?

With foster child care a family takes one or more children into their home, usually for a short period of time. Foster care is often necessary if natural parents are ill, out of work, divorced, imprisoned, or for a variety of other reasons. Frequently, foster children are adopted by their foster family. However, this must be legally designated by the natural parents. Foster care is paid for through the state or local social service department.

Burrhus Frederic Skinner (1904-) is a behavioral psychologist. He is interested in observing how, not why, people and animals behave as they do. Skinner believes that most types of behavior can be learned—or unlearned—and his techniques for teaching people new patterns of behavior are now being used in education and in psychotherapy.

COMMUNAL LIVING

A commune is composed of a group of people who have chosen to live together and equally share the responsibilities of the household. There are many different types of communes in existence and some of them are explored in this section of the chapter.

Communal living is not new. There were many communes in this country that existed as farm communities and industrial groups. They later developed into noncommunal enterprises such as Oneida Community Limited, which to this date is a successful commercial enterprise. The Oneida Community was founded by John Noyes in Putney, Vermont, in 1841. The group later moved to Oneida, New York. This commune was based on a complex system of marriage where each man and woman were married to each other. Noyes believed that this extended family system could eliminate selfishness from its members.

Walden Two is a fascinating book by Dr. B. F. Skinner that explores a utopian communal living arrangement. It pictures a society where human problems are solved by scientific technology that deals with human behavior. It shows some of the ways in which contemporary values may be obsolete. *Walden Two* operates under the assumption that the family is an ancient form of community, and society should not be based on blood ties. A commune of this type replaces the family economically, socially, and psychologically. Children are cared for in groups, and the goal of the commune is that every child feel that every adult is his or her parent. Though *Walden Two* presents us with a highly utopian communal structure, it offers an enjoyable and thought-provoking concept of living.

Communes have become more popular in recent times. Much of this popularity is associated with the "hippie" cults of the 1960s. Many of the young people of that era sought out communal life in an effort to escape the so-called "establishment." In most present-day communes, work, money, chores, and child rearing are shared by all the members.

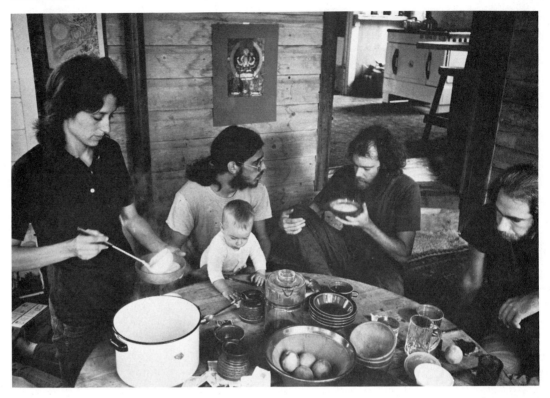

Communal living often exhibits similar characteristics from coast to coast. People together, simplicity of style, low threshold of consumerism, and (on the wall) inspiration from other cultures. This commune was photographed in upstate New York.

Individuals with an expertise in a particular area are called upon for their contributions. Some communes exist as artist colonies, where all members have a similar interest. Sexual relations may be exclusive involving only two people or may be partially exclusive. Sometimes the commune is open to sexual involvement with all members.

Studies have indicated that the life-span of communes is quite short. Some of the reasons for this include disputes concerning household duties and personal problems concerning sexual partners. In many cases, disputes develop because of jealousy. There are numerous financial problems. A commune that attempts to survive solely by farming or selling crafts will have a difficult time. Arguments may ensue concerning those who must work outside of the commune and the delegation of responsibilities to others. Pressure also comes from the outside. If a commune is established in an "unfriendly" area, residents often use political pressure to evict the commune members from their property. Many "outsiders" have a distorted view of

what a commune is all about and find it as a threat to their own survival. Communes are not usually "havens of sex and drugs." They are usually a group of young, educated persons who are looking for a new life experience. Have you ever belonged to or visited a commune? How would you feel if a commune formed a few miles outside of your community?

TRIAL MARRIAGE
OR LIVING TOGETHER

Trial marriage differs from living together in that in the former case two people are living together with the intention of getting married. Living together is a choice made by two people who do not necessarily plan to marry.

Not too long ago, cohabitation or living together was a reason for expulsion in some communities. Today, it is a relatively open and widespread situation. Studies have indicated that from 10 to 33 percent of college students have lived with someone or are presently living together. The percentage varies depending on location of the school, regulations, housing, and male–female sex ratios.

A study of college students at Cornell University was conducted by E. D. Macklin (*Psychology Today,* November 1974). In this study, 31 percent of those questioned had cohabited at some time. (Cohabitation according to this study was defined as sharing a bedroom with someone of the opposite sex for four or more nights a week for three or more consecutive months). Seventy percent of the cohabitants reported "emotional attachment" as the main reason for living together. Only ten percent of these individuals had definite marriage plans. These couples generally did not view their living together as a trial marriage. They thought they were not ready for the commitment of marriage. More than 90 percent of these students thought that the experience had been "successful, pleasurable, and maturing."

Living together outside of marriage is not limited to college students; it has also been chosen by many people as an alternative to marriage. Many couples spend years together without ever seeking a formal commitment. Many persons who do not wish to have children see no reason for legally getting married. Others enjoy the freedom of living together that they do not feel they would have if they were married. Of course, there are numerous persons who do live together and decide to marry. Cohabiting is generally accepted today and couples have little or no problems in obtaining housing or jobs because of it. Legal problems may arise, however, with property settlement if the couple decides to split-up or if one partner dies. It is *so* accepted that some people are wondering whether we are experiencing a complete reversal of attitudes. Are those who "opt" to marry looked down upon? Have you found this type of reversal among your friends? How do you feel about it?

Fewer people are involved in trial marriage than in cohabitation. This is true because many individuals drift into cohabitation without a lot of thought as to why they are

living together. It seems to be the natural course of events for many couples who are emotionally involved. However, trial marriage implies forethought and purpose.

Many individuals have expressed the belief that *all* marriages should be *trial* for the first year or two. A preliminary license would be issued and would not be permanent until both parties agreed to it at a later date. If they decide to separate, there would be no legal obligations to either party. Another suggestion along these lines is the renewable marriage contract. A couple would sign a contract that binded the marriage for a set number of years. When the contract expired, both parties would have to renew it, if they so desired. If not, the marriage would be terminated without any liability to either party. Do you think that preliminary or trial marriages and contract marriages are feasible ideas?

A novel educational experience dealing with marriage training is taking place at Parkrose Senior High School in Portland, Oregon. The program is called *Contemporary Family Life* and consists of a simulated marriage between two classmates. After a mock marriage ceremony, the students are confronted with a variety of problems that they might meet in a "real" marriage. Decisions must be made concerning jobs, where they will live, expenses, children, and a variety of other factors. Many students are surprised to find out some of the actual expenses involved in a marriage and establishing a household. The course is open only to seniors and more than three-quarters of the students elect to take the course. Do you think this would be a good experience for most young people?

HOMOSEXUAL MARRIAGE

In homosexual marriage two persons of the same sex live together as if they were married. Many homosexuals live with one partner for many years as in a traditional marriage. This mode of life has been discussed in the media in recent years because some persons have tried to make these marriages legal. Some gay activist groups have protested that homosexual marriages should have state licensure as do heterosexual marriages. However, this has not yet met with legislative approval.

Another aspect of this is homosexual parenthood. There are some homosexuals who have custody of children by previous marriages, have children because they want them, or seek to adopt children. There have been many breakthroughs in these cases, and in numerous custody cases children have been awarded to the homosexual parent. How do you feel about homosexuals gaining custody of their children or adopting children?

being single in a "married society"

How does it feel to be single in a largely "married society?" It is less difficult today than it was in past years. At one time, any unmarried woman over the age of 25 was thought to be an "old maid." However, men who were this age were called "swinging bachelors." The double sexual standard rears its ugly head once more!

The times and attitudes have changed, and women are often encouraged to "find themselves" before they marry. Women are marrying at later ages and not having to make excuses about it. Many couples are postponing marriage until their basic education and often advanced degrees are completed.

The single population consists of persons who have never been married, divorced persons, and those who are widowed. There are many social groups that cater to these individuals. Events are planned and groups are often separated by age. *Parents Without Partners* is one such group that has a dual

After he's gone: single parenthood.

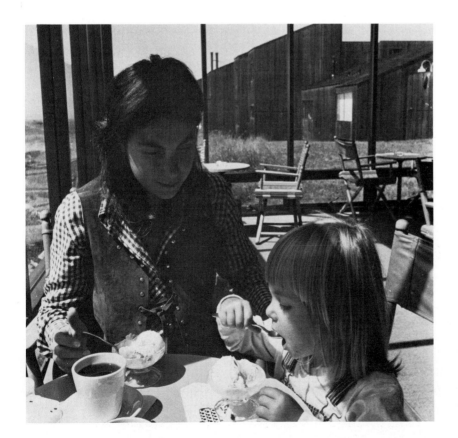

Parents Without Partners is an organization for people who have lost their spouses through death or divorce. The group sponsors lectures and discussions on the problems of the single parent and activities for the children. But perhaps its most important function is as a meeting place where the newly unmarried can be reintroduced to single life.

purpose. It is a social group but also brings together single persons with a common interest—children.

Sex for the single person is much more liberated and accepted today than in past years. Persons who are single can openly have sexual involvements without feeling inhibited. This is especially true in the larger urban areas. However, sex does present certain problems to some single individuals. Some persons think that the "label" of being single assumes sexual permissiveness. This is certainly not true among the majority of single persons. They may become involved in sexual relationships but do not wish to be promiscuous. This is often a very difficult problem for divorced women. Because they have been married, many men feel that they are open to all sexual involvement. Why do you think that many persons feel this way about divorced women? How could a divorced woman cope with this situation?

Single parenthood was briefly discussed in relation to homosexuals. However, single parents are rapidly increasing in numbers, and they are faced with some very difficult problems in adjusting their lives and the lives of their children to society. Who are the single parents? Some are divorced persons who have custody of their children, others are adoptive single parents, and others have borne children without any intention of marriage. The last two groups are relatively new in today's society.

The number of adoptive single parents has increased because of an easing of restrictive laws that prohibited single persons from adopting children. If one can establish that he or she is loving, economically stable, and can provide adequate care for a child, then it is very possible that adoption can take place. There are still laws, but they are less rigid than a few years ago.

Have you ever thought of intentionally having a child without being married? A few years ago this would not have occurred to most women. Women automatically thought that if they never married, they would never have children. This is no longer true for some

women. For a variety of reasons, these women do not wish to be married but they do wish to have children. There are many women who become pregnant unintentionally who also do not wish to marry, but do wish to keep their children. How do you feel about a woman raising a child as a single parent?

divorce

Studies indicate that Americans are getting married less and divorced more. In the four-year period 1970 to 1974, the nation's divorce rate increased as much as it had in the previous ten years. According to the Census Bureau, there were 63 divorced persons in 1974 for every 1,000 married persons living together. This compares with 47 in 1970 and 35 in 1960.

The divorce rate is increasing and the legal entanglements involved in divorce are, in some areas, lessening. For example, child custody was once almost automatically awarded to the mother—even if she was "unfit." It was extremely difficult to prove that any mother was "unfit." Today's laws have been liberalized so that many fathers are given custody of their children.

Alimony (the payment of money to the divorced spouse) has also been liberalized in the past few years. Women who can work are often unable to receive alimony or they receive it for a short period of time. Sometimes alimony is in the form of tuition and expenses so that a woman can become trained in a profession. Some men have sought and won alimony payments from women who were in a better financial position than they were.

Grounds for divorce (the legal reasons for asking for divorce) were once limited to adultery (sex outside of the marriage), incompatibility, and extreme cruelty. Different states have different grounds for divorce. However, some states have already adopted "no fault" divorce laws where neither party is found to be at fault in a marriage. California does not recognize the term divorce but refers to it as a "dissolution of the marriage." Marriages are dissolved because of *irreconcilable differences* and blame is placed on neither party. Do you feel that "no fault" divorce is an improvement over traditional divorce laws?

being happy regardless of marital status

It is important to be happy no matter what your marital status may be. How can one achieve this contentment with one's self? Much of this has already been discussed in the first part of this book, which dealt with personality adjustment and coping. Persons who have a healthy self-concept are able to adjust to most of life's situations and enjoy them. The "I'm OK, you're OK" philosophy is essential.

If you are having difficulty coping with your marital situation, there are a number of places to seek help. Married and unmarried individuals can derive much benefit from intensive therapy and from short-term behavioral modification therapy. In either case, one should carefully check the legitimacy of the therapist or group. There are many "fly-by-night" groups that are there for one purpose only—taking your money.

Marriage counseling is practiced by many trained sociologists, psychologists, and psychiatrists. It is important that both people realize that there is a need for counseling and are willing to try and save their marriage. Some types of counseling include the entire family in the counseling situations. Some problems are not necessarily exclusive to the adults but may be fostered by disagreements concerning the children.

Sex counseling became popular with the introduction of the Masters and Johnson technique. This technique requires the couple to learn to solve their sexual difficulties together through a carefully planned schedule of events that teach the couple how to relate sexually and emotionally. According to Masters and Johnson, most sexual problems such as premature ejaculation, impotence, and orgasmic dysfunction can be solved by certain techniques that are taught to the couple.

Sex counseling clinics have appeared in great numbers since the Masters and Johnson technique was published. It is important that a couple inquire about the legitimacy of the clinic and the credentials of the sex therapists.

THINKING IT OVER

1. What were some of the traditional reasons for marrying? Do these reasons exist today? If not, how have they changed?
2. Why are many young people disappointed in marriage?
3. How have the traditional roles of family members changed? Discuss some of the advantages and disadvantages of the extended family.
4. What types of "mixed marriages" exist? How do you think each type is accepted in today's world?
5. Discuss the meaning of marriage negotiation and marriage contracts.
6. What is the basic concept of "open marriage"? Do you think that this concept can work? Explain your answer.
7. What is meant by the term *group marriage?* What types of group marriages are most common?
8. Discuss some of the reasons why people may choose not to have children.
9. What is meant by the term *communal living?* Discuss some of the characteristics of a commune.
10. What is the difference between cohabitation and trial marriage? Which is more common among today's young people? Why do you think this is so?
11. What innovations have been suggested along the lines of a trial marriage? How do you feel about these alternatives to traditional marriage?
12. Is it easier to be single today in a married society? Explain your answer.
13. Discuss some of the legal aspects of divorce and how divorce laws have changed in recent years.

14. Where can an individual or couple go for help in coping with their marital situation? What should one look for in seeking help?

KEY WORDS

Alimony. Support money awarded to a spouse upon divorce.

Cohabitation. Living together without any plans of marriage.

Co-husband. A term used to describe a man in a group marriage.

Communal living. Individuals who live in groups and share the financial and household responsibilities.

Co-wife. Term used to describe a woman in a group marriage.

Fidelity. Sexual faithfulness to each other in a marriage.

Group marriage. A relationship between three or more persons that is like marriage but is not legal.

Homosexual marriage. A long-term relationship between two homosexuals that is not legally recognized.

Interclass marriage. Marriage between two persons of differing socioeconomic classes.

Interethnic marriage. Marriage between people of different ethnic backgrounds who may be of the same religion.

Intermarriage. Marriage between persons of different religions or racial or ethnic backgrounds.

Interracial marriage. Marriage between two persons of a different race who may be of the same religion.

Interreligious (interfaith) marriage. Marriage between two persons of different faiths.

Marriage contracts. A contract drawn up prior to marriage that discusses certain aspects of the marriage that require clarification.

Marriage counseling. Therapy to help couples and families who are having difficulties.

Marriage negotiation. A system of solving marital problems through assigned duties, rewards, and punishments.

Monogamous. Having one husband or wife at a time.

Multilateral marriage. Different relationships involved in a group marriage.

Open marriage. A marriage based on the premise that a husband or wife should try to maintain their own identities in marriage.

Polygamous. Having more than one husband or wife at a time.

Sex counseling. Therapy to help individuals cope with sexual problems.

Triads. Three-member group marriages.

Trial marriage. Living together in preparation for marriage.

Zero population growth (ZPG). This will occur when as many persons are born as those who die; the result is no growth in population.

GETTING INVOLVED
Books and Periodicals

Constantine, Larry and Joan. *Group Marriage.* New York: The Macmillan Co., 1973. One hundred group marriages are studied.

Mead, Margaret. *Sex and Temperament.* New York: Dell, 1967. Other societies have different notions about "masculine" and "feminine" behavior.

O'Neill, Nena, and O'Neill, George. *Open Marriage: A New Life Style for Couples.* New York: M. Evans, 1972. How and why to achieve less togetherness in marriage.

Peck, Ellen. *The Baby Trap.* New York: Pinnacle, 1972. To some people, children aren't bundles of joy.

Rogers, Carl R. *Becoming Partners: Marriage and Its Alternatives.* New York: Delacorte, 1972. The humanistic psychologist gives his views on love and marriage.

Skinner, B.F. *Walden Two.* New York: Macmillan, 1960. The behavioral approach to communal living.

Movies

Brief Encounter, with Celia Johnson, Trevor Howard, 1946. Noel Coward's tender account of two people who love each other but decide to remain faithful to their spouses. Distributed by Twyman, Walter Reade 16.

Diary of a Mad Housewife, with Richard Benjamin, Carrie Snodgress, 1970. Marriage to a male chauvinist can drive a woman up the wall. Distributed by Cine-Craft, Clem Williams, The Movie Center, Swank, Twyman, and Universal 16.

Divorce American Style, with Dick Van Dyke, Debbie Reynolds, 1967. Divorce, and its effects on lifestyle. Columbia Cinemateque, Clem Williams, Institutional, Macmillan, Modern, Mottas, Roa's, Swank, "The" Film Center, Welling, Westcoast, and Wholesome.

A Doll's House, with Claire Bloom, 1973. Ibsen's classic tale of one woman's liberation. Distributed by Paramount.

Georgy Girl, with James Mason, Lynn Redgrave, Alan Bates, 1966. About living together, abortion, etc. Distributed by Argosy, Budget, Cine-Craft, Charand, Columbia, Contemporary/McGraw-Hill, Clem Williams, Institutional, Macmillan, Modern, Mottas, Roa's, Select, Swank, Twyman, Welling, Westcoast, Wholesome, and Willoughby Peerless.

Scenes from a Marriage, with Liv Ullman, 1974. A realistic and sensitive portrayal of divorce. Distributed by Cinema V.

A Touch of Class, with Glenda Jackson, George Segal, 1973. The story of an extramarital affair. Distributed by Avco-Embassy.

Who's Afraid of Virginia Woolf? with Elizabeth Taylor, Richard Burton, 1966. The violence of a marriage gone sour. Distributed by Warner Brothers.

A Woman Under the Influence, with Gena Rowlands, Peter Falk, 1974. She's under the influence of her husband, and he doesn't understand her at all. Distributed by John Cassavetes.

The Women, with Norma Shearer, Joan Crawford, 1939. The way marriage, divorce, and the relationships between the sexes used to be—maybe. Distributed by Films Incorporated.

PART IV
PERSONAL FITNESS

11
PHYSICAL FITNESS

You have probably heard the term "physical fitness" countless times, but have you ever stopped to think about what it means? The term means different things to different people, but in this chapter we define it in a practical way that will have meaning to you as an individual. We also discuss what physical fitness is not. Many persons think in stereotypes when it comes to this subject. One can certainly be physically fit and not have bulging muscles. Physical fitness is desirable for both men and women, and gracefulness and coordination are all a part of fitness.

In this chapter you will learn about the concept of total fitness and how it applies to your every thought and action. You will also learn about the Krauss–Raab effect, which is related to a lack of physical exercise. It is common in our country as well as other industrialized nations. A recent study of the fitness of adult Americans is both enlightening and frightening. You will find out if you are a part of the average American population when it comes to fitness and participation in exercise.

The components of fitness are discussed and their interrelationship is stressed. It is very difficult to look at any component of fitness alone, because they are all interdependent. Certain types of training, including an exercise plan that is currently being used by the United States Air Force, are explained and their benefits to the circulatory and respiratory (C-R) systems are stressed. The benefits of exercise training to the increased efficiency of the C-R system is also explored.

Questions that might arise concerning you and physical fitness are explored. Jogging, cycling, exercise clubs, heart disease, and tension are discussed in relation to fitness programs.

While reading this chapter, think about the following concepts:

■ Physical fitness varies with the life style of the individual.

■ Total fitness should be the goal of anyone interested in good health.

■ Fitness is individual, and fitness programs should be geared to the needs of the individual.

■ The components of physical fitness are interrelated.

■ Fitness programs should be enjoyable, recreational, and beneficial to good health.

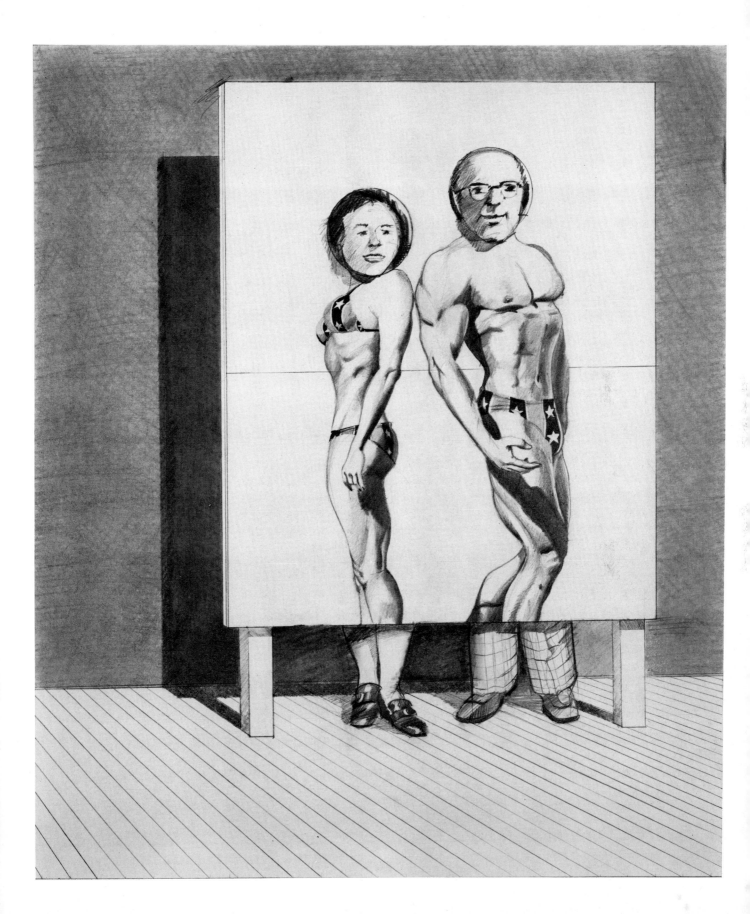

Have you ever thought about the term "physical fitness"? If you ask five people what it means, you will probably get five very different answers. Physical fitness varies with the life style of the individual. The office worker, construction worker, housewife, and athlete will all have different levels of fitness. Some housewives are more physically fit than workers who have strenuous jobs. This is because they work at it and try to develop a total fitness. This concept is explored later in this chapter. One can say that physical fitness has many interrelated components, and these components may be at different levels of development in each individual.

what is physical fitness?

Physical fitness is commonly defined as the level of physical energy that will enable one to comfortably perform his or her daily routine and have enough in reserve to meet unexpected emergencies. There have been many tests used to "measure" physical fitness; however, no one test can evaluate all of the aspects of a physically fit individual. Many tests tend to measure athletic ability (muscular strength and training) rather than general physical fitness.

Being able to run long distances at great speed or the ability to lift heavy weights is *not* what we mean by physical fitness. This may represent one aspect of physical fitness but not all of the components. Physical fitness does not mean that one has to resemble "Mr. America" and have bulging muscles all over one's body. There are probably many "Mr. America" types who are not at all physically fit. Physical fitness is also *not* an undesirable trait for girls and women. Many physically fit individuals, such as ice skaters Peggy Fleming and Dorothy Hamill and the gymnast Kathy Rigby, are lithe, graceful young women. The components of physical

fitness will help us better understand what is included in physical fitness. These components are discussed in a later section of this chapter.

TOTAL BODY FITNESS

Total body fitness should be the goal of everyone interested in their health. Total fitness may be defined as physical as well as mental and social fitness. A totally fit person feels well and is both physically and emotionally able to cope with his or her life. Refer to Chapters 1 to 4 in order to review some of the concepts related to personality adjustment and coping skills.

In total fitness, the three aspects of physical, mental, and social adjustment are interrelated. For example, an individual who is physically fit may be socially maladjusted and/or mentally exhausted. This individual could not be called totally fit. Very often when one of these aspects is malfunctioning, then everything "falls apart." After a bout with midterm exams, have you ever felt like collapsing for a few days? You may have been tired, emotionally drawn, and tense or nervous about your grades, malnourished from skipping meals, and generally out of shape from a lack of physical exercise. You would be totally unfit at this point. Each aspect would have to be rebuilt in order to feel well and fit once again.

PHYSICAL FITNESS OF AMERICANS

Many Americans suffer from a disease you may not know about. It is called the Krauss-Raab effect or hypokinetic disease. The concept of hypokinetic disease was defined by Krauss and Raab as "the whole spectrum of inactivity—induced somatic and mental derangements." This simply means that physical inactivity can produce a wide range of physical and mental problems.

Hans Kraus and Wilhelm Raab are two American physicians who stress the need for physical activity. Their 1961 book *Hypokinetic Disease* (Springfield, Ill.: Charles C. Thomas, o.p.) points out that lack of exercise may actually lessen one's ability to move.

Physical fitness, attractiveness, and professionalism combine in the woman athlete: Billie Jean King.

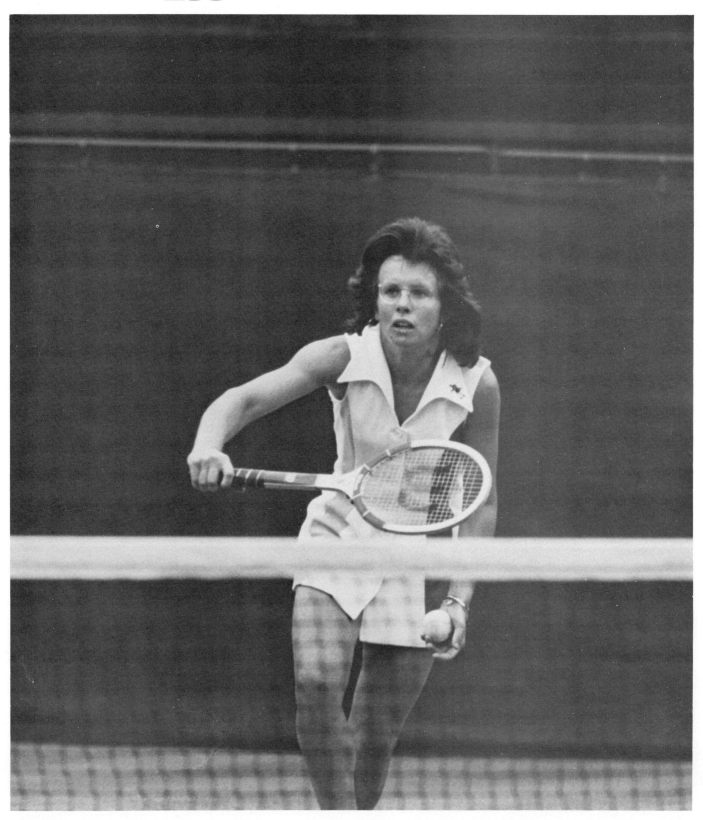

Although other factors, of course, are also related, statistics indicate that heart disease is twice as frequent in the sedentary (inactive) individual as in the active one. Other diseases that appear more frequently among sedentary individuals include diabetes, duodenal ulcers, low back pain, and numerous other internal problems. Lack of physical exercise parallels emotional difficulties in many cases. Physically active individuals show better adaptability to stress, less neuromuscular tension, less fatigability, later aging, less obesity, lower blood pressure and pulse rate, and great respiratory capacity than those who are not physically active.

American youth and adults have lower fitness levels than do their European counterparts. What are some of the reasons for this lower level of physical fitness? One of the major reasons is automation. There are very few things in the United States that are not operated, at least to some degree, by automation. We are a population of drivers. When was the last time you walked any distance to get somewhere? Children are bused or driven to school, sometimes from distances less than one-half mile away. The local grocery may be around the corner, but few people will walk to get there. The housewife has more conveniences than she needs and because of them her exercise is also limited. The less one does the greater the effort that has to be put forth in doing even simple chores. Jobs have also become automated; machines perform many functions that were once physically performed. How has automation affected your physical fitness?

The "Monday morning quarterback" is the individual who watched television for most of his or her exercise. This person knows every football play but his total exercise for the weekend may be reduced to a few well-timed dashes to the refrigerator. Spectator sports are among the most popular recreational outlets of Americans. Americans watch sporting events on televisions, at stadiums, and in schools. Only a small percentage of these people ever participate themselves in a *regular* program of exercise. The word *regular* should be stressed—a once-a-month tennis

game or throwing a basketball around with some friends will not build one's physical fitness.

Many Americans of all ages find excuses for not being involved in a regular fitness program. "It is too difficult," "there is not enough time," or "who needs it" are a few commonly voiced objections. Each of these statements can be answered. Physical fitness programs are not difficult. There are all types of simple exercise patterns that include activities that most people will enjoy. Time is only needed in very small amounts. A good fitness program could be accomplished by a half-hour of activity daily. Do you really need physical activity? This question has already been answered for you. Physical fitness is a part of total health; without it you are not functioning up to your potential. The way you usually feel will reflect your levels of physical and total fitness.

A recent poll of adult physical fitness in the United States indicated some startling findings in relation to the fitness of the American adult population. The survey was conducted by Opinion Research Corporation of Princeton, New Jersey, for the President's Council on Physical Fitness and Sports. The survey involved interviews with 3,875 men and women aged 22 and over. Some of the major findings of this survey are given here for your consideration.

Forty-five percent of all adult Americans (roughly 49 million of the 109 adult men and women) do not engage in physical activity for the purpose of exercise.

Those who are sedentary tend to be older, less well educated, and less affluent than those who do exercise.

Fifty-five percent of American adults do no exercise at all, but 57 percent of American adults believe they do get enough exercise. (It is interesting to note that those who do not exercise are more inclined to believe they get enough exercise than those who do exercise.)

Of the 60 million adults who do engage in

The President's Council on Physical Fitness and Sports is a government agency that develops and supports programs to increase the fitness of the American people. One of their recent surveys showed that 55 percent of adults do exercise, and that the most popular exercises are walking, bowling, bicycling, and swimming.

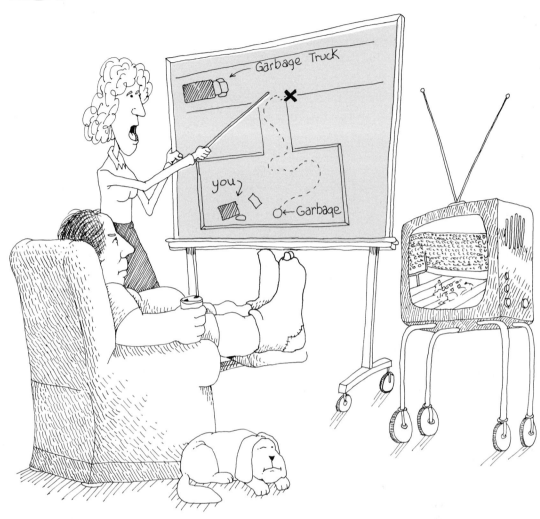

Getting the "quarterback"
to empty the garbage.

some exercise, the majority of them walk
(44 million), 18 million ride bicycles, 14
million swim, 14 million do calisthenics,
and 6.5 million jog. These activities are
done for exercise as opposed to recreation.

The study also indicated that those adults
who had participated in school sports (high
school or college) were more regularly involved in physical activity than those who
were relatively inactive while in school. The
persons least likely to be exercising today
are those who had no physical education in
school or college.

What do you think is the major reason that
people give for exercising? Concern for
health is the answer. Most individuals surveyed responded that "exercise is good for
your heart" or "helps you to breathe better."
One-fourth of those who exercise do so in
order to lose weight and about the same
number do so for relaxation and enjoyment.
Men are more likely to exercise for reasons
of health; women are more likely to do so
in order to lose weight. Why do you think
this is so?

From this survey one can easily see that
American adults are not physically fit (although many think they are). The President's
Council on Physical Fitness and Sports defines regular exercise as activity engaged in a

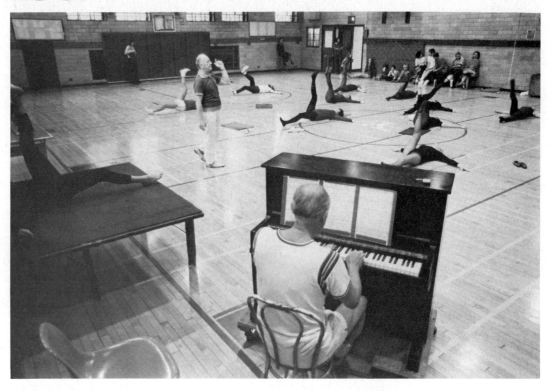

Keeping the body in tune.

minimum of three times a week. Many individuals may run or jog once in a while for a short period of time (ten minutes or less). This does not constitute regular exercise and will not develop fitness. The components of physical fitness and some exercise programs that utilize these components are discussed in the following sections.

components of physical fitness

The components of physical fitness are interrelated. One component is dependent on another in order to achieve total fitness. An individual who has developed his or her muscular strength may have not developed adequate circulatory-respiratory endurance. This person would not be considered physically fit. In this section, these and other components are discussed and their interrelationship is stressed.

MUSCULAR STRENGTH

Muscular strength may be defined as the

force muscles exert in a single effort or contraction. This type of strength can be measured by such instruments as a dynamometer or tensiometer. These devices measure the force of a muscular contraction. Muscles develop strength if they are subjected to tension in progressively increasing amounts. Muscular strength is an essential component of physical fitness.

There are two types of muscular contractions that all of you have probably heard about. One is isometric contraction and the other is isotonic contraction. In isometric muscle contraction there is little or no movement. In this type of contraction, the resistance (weight to be lifted) is too great to overcome and contractions are produced that are termed "tension" or "static" contractions.

Isometric contraction of muscles will improve muscular strength if done in sufficient amounts of time. Contractions should be held for five to eight seconds and repeated five to ten times a day. It is important that all muscle groups be exercised so that unequal strength does not occur. Muscular endurance and flexibility is *not* developed by isometric contraction. Isometrics tend to be dangerous for older or untrained individuals because such contractions, if overdone, can cause a definite elevation of the blood pressure.

An isotonic contraction is produced by raising and lowering a moderate load (such as a weight). In an isotonic exercise program, one can do a combination of exercises having different weights to be lifted and times of repetition. Muscular strength is developed most beneficially when the weight to be lifted is heavy and the number of repetitions of weight lifting is low.

The development of both isometric and isotonic strength is important. However, isotonic strength is more beneficial in a general type of fitness program. Most of the movements we do daily are of the isotonic type. Isotonic exercise also strengthens the circulatory-respiratory system. In addition, isotonic exercises can be planned to cover all of the body's muscle groups. Areas that need greater strength can be concentrated on by doing certain exercises. These exercises can usually be performed easily at home and can become part of an individual's daily routine.

The value of muscular strength in work and recreational activities is obvious. However, lack of muscular strength, particularly in certain areas of the body, may result in physical discomfort. This is thought to be true in the case of dysmenorrhea (menstrual cramping) and in low back pain. Both of these conditions are thought to be related to weakness of the abdominal muscles.

There has always been some disagreement by experts in the field concerning the merits of isometric and isotonic exercises. In a recent edition of the *Physical Fitness Research Digest* (January 1974), some of the conclusions pertaining to the comparative merits of these exercise forms were given. The findings are as follows:

Motivation is generally superior with isotonic

exercises because they are self-testing in nature.

Both isotonic and isometric forms of exercise improve muscular strength. Most studies do not favor one method over another; however, some individuals in this area have reported greater gains from using the isotonic form of exercise.

Muscular endurance is more effectively developed through isotonic exercise. Recovery from muscular fatigue is faster following isotonic exercise.

Isometric training increases blood pressure and can have other undesirable cardiocirculatory effects on heart patients and unfit individuals.

Think about some of the things you do every day. Are they isotonic or isometric in nature? For example, shutting a stuck window or shoveling snow are *isotonic* while ironing or clapping hands is *isometric*. What other examples can you give from your daily routine?

MUSCULAR ENDURANCE

Muscular endurance may be defined as the ability of a muscle to continue to work for a prolonged period of time. In isometric muscular endurance, one must hold a static contraction for a prescribed length of time. In isotonic muscular endurance, one must be able to repeat a movement of low resistance for a prescribed number of times (such as doing sit-ups). Both isometric and isotonic endurance are slowly built up over a period of time in planned exercise programs. There are certain tests of muscular endurance that can be applied, depending on the exercise program in which you are involved.

MUSCULAR POWER

Muscular power may be defined as the strength of muscles and speed of movement. Although many persons do not consider muscular power to be a direct component of fitness, it is important in performing effi-

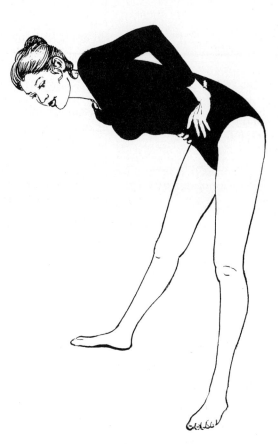

(a) Isotonic exercise.

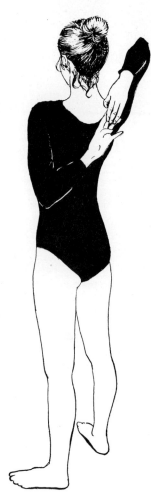

(b) Isometric exercise.

cient and effective movement. Almost every-thing we do is to some extent dependent on muscular power. The way you throw a frisbee or return a tennis ball is dependent on your individual muscle power.

FLEXIBILITY

Another essential element of physical fitness is flexibility. It is usually defined as the range of motion at a joint. Flexibility is not general but rather specific to each joint of the body. The flexibility of the joints will determine the general flexibility of the body. This body flexibility is the capability of the body to move freely in all directions and in a variety of body movements.

Certain factors limit the flexibility of joints. Crippling diseases such as arthritis and bursi-tis will inhibit joint flexibility. Injury to tissue in and around a joint will also inhibit flex-ibility. These types of injuries are common to certain sports. There are a number of tennis players who complain of tennis elbow and football players are frequently being operated on for knee injuries.

A lack of exercise can also reduce joint flexibility and in so doing contribute to inad-equate body flexibility. Insufficient exercise tends to result in a shortening of muscles and tendons around a joint. Shortening and general weakening of these muscles and tendons are one of the major causes of low back pain. In a recent study of more than

5,000 persons who complained of low back pain, only 1,000 were able to pass simple tests of muscular strength.

You may wonder if an individual can be *too* flexible. The answer is "yes." Too much flexibility may leave the joints susceptible to injury. The amount of flexibility needed, like fitness in general, is an individual matter. One needs enough to perform necessary daily tasks of bending and stretching (tying shoes, zipping zippers) and, to meet emergency situations, to perform movements requiring sudden muscular strength.

CIRCULO-RESPIRATORY ENDURANCE

Circulo-respiratory (C-R) endurance pertains to the ability of the heart and circulatory system, working with the respiratory system, to supply the active cells with oxygen and remove waste products during exercise. Stress is placed on the circulo-respiratory system in general physical activity such as running and jogging. Swimming, cycling, and many other activities also place stress on the circulo-respiratory system and, if done systematically and frequently, will improve the endurance of these systems.

There are two types of physical training that are related to oxygen intake. Anaerobic exercise is exercise without oxygen, while aerobic exercise is exercise requiring oxygen. Of course, all of life is dependent on oxygen consumption. Here we are actually referring to the amount of oxygen consumed and the degree to which the C-R system is involved in the exercise performed.

Exercise that is anaerobic usually falls into two classes: those exercises that require oxygen but are cut short voluntarily by the individual, and those exercises that demand too much oxygen so that the individual cannot complete them. An example of the first type is when you run a few seconds, then stop to "catch your breath." Here you have voluntarily stopped an exercise that could have put stress on your circulatory and respiratory systems. You may have stopped because you physically could not complete the running or because you did not wish to

run any longer. In the second class of anaerobic exercise, you may run a 100-yard dash and be forced to stop because you cannot take in enough oxygen. The only way to recover the oxygen you need is to stop the exercise. If a person slowly builds up his or her C-R endurance in a systematic manner, then exercises requiring oxygen consumption are much more efficient and easier to perform.

Aerobics are usually thought of as exercises that stimulate both the heart and lung activity long enough to produce beneficial changes in the body. There are many types of aerobic exercise, including walking, bicycling, and running long distances. Can you suggest other aerobic exercises that require C-R involvement?

All aerobic exercise makes the body work hard and in so doing increases the oxygen needs of the body. This is sometimes referred to as aerobic capacity. Aerobic capacity is dependent on the ability to breathe large amounts of air, deliver large volumes of blood, and to efficiently supply oxygen, as needed, to all parts of the body. Aerobic training is discussed in more detail in the following section of the chapter where the aerobics plan of Dr. Kenneth H. Cooper is explored.

Dr. Kenneth H. Cooper, a lieutenant colonel in the United States Air Force and a physician, has written and co-authored a number of books concerned with aerobics. His first book, *Aerobics,* was published in 1968 and resulted from studies to determine the effects of exercise on the human body, especially as it affected pilots and astronauts. More than 5,000 subjects were studied prior to the publication of *Aerobics.* Dr. Cooper concluded that the element which separates the "fit" from the "unfit" is the body's ability to deliver oxygen and that, in most cases, the energy demands of the body surpass one's capacity to produce oxygen.

Dr. Cooper frequently refers to the training effect in his books. This is defined by him, "as the changes induced by exercise in the various systems and organs of the body."

Kenneth H. Cooper almost singlehandedly started the fad for jogging. When he was in the Air Force, Dr. Cooper was asked to work out an exercise program for military men, and so he developed his "aerobics" system. Aerobics consists of exercise that increases the body's use of oxygen and strengthens the heart and lungs. According to Dr. Cooper, this is much more important than mere muscle building. That's why jogging—and swimming, and bicycling, and walking—are good for you.

This effect includes some of the following points:

A strengthening of the respiratory muscles and an increase in the rate air flows into and out of the lungs.

An improvement in both the strength and pumping efficiency of the heart. More blood is pumped with each stroke and there is an increased capability of oxygen transportation to the heart and other body parts.

Generally improved muscle tone and blood circulation. Blood pressure is frequently lowered, reducing the work load of the heart muscles.

An increase in the total amount of blood circulating in the body, increase in red blood cells and oxygen-carrying capacity of these cells.

The results of the training effect have been indicated scientifically in Dr. Cooper's studies. All of these effects have been documented numerous times in his and other laboratories. In his books he refers frequently to tests that "prove" the training effect.

Cooper stated in his book, *Aerobics,* that there are two basic conditions necessary for the training effect to take place. It will take place if the exercise is vigorous enough to produce a sustained heart rate of 150 beats per minute or more. In this case, the training effect would take place about five minutes after the exercise has started and will continue as long as the exercise is performed. The second principle says that if the exercise is not vigorous enough to produce or sustain a heart rate of 150 beats per minute, but is still demanding oxygen, the exercise must be continued considerably longer than five minutes, the total time required is dependent on the oxygen consumed.

The next question you may ask is how an average person knows his heart beat rate or the amount of oxygen consumed. The answer is found in Cooper's point system. Different activities were analyzed for the amount of oxygen they consumed and the increase in heart rate. Some exercises are more vigorous and demand greater amounts of oxygen than others. For example, if you walk a short distance daily, this would be considered an anaerobic exercise. An insufficient amount of oxygen is utilized and the exercise would not receive any points according to this system. However, if one were to walk a prescribed distance in a set time on a daily basis, then he would be doing an aerobic exercise. Cooper outlines different categories of exercise programs, distances, goal times, and frequency. He also assigns a point value to each of these programs. He has concluded that a man needs a total of 30 points a week in order to achieve and maintain the training effect and thus become a physically fit individual.

An example of Cooper's point system is as follows:

Running 1 mile in less than 8 minutes

Swimming 24 laps (600 yards) in less than 15 minutes

Cycling 5 miles in less than 20 minutes

Stationary running for a total of 12½ minutes

Handball played for a total of 35 minutes

Each of these exercises is worth five points. If they are done daily, six times a week, they would result in 30 points and would produce the training effect. Since points should be earned over a week's time, the individual should exercise daily. To earn 30 points in one day and do nothing for the rest of the week would not maintain the training effect. There are a variety of exercise programs and levels, and it is fairly easy to earn 30 points doing something that you enjoy. If you wish to pursue this program of exercise, read Dr. Cooper's book on *Aerobics* (available in paperback from Bantam Books).

Dr. Cooper followed *Aerobics* by another book published in 1970 entitled *New Aerobics.* This book follows the outline of the original *Aerobics* but expands it to include age adjustments, wider range of exercise options, and comprehensive data tables. It also discusses different exercise programs for women and problems that are often experienced by women that can be alleviated by exercise programs. In pursuing any of the *Aerobic* programs, it is essential to closely follow the author's plan and not exceed your capabilities. This is true for all persons, but particularly important for those who are older, not physically fit, and/or suffering from heart disease, obesity, or other chronic medical problems.

The latest book on aerobics is entitled *Aerobics for Women* and is co-authored by Mildred Cooper and her husband, Dr. Kenneth Cooper. They felt that the previous books did not give adequate coverage to exercise programs for women. Research has shown that a woman's aerobic capacity is smaller than the capacity of most men. Most women's hearts are also smaller as are their lung capacities and amounts of circulating blood. It was concluded that women need to earn approximately 24 points a week (instead of the 30 earned by men) in order to achieve the training effect. In this book, there are progressive, age-adjusted aerobic exercise programs, caloric value charts, exercise selector for burning up specific caloric amounts, exercise "menus," and new point evaluations that pertain to many activities that women perform in their daily routines.

What are the benefits of aerobic training in increasing the efficiency of the circulo-respiratory systems? There is an increase in the size and power of the heart muscle, enabling it to pump more blood per stroke and an increase in stroke volume. An "enlarged heart" from exercise is a heart that is powerful and has an increased number of capillaries that aid in coronary (heart) circulation. This type of "enlarged heart" is just the opposite of a heart enlarged as a result of disease. The disease-caused enlarged heart has thin walls and an average or below-average number of capillaries.

Aerobic training also increases the number of capillaries in the skeletal muscles as well as in the heart muscle. The improved circulation throughout the body allows for a more efficient performance of physical as well as mental tasks. Specifically, an increased number of capillaries in the heart helps to prevent serious heart attacks and makes recovery from heart attacks both easier and quicker. An increase in the capillaries of the lungs facilitates efficient exchange of oxygen and carbon dioxide. There is also an increase in the number of red blood cells, allowing more oxygen to be carried to the muscles. Of all the components of fitness, the circulo-respiratory element is extremely important because of the effect on the heart and circulation.

what does physical fitness mean to you?

Now that you are familiar with the components of physical fitness, you may be wondering how these components can be applied to making yourself physically fit. There are numerous types of exercise programs that attempt to achieve fitness as well as weight control, reduced tension, and general well-being. In this section some of these aspects of fitness are discussed.

HOW MUCH AND HOW OFTEN SHOULD ONE EXERCISE?

Each person has individual limits in exercise as well as other aspects of his or her life. It is accepted among medical professionals that exercise is an essential ingredient to health. The American Medical Association has recommended that individuals should exercise between one-half hour and an hour a day. This would be a minimum requirement. Exercise must be done on a daily basis so that satisfactory levels of strength, endurance, and flexibility are achieved. It is also essential that one put his or her whole self into the exercise programs so that vigorous breathing and heart action takes place.

If you are about to begin an exercise program, you should not look for immediate changes in weight loss or in general health. Exercise takes a while to work and if you are persistent, you will notice a gradual feeling of well-being. You will probably sleep more soundly and awake feeling fresh and ready to start the day. These expressions may sound "corny" but many individuals feel just this way after being involved in a fitness program. If you have been involved or are presently involved in a fitness regime, how do you feel? Has the program changed you in any way? If so, how has it changed you?

WHAT SHOULD ONE DO BEFORE BEGINNING A FITNESS PROGRAM?

It is advisable that anyone who is planning to start an individual fitness program should obtain a complete medical examination. This is true for people of all ages and is stressed because many individuals are not aware of physical conditions that may cause serious problems during strenuous exercise. Many individuals have suffered heart attacks or strokes while jogging or during an active tennis game.

Certain physical conditions must be carefully considered when planning an exercise program. If you are overweight, have high blood pressure or heart disease (or a family history of either), or are middle-aged, then your physician should help you to plan an exercise program. Physical exercise is important to individuals with these and other conditions, but it must be appropriate to the individual.

FITNESS PROGRAMS YOU MIGHT ENJOY

There are many fitness programs that young people are "into" today. Cycling, jogging, running, and yoga are only a few. If you do any of these on a regular basis, there are certain warm-up and conditioning exercises that will improve circulation, muscle tone, strength, posture, and will also contribute to flexibility and coordination. These "conditioners" can be found in any exercise manual and include such common exercises as stretching, bending, knee pulls, pull-ups,

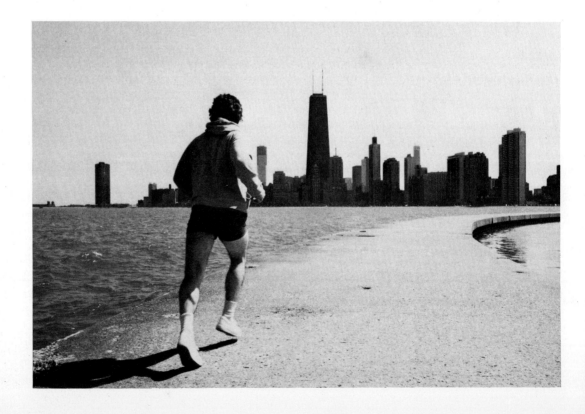

torso twisting, push-ups, and arm circles. You may already be familiar with many of these exercises.

Jogging is a slow running pace. It is often alternated with periods of walking so that a person can catch his or her breath. This activity became popular in the late 1960s after the publication of *Jogging* by Dr. W. E. Harris, W. J. Bowerman and J.M. Shea. This book presents a detailed jogging program. Many individuals enjoy jogging as a group and on some college campuses it is a social event. Groups of students will meet daily at a set time (usually early morning) and will jog together for a half-hour or longer. This time is usually spent in walking and jogging.

In any beginning program in jogging, one must gradually work up to a goal. Most programs start at a few minutes of jogging and walking for a total distance of one-half mile in a week. The book *Jogging* and other books or your physical education instructor will be very helpful in setting up a jogging program.

There are certain jogging guidelines suggested by the President's Council on Physical Fitness and Sports. They are given here for your consideration.

How to Jog. Run in an upright position, avoiding the tendency to lean. Keep your back as straight as you can and still remain comfortable, and keep your head up. Don't look at your feet.

Hold your arms slightly away from your body, with elbows bent so that the forearms are approximately parallel to the ground. Occasionally shaking and relaxing the arms and shoulders will help reduce the tightness that sometimes develops while jogging. Periodically taking several deep breaths and blowing them out completely also will help you to relax.

It is best to land on the heel of the foot and rock forward so that you drive off the ball of the foot for your next step. If this proves difficult, try a more flat-footed style. Jogging only on the balls of the feet, as in sprinting, will produce severe leg soreness.

Keep your steps short, letting the foot strike the ground beneath the knee instead of reaching to the front. Length of stride should vary with your rate of speed.

Breathe deeply, with your mouth open. Do not hold your breath.

If, for any reason, you become unusually tired or uncomfortable, slow down, walk, or stop.

What to Wear. Select loose, comfortable clothes. Dress for warmth in the winter, for coolness in the summer. "Jogging suits" or "warmups" are not necessary, but they are extremely practical and comfortable, and they can help create a feeling of commitment to jogging.

Do not wear rubberized or plastic clothing. Increased sweating will not produce permanent weight loss, and such clothing can cause body temperature to rise to dangerous levels. It interferes with evaporation of sweat, which is the body's chief temperature control mechanism during exercise. If sweat cannot evaporate, heat stroke or heat exhaustion may result.

Properly fitting shoes with firm soles, good arch supports, and pliable tops are essential. Shoes made especially for distance running or walking are recommended. Ripple or crepe soles are excellent for running on hard surfaces. Beginners should avoid inexpensive, thin-soled sneakers. Wear clean, soft, heavy, well-fitting socks. Beginners may want to wear thin socks under the heavier pair.

Where to Jog. If possible, avoid hard surfaces such as concrete and asphalt for the first few weeks. Running tracks (located at most high schools), grass playing fields, parks, and golf courses are recommended. In inclement weather, jog in school, recreation centers, in protected areas around shopping centers, or in your garage or basement. Varying locations and routes will add interest to your program.

When to Jog. The time of day is not important, although it is best not to jog during the first hour after eating, or during the middle of a hot, humid day. The important thing is to commit yourself to a regular schedule. Some believe that people who jog early in the morning tend to be more faithful than those who run in the evenings. Persons who jog with family members or friends also tend to adhere to their schedules better. However, companionship—not competition—should be your goal when jogging with someone else.

Illness or Injuries. Take care to prevent blisters, sore muscles, and aching joints. If you develop an illness, ask your physician about the advisability of continuing to jog. Any persistent pain or soreness also should be reported.

Cycling is an enjoyable and relaxing way of exercising. The energy crisis, too many

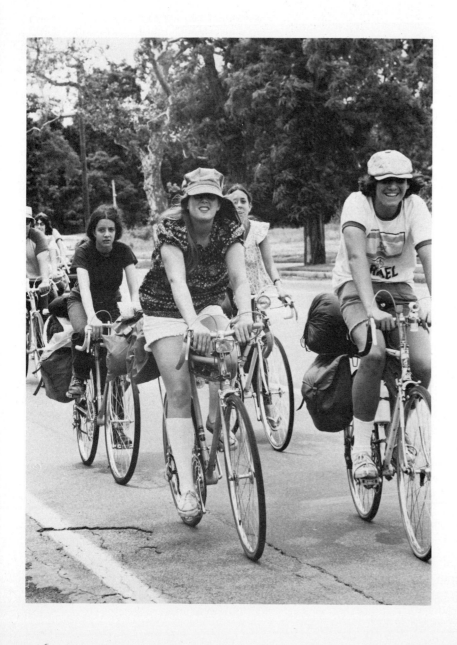

automobiles, and pollution has made cycling both a healthy and practical thing to do. Cycling is an excellent exercise to stimulate the circulatory and respiratory systems. It is also an excellent way to lose pounds and inches. It is a social sport where groups can exercise together or become involved in bicycle trips that often tour for many days at a time. As with other exercise programs, one must work up to a number of set goals in order to increase endurance. The book *Cycling* by Roy Ald may be helpful to you in planning an exercise program based on cycling.

A number of people have become interested in health clubs, spas, exercise clubs, or other such groups. They are usually advertised in a glorified manner that promises extensive weight loss in addition to a fitness program. Some of these clubs are legitimate and if you follow all of their instructions to the letter and carefully watch your diet, you will lose weight. However, others are "fly-by-night" enterprises that go out of business with great frequency and leave you holding a year's contract that has been paid in full. It is best to check the company out with the Better Business Bureau in your area prior to signing any contract for such an exercise program.

EXERCISE AND HEART DISEASE

Coronary heart disease kills more than 700,000 Americans every year. The subject is discussed in detail in Chapter 15. There are many factors that contribute to heart disease of this type, and a lack of physical activity has been indicated as a definite risk factor. Comparisons of sedentary individuals to those who are active indicate that the risk and actual heart attack rate is decidedly greater among the sedentary individuals. In a recent study by a United States Health Service team in Framingham, Massachusetts, results indicated that the most sedentary men in every age group had an incidence of coronary heart disease that was twice that of those persons who were at least moderately active.

One can assume that exercise is related to disease prevention as well as a general feeling of well-being. Studies indicate that a moderate level of physical activity throughout life is one of those factors that act to inhibit coronary heart disease. Do you know any one who has recently suffered from a heart attack? If so, had he or she been engaged in some type of fitness program prior to the attack?

EXERCISE AND RELAXATION

Exercise should be performed with a relaxed attitude. There are many types of exercise programs that are both recreational as well as healthful. If an exercise program is extremely rigid and not enjoyable, then it is self-defeating. Try to find an activity or group of activities that are enjoyable to you. Frequently, a group activity is the answer. Even push-ups are more fun when there are ten or more people grunting and groaning along with you.

There are many exercise techniques that can help to relieve tension and allow you to feel relaxed. In any of these exercises, it is important to forget the world around you and concentrate only on yourself—your body. It is best to be alone and in a quiet room. Soft music may be helpful to make you forget about extraneous thoughts. Try to sit quietly and think of something pleasant. Then think about your body and consciously try to relax those areas that are tense. Sometimes it is easier to lie flat on the floor and slowly think of each part of your body and try to relax it. Some persons find themselves almost falling asleep after this exercise. Sometimes, it is helpful to imagine you are a rag doll and that every part of your body is free and loose.

As you can see from the above exercise techniques, *exercise* does not always mean a strenuous activity. There are all forms of exercise; some exercises originate in the mind and then are extended to the body. Whatever exercise program you choose, it should be enjoyable and beneficial to you as an individual for that is the true goal of a fitness program.

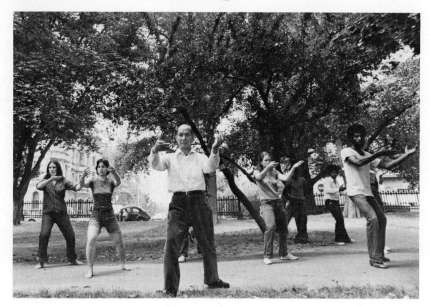

Exercise from China: the nonstrenuous harmony of body and mind in *T'ai ch'i chuan.* Here a T'ai ch'i master practices with his pupils in Boston.

THINKING IT OVER

1. Why is it difficult to define the term *physical fitness?*
2. How would you define the term physical fitness? How does your definition differ from that of the text?
3. What is meant by the term *total body fitness?* Do you think that most individuals consider *total fitness?* Explain your answer.
4. What is hypokinetic disease? What types of individuals would be most prone to to the effects of this disease?
5. Discuss the results of the recent adult physical fitness survey. Do you agree or disagree with these results? Explain your answer.
6. Discuss some example of how automation interferes with physical fitness.
7. Why is it difficult to separate the components of fitness?
8. Discuss the differences between isometric and isotonic exercise. Give examples.
9. Explain how muscular strength and muscular endurance differ from one another.
10. Discuss the meaning and factors that affect flexibility.
11. What is circulo-respiratory endurance? What are some of the benefits to C-R efficiency that are obtained from aerobic training?
12. Discuss Dr. Cooper's *Aerobics* and the benefits of such a program.
13. What should an individual do before he or she begins to exercise regularly?
14. Discuss jogging and some of the guidelines that should be followed in participating in this activity.
15. What are some of the exercise techniques that can be utilized in reducing tension? Can you add any techniques to those discussed in the text?

KEY WORDS

Aerobic training. Training that utilizes oxygen and increases the effiiciency of the C-R systems (also a method of training introduced by Dr. Kenneth H. Cooper).

Anaerobic training. Training that does not increase the efficiency of the C-R systems (without oxygen).

Circulo-respiratory endurance. Adjustments of the circulatory and respiratory systems to moderate contractions of large muscle groups for relatively long periods of time.

Dynamometer. A calibrated instrument that measures muscular strength.

Flexibility. The range of motion at a joint.

Hypokinetic disease (Krauss–Raab). A number of conditions linked to a lack of physical exercise.

Isometric strength. A contraction against a resistance that is too great to overcome.

Isotonic strength. Lifting an object through a range of motion.

Jogging. A rapid rhythmical walking or slow run that is excellent for C-R endurance.

Krauss–Raab effect. See *hypokinetic disease.*

Muscular endurance. The ability of muscles to perform work, either by sustained muscular contractions (isometric) or by continuing to raise and lower a submaximal load (isotonic).

Muscular power. Strength of muscles and speed of movement.

Muscular strength. Strength of muscles as determined by a single maximum contraction that may be measured by calibrated instruments.

Physical fitness. A level of physical energy that will enable one to comfortably perform his daily routine and have enough in reserve to meet unexpected physical emergencies.

Tensiometer. A calibrated instrument that measures muscular strength.

Total body fitness. Mental, social, and physical fitness.

GETTING INVOLVED

Books and Periodicals

Ald, Roy, *Cycling.* New York: Grossset and Dunlap, 1968. A complete discussion of the sport and exercise of cycling.

American Association for Health, Physical Education, and Recreation; and the American Medical Association. *Exercise and Fitness.* Washington, D.C.: 1964. Authoritative advice about keeping fit.

Bowerman, William J., W. E. Harris, and James M. Shea. *Jogging.* New York: Grosset and Dunlap, 1967. Jogging in detail, with a complete jogging program.

Cooper, Kenneth H. *The New Aerobics.* New York: M. Evans, 1970. Exercising the circulatory system as well as the muscles.

_____ and Cooper, Mildred. *Aerobics for Women.* New York: Bantam, 1973. Aerobics adapted to the female body.

Physical Fitness Research Digest, published quarterly by the President's Council on Physical Fitness and Sports. A series of reports about recent trends in physical fitness.

Rossman, Isadore, and Obeck, Victor. *Isometrics: The Static Way to Physical Fitness.* New York: Stravon Educational Press, 1966. Exercise without exertion.

Royal Canadian Air Force. *Royal Canadian Air Force Exercise Plans for Physical Fitness.* New York: Essandess, n.d. Popular exercise program.

Movies

The Loneliness of the Long Distance Runner, with Tom Courtenay, Michael Redgrave, 1962. A young man is forced to trade in on his sports talents. Distributed by Clem Williams, Twyman, and Walter Reade 16.

The Fitness Challenge. Why keeping fit is important. Distributed by the American Osteopathic Association.

12
NUTRITIONAL NEEDS AND THE FOODS YOU BUY

Can you be totally healthy without adequate nutrition? This is one of the subjects explored in this chapter. The chapter examines why it is necessary for humans (and most animals) to eat food. The word "calories" is defined and related to the food we eat.

Nutrients are the basic components of food. In this chapter, you will learn about the basic nutrients and how they are utilized by the body. Controversies that presently exist concerning nutrients are explored and discussed. Cholesterol, vitamins, and food supplements are also discussed.

What is a balanced diet? Many people have heard the term but have either forgotten or never knew what was meant by it. A balanced diet consists of food from the four basic food groups. These groups and how they should be used to select a balanced diet are discussed.

The food you buy is an interesting topic that includes such areas as why we buy certain foods, advertising of food products, planning menus, and the nutritional needs of pregnant women, children, teenagers, and adults. The final topic of this chapter examines nutritional misconceptions (additives and organic foods) and nutritional myths. This chapter will give you a basic understanding of nutrition and how you can provide for your own nutritional needs in the most efficient and economical way.

While reading this chapter,

think about the following concepts:

■ Good nutrition is essential for good health.

■ All living things need food.

■ One's diet must be balanced in order to be nutritious.

■ Vitamins and food supplements are generally not needed if one has a balanced diet.

■ The food one buys is often influenced by factors other than nutritional needs.

■ Nutritional needs vary for different age groups and physical conditions.

■ Nutritional misconceptions and myths definitely exist today.

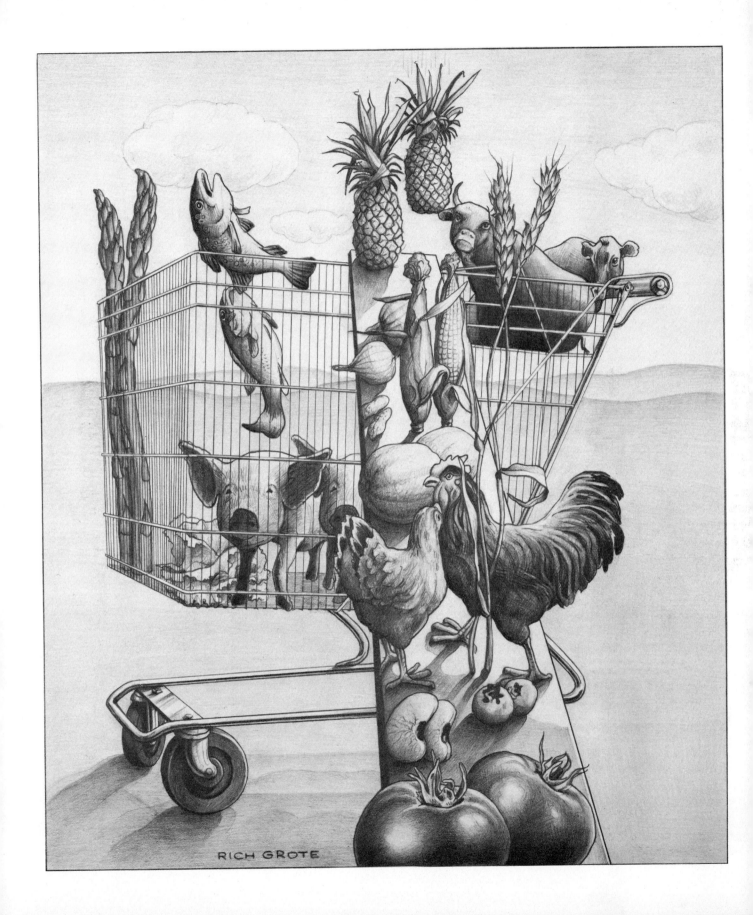

RICH GROTE

Do you eat many of the foods that are advertised on television? If you do, your nutrition is probably inadequate. In a recent massive computer study of network television advertising, 473 food products advertised during a four-month period in 1971 were "scored" as to their nutritional content. Products were given numerical ratings based on the presence or absence of vitamins, minerals, proteins, and other nutrients. They were also rated on nutrients added or left out during processing. The highest possible score was 100, the lowest score was minus 200. The television-advertised products rated below zero according to this study.

What do you think are the implications of such a study? One can conclude that a great deal of money is being spent on the production and advertising of food substances lacking in nutritional value. In fact, annual spending on food advertising is estimated to be more than 3.5 billion dollars. People are responding to such advertising and buying many "junk" foods—those without nutritional value. Many people are unaware of what comprises a nutritionally balanced meal. In this chapter, you will become familiar with the subject of nutrition and become aware of what to look for when purchasing food products.

food and nutrition

Good nutrition is essential to good health. One cannot be *totally* healthy unless one has good nutritional habits, and a healthy, attractive appearance is linked to nutrition. Many physical conditions such as heart disease, diabetes, vitamin-deficiency diseases, and other physical problems can be controlled under dietary supervision. A knowledge of nutrition is essential to good health and to disease control and prevention.

All living things need food in order to survive. Food is necessary to support growth, repair wearing tissue, supply energy, and ensure proper physical and mental functioning. Nutrition is necessary *before* birth as well as *following* birth. Prenatal nutrition (before birth) is an important factor in the growth and development of the fetus. This is discussed in more detail later in this chapter.

Food supplies calories. These are units of food energy that provide the necessary energy for activity and heat production. You are probably familiar with the word *calorie* from diet books that tell one how many calories are contained in a certain amount of a food product. Excess calories are stored in the body in the form of fat. This fat is actually an energy reserve that the body can use when it needs to produce more activity or heat. However, one can have *too* much of an energy reserve of fat and that may lead to obesity (a condition where one is considerably overweight). Obesity and weight control are discussed in Chapter 13.

nutrients found in food

Nutrients are the substances found in foods that the body can utilize to produce energy, build and repair tissue, and regulate body functions. Some foods contain many nutrients in adequate quantities, where other foods are completely lacking in nutrient value.

Nutrients may be divided into the following groups: carbohydrates, fats, proteins, minerals, water, vitamins, and fibers. Each of these essential nutrients is found in many food products (see Table 12-1). However, some foods have a greater nutrient value than others. When choosing foods to supply certain nutrient values, one should try to choose those that are highest in nutrient content.

PROTEINS

Proteins are the basic material that makes up the cells of the body. They are needed for growth, maintenance, and repair of body tissue. Proteins contain carbon, hydrogen, oxygen, nitrogen, and usually sulfur. They may also contain some iron, phosphorus, iodine, and copper. During digestion, food proteins are broken down into amino acids which are the basic chemical compounds that make up proteins. The amino acids are often referred to as *building blocks* because no body tissue can be built without them. Some amino acids can be produced by the body, while others, called the essential amino acids, must be derived from certain foods. Those amino acids not used in building tissue are used as a source of energy.

There are eight essential amino acids. These amino acids must be furnished in the diet because the body cannot manufacture them. Proteins that contain many of the essential amino acids that are high in nutritional value include:

1. eggs and dairy products
2. meat, fish, and poultry
3. beans, grain, cereals, and nuts

Eggs and dairy products are good sources of protein. Milk does not have a large amount of protein, but the protein it does have is of an excellent quality. Most foods that are high in protein contain considerable amounts of water and fat (except for bean products) and little or no carbohydrates. Meat, fish, and poultry are excellent sources of protein; cereals and other grain products yield somewhat less protein and do contain carbohydrates. One should consume a combination of foods and animal and plant protein that contain the essential amino acids.

Think about your food intake so far today. Have any of the foods been high in protein content? Do you *think* about what you consume during your meals and do you make an effort to supply the nutrients that your body needs each day?

CARBOHYDRATES

Most of you who have had to diet are probably familiar with the word carbohydrate. Carbohydrates are the food substances to watch out for when trying to shed those excess pounds. What makes up a carbohydrate? Chemically a carbohydrate is composed of carbon, hydrogen, and oxygen. Starches and sugars are carbohydrates. They are the most economical sources of body energy that are available. Carbohydrates are

essential to the functioning of the body. They serve as sources of energy and are important in the maintenance of body temperature. They are necessary for the normal burning of fat and are a source of energy for the central nervous system.

Common sources of carbohydrates include cereals and their products such as bread and baked goods, breakfast cereals, rice, and noodles, most vegetables and fruit, as well as sugar and honey. Milk and most milk products also contain a certain amount of carbohydrates.

An excess of carbohydrates is converted into fat and stored as fatty tissue. Too many carbohydrates may cause obesity, and other problems that result from too much sugar in the body may also become evident. These problems include dental caries, increased triglyceride levels, and irritation of the digestive lining (which may aggravate ulcer conditions). A high *triglyceride level* is recognized as a contributory factor in heart disease. Triglycerides—fats found in high-carbohydrate foods—may clog the coronary arteries and increase the chance of blood clotting. Cholesterol (a fat product) is linked to heart disease in a similar way. It is discussed in a later section of this chapter.

Some people go on low-carbohydrate diets in order to lose weight. This is acceptable as long as there is some carbohydrate in the diet. People who are accustomed to eating adequate or excessive carbohydrates may need more than other people when they begin to restrict their carbohydrate intake. Insufficient carbohydrate intake can result in excessive protein breakdown.

Do you eat a lot of carbohydrate foods? Many Americans do. In fact the per capita consumption of sugar is said to exceed 1.5 pounds of sugar per week. Much of this sugar is found in soft drinks, as refined sugar, in alcohol, and in other foods. These foods are considered "empty" because, except for the calories they provide, they are completely lacking in nutritional value. Think about the number of "empty" calories you consume in a day. If you tend to gain weight easily and are not very active physically,

Table 12-1

Nutrient	Foods That Supply Important Amounts	Some Reasons Why You Need It
Protein	Meat, fish, poultry, eggs All kinds of cheese Milk Cereals and breads Dried beans and peas Peanut butter, nuts	To build and repair all tissues in the body To help form substances in the blood which are called "antibodies" and which fight infection To supply energy
Carbohydrate (sugar and starch)	Breads and cereals Potatoes and corn Dried fruits, sweetened fruits Smaller amounts in fresh fruits Sugar, syrup, jelly, jam, honey	To supply energy
Fat	Butter and cream Salad oils and dressings Cooking and table fats Fat meats	To supply a large amount of energy in a small amount of food To help keep skin smooth and healthy by supplying substances called "essential fatty acids" To carry vitamins A,D,E,K
Vitamin A	Orange fruits, dark green and orange vegetables Butter, whole milk, vitamin A fortified lowfat and skim milk, cream, cheddar-type cheese, ice cream Liver, eggs	To help keep skin smooth and soft To help keep mucous membranes firm and resistant to infection To protect against night blindness and promote healthy eyes
Vitamin C or Ascorbic acid	Citrus fruits—lemon, orange, grapefruit, lime Strawberries, cantaloupe Tomatoes Green peppers, broccoli Raw or lightly cooked greens, cabbage White potatoes	To make cementing materials that hold body cells together To make walls of blood vessels firm To help resist infection To help prevent fatigue To help in healing wounds and broken bones

these "empty" calories can begin to add up in the form of extra pounds of fat.

FATS

Fat is primarily a source of energy. Fats produce more than twice as much energy as proteins or carbohydrates. Fats are made from a combination of fatty acids and glycerol. They contain the elements of carbon and hydrogen (in large amounts) and a small amount of oxygen. Approximately 40 percent of the American diet is based on calories from fats. Americans also eat more animal fats than plant fats.

Fats are essential, in the proper quantity, to good health. Besides being a rich source of energy, fats provide padding around the vital organs of the body. The fat layer protects these organs and also acts as an insulation to help keep in body heat. Fats slow

Nutrient	Foods That Supply Important Amounts	Some Reasons Why You Need It

Thiamin (B_1), Riboflavin (B_2), and Niacin	Meat, fish and poultry
	Eggs, dried peas and beans
	Milk, cheese and ice cream
	Whole grain and enriched
	  breads and cereals
	White potatoes
		To play a central role in the
		  release of energy from food
		To help the nervous system
		  function properly
		To help keep appetite and
		  digestion normal
		To help keep skin healthy

Calcium	Milk Cheese, especially cheddar-type Yogurt Ice cream Turnip and mustard greens Collards, kale, broccoli Canned sardines, salmon	To help build bones, teeth To help make blood clot To help muscles react normally To delay fatigue and help tired muscles recover

Iron	Liver
	Meat, eggs, and dried legumes
	Enriched and whole grain bread,
	  cereals
	Green leafy vegetables
	Raisins, dried apricots
		To combine with protein to make
		  hemoglobin, the red substance
		  in the blood that carries
		  oxygen to the cells

Vitamin D
or
The sunlight vitamin
	Vitamin D milk
	Fish liver oil
	Sunlight (not a food!)
		To help the body absorb calcium
		  from digestive tract
		To help build calcium and
		  phosphorus into bones

Vitamin B_6
 	
Folic acid (Folacin)
 	
Vitamin B_{12}
	Vitamin B_6—meats, potatoes
	  dark green leafy vegetables,
	  whole grains and dry beans
	Folacin—green vegetables, whole
	  grains and dry beans
	Vitamin B_{12}—milk, cheese, eggs
	  and meats
	All three B-vitamins—organ meats
		To help prevent anemia
		To help enzyme and other
		  biochemical systems function
		  normally

Iodine	Seafoods
	Iodized salt
		To make thyroxine, an essential
		  hormone that regulates
		  metabolic rate
		To prevent (simple) goiter

Adapted from "A Girl and Her Figure," by Ruth M. Leverton, Copyright National Dairy Council, 1955, 1970, 1975. National Dairy Council, Chicago 60606.

digestion and give one the feeling of being "full" for a longer period of time. Fat carries the fat-soluble vitamins A, D, E, and H. Essential fatty acids are necessary for body functions. Fats also add flavor to many foods.

Cholesterol, though potentially harmful in large amounts, is essential to the production of many hormones.

As we have learned fat is essential to normal body functioning; however, too much fat can be harmful and in some cases life-threatening. Excess fat in the diet may result in obesity. Obesity can cause additional demands on the heart and other body organs.

People who are obese are more prone to such conditions as heart failure, diabetes, and kidney failure. They are also more likely to have a shorter life span and face a greater risk during surgery. Excess fats may slow digestion and absorption of food for too long a period of time. Excess fat also contributes to circulatory disease, especially coronary artery disease.

The term cholesterol is a familiar one to most of us. It is commonly used today in advertising, and most people are aware that it is a contributory factor in heart disease. What is cholesterol? Cholesterol is a fatty alcohol found in animal and dairy fats, egg yolks, and in cocoanut oils and chocolate. Cholesterol is a normal component of the blood and is essential to the growth and functioning of body cells, nerve cells, and nerve tissue. Although cholesterol is vital to body functioning, in excess it can cause problems. One condition that it is linked to is atherosclerosis (coronary artery disease). In atherosclerosis, deposits of cholesterol and other substances form inside the coronary arteries (the heart's circulatory system) and begin to close up these passageways. Eventually the artery may be completely blocked off and a blood clot may form. This would be called a heart attack. This subject is discussed in detail in Chapter 14.

What are the sources of fats in foods? Common sources include meats, butter, cream, cheese, whole milk, mayonnaise, egg yolks, and peanut butter. Other foods high in fat are lard, oils, cocoanut, chocolate, and nuts.

You may have heard the terms *saturated, monounsaturated,* and *polyunsaturated.* These terms are used to describe the kinds of fatty acids found in foods. There are about 20 different kinds of fatty acids. Those foods that contain polyunsaturated fatty acids are also low in cholesterol. Some foods in this group include corn, cottonseed, safflower,

soybean, and sunflower oils; walnuts; margarine, fish and mayonnaise, and salad dressings prepared with the previously mentioned oils.

As with the other nutrients discussed, fats play an important role in body functioning. When you go on a diet, do *not* restrict *all* fat intake. Avoid dietary extremes and make sure that any diet includes all of the essential nutrients. Your doctor should be consulted before beginning any dietary program.

MINERALS

Minerals are essential to building bones, teeth, muscles, blood, and nerve cells. They help in the regulation of water and acids and bases in the body. It is important that they be supplied daily as they are excreted from the body at a rapid rate.

Minerals are important in the formation of bones and teeth and in the building of new tissues. Mineral-rich foods are essential during growth, pregnancy, and if the mother is breast-feeding her baby. Some of the most critical minerals include: calcium, phosphorus, iron, iodine, sodium, fluorine, and potassium. Each of these minerals, their functions, and food sources is briefly discussed.

CALCIUM

Calcium is essential to the building of bones and teeth. About 99 percent of the total body calcium is found in these structures. Calcium gives bones and teeth their strength and rigidity. Other functions of calcium include: (1) muscle contraction; (2) blood clotting; (3) maintaining acid–base balance; and (4) response of nerve fibers and nerve cells. The primary food sources of calcium include milk products, green leafy vegetables (except spinach), broccoli, cauliflower, and cabbage. Small amounts are found in citrus fruits and bread. A lack of calcium can result in poorly formed bones and teeth, slow blood clotting, and rickets (a disease of children where bones are malformed and brittle).

PHOSPHORUS

Phosphorus has many functions in the human body, including maintenance of acid–base balance, adding rigidity to bones and teeth, utilization of carbohydrates and their conversion to energy, and as a component of every body cell nucleus. Phosphorus is found in milk, cheese, meats, egg yolks, fish, nuts, and certain cereals. Diets that are adequate in protein and calcium are also usually adequate in phosphorus.

IRON

Iron is an essential component of hemoglobin (a part of the red blood cells that unites with oxygen). Iron is essential to the production of new red blood cells and is stored in the liver, bone marrow, and spleen. A deficiency in iron can result in anemia (a condition where there are too few red blood cells), red blood cells of irregular shape, or cells that do not have sufficient hemoglobin. Sources of iron include liver, red meats, yellow fruits, enriched cereals, potatoes, and tomatoes.

IODINE

Iodine is essential in the functioning of the thyroid gland. Insufficient iodine may result in an enlarged thyroid gland, low energy level, sluggish metabolism, stunted growth, and retardation. Sources of iodine include sea foods and iodized salt.

SODIUM

Sodium is essential to body functioning. It makes up a portion of the fluid found outside of the cells. It also helps to maintain acid–base equilibrium, nerve function, and water balance. Some individuals may have edema (a condition where too much water is stored in the body). For these individuals, low-sodium diets may be prescribed. This type of diet will reduce excess body fluid. Sodium is found in table salt, baking soda, baking powder, milk, cheese, egg white, meat, carrots, spinach, and beets. In some areas, the drinking water is high in sodium content.

FLUORINE

You may be familiar with this mineral because it has been the subject of controversy in recent years. Fluorine has been added to the drinking water of some communities because research has indicated that it protects teeth from decay. However, too much fluorine has been known to cause mottling or discoloration of the tooth enamel. In general, one can say that fluorine strengthens teeth and makes them more resistant to mouth bacteria. In fact, some dentists give children fluoride applications to strengthen their teeth and some children's vitamins contain fluorine. Fluorine may be found in the water supply and in small amounts in certain foods.

Does your community have a fluoridated water supply? Find out if it does. If it doesn't, try to determine why. When such questions appear in referenda they are often rejected by the public because the population may not be aware of the significant value of fluoride.

POTASSIUM

Potassium is found in the body fluids and is essential for normal functioning. It is important as a regulator of water balance, acid–base balance, carbohydrate metabolism, nerve function, and muscle contraction. Potassium is found in many foods, including whole grains, beans, prunes, oranges, bananas, and raisins. Most people receive adequate amounts of potassium in a well-balanced diet. However, there are some conditions that produce potassium deficiencies. Some of these conditions include severe burns, diarrhea, vomiting, and prolonged use of drugs called diuretics (drugs used to remove excess water from the body). Some individuals wrongly use diuretics for purposes of weight reduction. They should only be used under a doctor's care for a specific physical condition.

VITAMINS

Vitamins are compounds needed in small

amounts for normal growth, development, and body functioning. Vitamins of different types are found in many different foods but all essential vitamins are not found in one specific food. Each vitamin has a specific function. Most balanced diets contain an adequate vitamin supply, and few people need additional vitamin supplements. (This fact is explored later in this section.)

There are two basic groups of vitamins: (1) the fat-soluble vitamins and (2) the water-soluble vitamins. The fat-soluble vitamins include A, D, E, and K and they are: (1) usually not destroyed by cooking; (2) can be stored in the body; (3) and are destroyed by aging. The water-soluble vitamins are C and B complex and they are: (1) usually affected by cooking; (2) have little or no body storage; and (3) can be lost in the discarded cooking or soaking water. Fat-soluble vitamins are usually found in liver, eggs, butter, and meats. Water-soluble vitamins are found in fruits, vegetables, grains, beans, and lean meats. Milk contains both types of these vitamin groups.

Vitamins have been the subject of controversy for many years. Many experts in vitamin research feel that their studies indicate that people can improve certain conditions with high dosages of particular vitamins. For example, Linus Pauling, a well-known and respected scientist, has presented data that indicates high dosages of vitamin C will prevent colds and can prevent or improve other conditions. However, this theory is still being debated. In recent studies, subjects who believed they were being given vitamin C, but were really given placebos (sugar pills), reported fewer colds; those who had

Vitaminman!

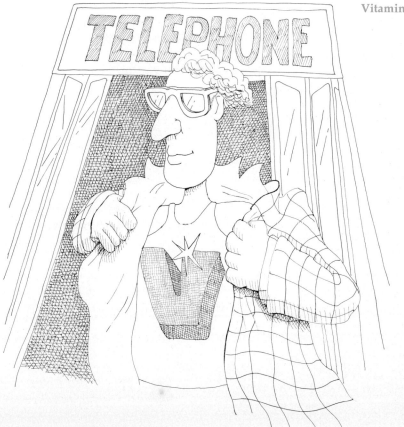

received vitamin C reported no change in the number of colds.

Do we need extra vitamins in our diet? The simplest, purest, and most economical way to obtain sufficient daily vitamins is to select foods from each of the four basic food groups: milk, meat, vegetables, and fruit, and the bread–cereal group. Only in specialized conditions do people need to take multivitamin supplements or high dosages of a specific vitamin.

Too much of any one vitamin can do more harm than good as illustrated by the fact that Poison Control Centers are reporting more than 4,000 cases of vitamin poisoning each year. About 3,200 of these cases involve children. Two vitamins that have been found to be very dangerous in excess amounts are vitamins A and D. Excessive amounts of vitamin A taken over a long period of time can increase pressure within the skull and may mimic a brain tumor. It may also retard growth in children, cause dry and cracked skin, headaches, and bone pain. Excessive doses of vitamin D have been known to retard mental as well as physical growth in children. Overdoses can also cause nausea, weakness, constipation, hypertension, and death.

Because of these findings, the Food and Drug Administration (FDA) prohibits, except by prescription, any daily recommended intake of a tablet or capsule of more than 10,000 IU (International Units) of vitamin A and 400 IU of vitamin D. The strength and labeling of each package is also controlled. Presently, a controversy exists as to whether large dosages of other vitamins should be restricted by prescription or amounts to be sold at one time. Many people feel that they have the right to buy as much of a product as they want in order to follow a particular dietary regimen. However, the FDA feels that people must be made aware of the harmful effects of excess vitamins. Research is now being conducted to identify how much of a vitamin is too much, conditions that may be helped by large dosages of a vitamin, and how a specific vitamin affects all of the body systems.

Do you respond to vitamin advertising on television? The ads usually show healthy-looking men or women of middle age who watch their weight, exercise, eat right, and take "brand X" vitamins or vitamin supplement. The vitamin, of course, is precautionary or "just to be sure." The implication is that they wouldn't look or feel as they do if they didn't take that little pill every morning. Do you take a daily multivitamin or large dosages of certain vitamins? If so why do you do so? If not, why have you made this decision?

The same problem exists with children's vitamins. They come in all colors and shapes from bunny rabbits to monsters. Does the child really need this vitamin? If the parents spent the money on the basic foods, vitamins would not be necessary at all. Most children's diets are adequate to supply their vitamin needs. In fact, the children who least need the extra vitamins (those from middle class and upper-middle class homes) are the ones who are probably taking these highly advertised products. Problems of children's vitamins include: (1) vitamin poisoning; (2) a dependency on vitamins that may continue into adulthood; (3) looking to pills for protection; and (4) excess sugar that can affect teeth.

There are many books available that will tell you how much of a food contains a certain number of vitamin units. However, as previously stated a balanced diet will provide all the essential vitamins.

WATER AND FIBER OR ROUGHAGE

Many of us do not think about water as being essential to our health. However, water composes about 70 percent of the human body and we lose from two to three quarts daily in the form of perspiration, vapor from the lungs, urine, and in the feces. The reason we don't think about water is that it is commonly found in most foods and drinks and our sensation of thirst usually informs us when more is needed. Water requirements vary and may be dependent on the individual, environmental temperature, and amount

Poison Control Centers exist in many communities. They are usually affiliated with local departments of health, hospitals, or medical schools, and their goal is to reduce deaths from poisoning. Available by telephone 24 hours a day, the centers give first-aid instructions to victims of accidental poisonings; and many centers also provide treatment information to physicians.

The Food and Drug Administration (FDA) is a federal agency charged with protecting the population against unsafe foods, drugs, and other substances. The agency is also responsible for developing standards of good nutrition. The labels you see on food nowadays—those that list the percentage of "recommended daily allowances" of nutrients the products contain—are based on FDA research.

of physical activity. Most individuals need about four to six glasses of water per day or equivalent water in foods or other drinks.

Fiber of roughage (sometimes called bulk) is needed for the proper functioning of the intestines. This material acts as a stimulus to the intestines and allows for normal bowel movements. Bulk is found in the outer coating of grains, in vegetables, and fruit. Cellulose is a fibrous material found in many plants. It is not digested and helps stimulate the intestines.

need for a balanced diet

When you first heard the word "nutrition," its definition was probably followed by a listing of the four basic food groups. Do you remember them and do you think about them when planning your meals? If someone else plans your meals, have they included foods from each of these groups in your daily diet?

If you are eating at a university cafeteria, foods from each of these groups is probably available, but are you choosing them?

THE FOUR BASIC FOOD GROUPS

There are four basic food groups that will supply an adequate nutritional diet if foods are chosen from each group daily. The groups are as follows:

1. *Milk and milk products* (two or more servings daily). Milk products include fluid whole, 2 percent homogenized, skim, buttermilk, evaporated skimmed, instant nonfat dry milk. Cheese products include cottage, cream, cheddar-type cheeses. Ice cream, cream, sour cream, and other dairy products are all in this group.
2. *Meat and meat substitutes* (two or more servings daily). Meat products include

The four basic food groups.

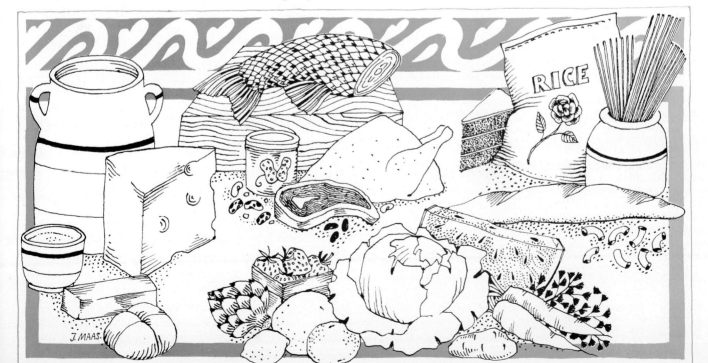

meat, poultry, and fish. Substitutes for meat include dried beans, peas and lentils, eggs and cheese, peanuts, peanut butter, and nuts. The substitutes, like meat products, are high in protein value as well as vitamin content.
3. *Fruits and vegetables* (four or more servings daily). Included in this group are citrus fruits, fruit juices, or vegetables; dark green and bright yellow fruits or vegetables; and potatoes.
4. *Breads and cereals* (four or more servings daily). Breads that are whole grained or enriched, crackers, and baked goods are all included in this group. In addition, cereal, corn meal, grits, rice, macaroni, spaghetti, and noodles are a part of this group.

A variety of foods from each group are necessary to supply the nutrients essential to normal growth, development, and bodily function. In certain conditions, such as heart disease, diabetes, obesity, and ulcers, special diets are necessary to prevent the condition from becoming worse. Infants, children, and older people also need diets that are suitable for their age. Some of these specialized diets are discussed in the section, "The Food You Buy." In that section, meal planning is also discussed.

VITAMIN OR FOOD SUPPLEMENTS

Vitamin or food supplements usually combine a variety of vitamins and other compounds that are taken as a supplement to one's daily diet. Sometimes these supplements become faddist and are very popular for a brief period of time. For example, recently a combination of kelp and lecithin, which is sold over the counter as are most food supplements, came in vogue as a weight-reduction aid.

Are these supplements useful in any way? The answer is generally "no." They are not necessary if one follows a balanced diet. Recent regulations established by the FDA included food supplements. Some of these

regulations are cited below for your consideration.

1. No food or dietary supplement, because of the presence or absence of certain vitamins or minerals, may claim or suggest it is sufficient in itself to prevent or cure disease.
2. No food or dietary supplement may imply that a balanced diet of conventional foods cannot supply adequate nutrients or imply that transportation, storage, or cooking of conventional foods may result in an inadequate or deficient diet, thus suggesting that everyone needs a dietary supplement.
3. No food or dietary supplement may claim that inadequate or deficient diet is a result of the soil in which a conventional food is grown.
4. All dietary supplements must list the source of their ingredients, but no supplement may claim superiority for either a natural or synthetic source. Rose hips, a part of the rose blossom, for example, cannot be promoted as a better or safer source of vitamin C than ascorbic acid tablets. (Vitamins and minerals are the same in chemical structure regardless of natural or synthetic origin.)

How do you feel about vitamin and food supplements? Do you agree or disagree that they are usually not necessary if one eats a balanced diet? Explain your viewpoint and be prepared to back it up with research material.

food you buy
What kinds of foods do people buy? When walking down the aisles of a food market, what influences our purchases? There are many reasons why we select certain foods and reject others. Most people will buy foods, to some extent, in order to satisfy basic nutritional needs. Foods are also chosen because they are economical; this is especially true if one is on a limited food budget, which most people are today.

Vitamin Supplements tend to disappoint people who are looking for a quick cure or a magic change in their bodies. In fact, abnormally large doses of vitamins can cause physical damage. For most people, a balanced diet provides a sufficient amount of vitamins—and besides, it's less expensive than vitamin supplements.

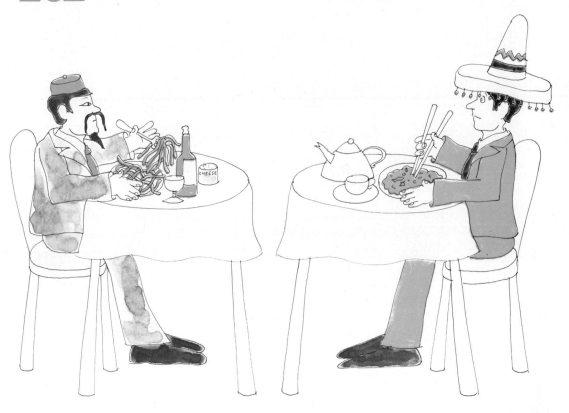

Individuals will also buy foods that are easy to prepare or are necessary for special diets.

FACTORS THAT INFLUENCE FOOD SELECTION

Think about some of the foods that you and your family enjoy. Many of them may be ethnic in origin. People from Spanish, Italian, Jewish, Oriental, and other backgrounds may purchase certain foods that they were accustomed to eating in their parents' homes. It is difficult to break these eating patterns and *not important* to break them if the necessary nutrients are being provided.

Unfortunately, many people either are not aware or cannot afford to provide adequate diets for themselves and their families. In a recent National Nutrition Survey, more than 80,000 people in ten states were interviewed. One-fourth of those people were living below the poverty level and were suffering from malnutrition. Though inexpensive, nutritional food is available; many people do not have sufficient funds to purchase these foods. Malnutrition is a problem in the United States as well as in other countries that we typically think of as having this problem.

There is also a problem of over nutrition in the United States. This does not necessarily mean better or superior nutrition, but too much food that results in obesity. Many obese people are fat but not nutritionally healthy. They snack on junk foods and eat foods high in carbohydrates, which are inexpensive but high in calories.

What can be done to correct these nutritional problems? People's eating patterns can be changed only through education. People must be reeducated on all levels: parents, teenagers, and children. Children may be taught nutrition in school, but it is useless if not followed in the home. Adults, especially those in low-income families, must be taught what nutritional foods can best be bought for the amount of money that they have to spend on food.

Advertising is another important factor in what we buy. If you have ever made a trip to the supermarket with a few children you know that the shopping cart will be filled with all the foods advertised on television that day. Adults, too, react to advertising,

especially to diet foods, fad foods (to be discussed later), and junk foods. A great deal of money can be saved by ignoring advertising and buying the basics.

PLANNING A BALANCED MENU

If you have never had to plan meals, you may not realize that it can be easy if you follow a few basic steps. First, you should consider the importance of all three meals

Old-world flavors survive in the land of the frozen dinner with hardly a generation gap.

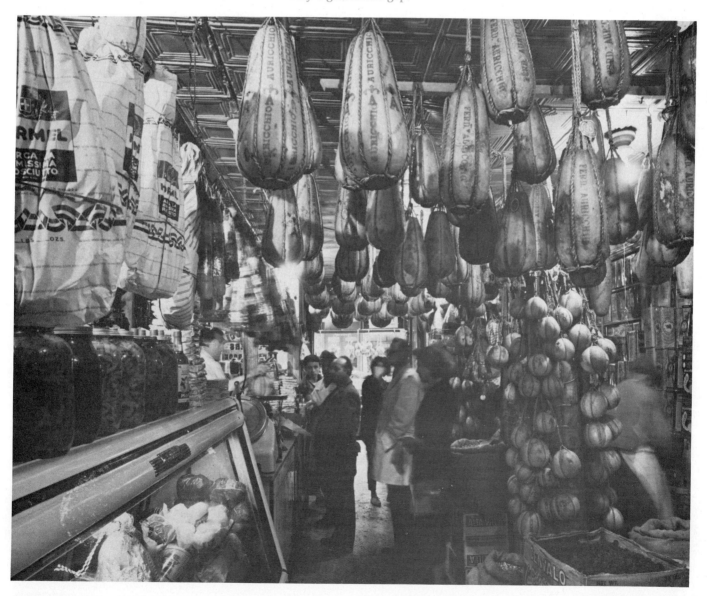

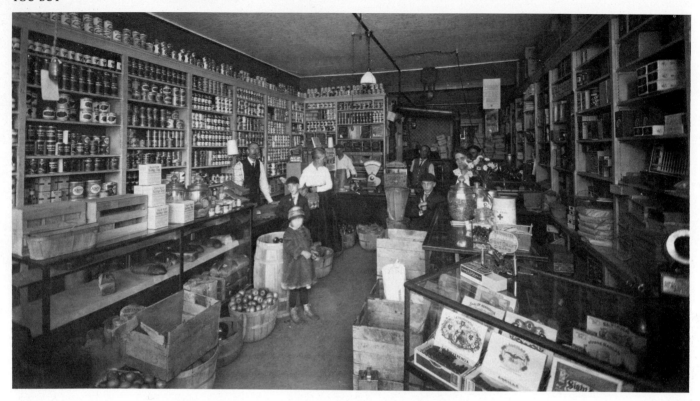

in satisfying the four basic food requirements. Each meal should provide three of the basic four groups. A good source of protein (meat or milk group or both) should be served at each meal. Second, one should provide for a variety of foods that include color, texture, flavor, and satisfy hunger. Too much of one type of food should be avoided. Leftovers should be used in another form or a couple of days later rather than on the next day. Third, foods should be both economical and attractive.

In menu planning you should also consider the people who are going to eat the meals. If there are small children in the family then plainer, lighter foods may be desirable. Active people need more calories than sedentary individuals, and teenagers generally need high-calorie foods. If one or two meals are very heavy then a lighter meal may be desirable as the third meal. Many people tend to eat a light breakfast and lunch and a heavy dinner.

What about breakfast? If you are like most adults, coffee often *is* breakfast. Is this nutritionally wise? As you may have expected, the answer is "no." Research in this area indicates that breakfast is an essential meal and that people who skip breakfast often show a decrease in mental alertness and an increase in fatigue and muscle tremor. In addition, people who skip breakfast tend to eat fattening snacks or heavy lunches and dinners. It is best to distribute one's total food intake over the three meals and try to eat one-third of the daily calories at breakfast. Protein foods have been found to satisfy one's hunger for a longer period of time. Breakfast is thought to be so important that many schools and a number of large corporations are offering breakfast to their students and employees at little or no cost.

What about the economics of meal planning? With the price of food continually increasing, this is an important factor to consider. For example, protein requirements can be satisfied without meat if one buys skim milk, cottage cheese, peas and beans, peanut butter, dairy products, and eggs. Instant nonfat dry

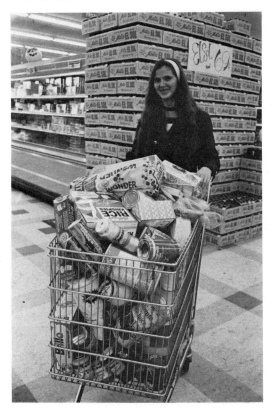

Fifty years ago the food shopper had a limited selection of groceries, but today the choice is tremendous and advertisers spend millions to influence the consumer.

milk is as nutritious as fresh milk but much less expensive. Other factors to keep in mind include:

1. Buy foods that are in season. They are cheaper and can be canned or preserved for future use.
2. Buy quantities of staple items when they are reduced in price.
3. Plan a week's menu in advance—allow for the use of some foods in two or more meals and use leftovers.
4. Buy large quantities of food that are cheaper in price and can be frozen (meats) or kept without spoiling.
5. Read labels—be aware of what you are buying, the amount contained, and the quality.
6. Store labels are usually as good as name brands and a lot less expensive.
7. Look for outlets that sell day-old bread and other baked goods.
8. Avoid food shopping when you are hungry—hungry people buy more, much of which they do not need.
9. Write a shopping list. Do not buy impulsively. This is an easy way to fill up on expensive extras.
10. Store foods properly and learn correct storing, freezing, and canning procedures. These facts are available from local and state agriculture departments.

Snacks should also be considered. If you are watching your weight, it is best to avoid them completely or snack on carrot or celery sticks, small amounts of natural cheese, or skim milk. Snacks are often expensive and lacking in nutrition. The mealplanner should provide nutritious snacks that can also be used as a part of the meal. Leftover meats, vegetables, and soups are nutritious, filling snacks.

NUTRITIONAL NEEDS DURING PREGNANCY

Nutrition during pregnancy is important to both the woman and the child. One does not have to eat for two in quantity but should

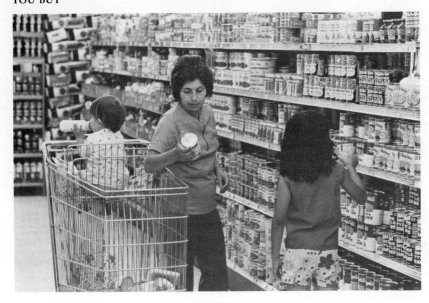

The educated shopper.

eat for two nutritionally. A woman who is well-nourished prior to pregnancy is likely to have few nutritional problems during pregnancy. Teenagers have been found to have the least adequate diet and during pregnancy may continue poor eating habits. Prenatal care at a very early stage in pregnancy is essential to inform pregnant women concerning nutrition, weight gain, and vitamin supplements.

A woman should gain between 20 and 25 pounds during pregnancy. Recent research indicates that too little weight gain can result in low birth weight or premature infants. Too much weight gain can cause complications during pregnancy, and it may be very difficult to lose those extra pounds after the baby's birth.

There is an increased need for nutrients during pregnancy. Milk is especially important, and between three and five cups of milk should be taken daily. In addition there should be at least three servings of meat or meat products, five servings of vegetables and fruit, and four or more servings of bread and cereals daily. The mother who chooses to breast-feed should follow her pregnancy diet but increase the intake of milk to at least five cups. Most doctors will prescribe vitamins for the pregnant mother to ensure

at this crucial time that sufficient vitamins are in the diet.

INFANTS AND CHILDREN

Infants and children need special diets because of the rapid growth that takes place in the early years. Malnutrition in these developmental years can retard growth, cause mental retardation, and result in poor bone formation and a variety of other nutrition-based problems.

Infants (up to the age of two) usually triple their weight in the first year. To triple one's weight requires good nutrition and high-calorie food. Breast milk is very adequate as the only food during the early months. Fortified milk-formulas are also used to nourish the young infant. Later in the infant's life, solid foods are slowly added to the diet.

Between the ages of two to ten years a child eats a variety of foods. It should be remembered that a child's stomach is not a bottomless pit. Many parents make the mistake of "piling" the food on the plate and "turning the child off" to eating. It is better to serve small amounts that the child can easily eat and have him ask for seconds if he is still hungry. It is also important that mealtime be happy, peaceful times where eating is relaxed and not rushed. Arguments and problems should be avoided during this time.

Teenagers are noted to have the poorest diet of any age group. They tend to grab meals on the run or skip them entirely. Much of their calorie consumption comes from snacking "junk" food which has little or no nutrient value. Many teenage girls and boys go on fad diets without a doctor's supervision. In the teenage years, growth and maturation reach their peak. Good nutrition is essential at this age as it is throughout life.

ADULTS

Adults also tend to neglect their nutrition. Many are "too busy" to eat proper meals. Others are always trying to lose weight and sacrifice nutrition for quick weight-loss diets. Unfortunately, as one gets older he is more likely to feel sluggish and suffer from physical conditions that require a specialized diet.

Adults have an additional problem that most teenagers do not encounter. This problem involves weight gain that usually results from consuming too many calories and not participating in enough exercise. Most adults must reduce their caloric intake between the ages of 25 and 30. If they continue to eat as they did at a younger age, they may find themselves gaining weight. Good nutrition is vitally important to the adult and should not be overlooked because one has "stopped growing" or "has no time to eat."

Older persons frequently need specialized diets. Most older people do not need as many calories as they did during middle age. Physical activity may be sharply reduced and people of this age group generally tend to be more sedentary. Special diets may be necessary for digestive ailments, heart disease, diabetes, emotional problems, and other conditions. Many older people prefer to eat four or five meals. It is important that older people, especially those who live alone, get adequate meals. Some communities have established meal services where elderly, often incapacitated individuals are brought nourishing meals. Does your community have any such programs for the elderly?

nutritional misconceptions

As in every field, nutrition has its share of misconceptions. Many nutritional misconceptions are based on faddism, often created by groups of people who use and publicize a type of food or diet. Other misconceptions are based in myths handed down from generation to generation and accepted as truth. Some of these misconceptions and myths are briefly discussed here.

ADDITIVES IN FOOD

You are probably familiar with the word additive, but do you know what it means? Food additives are substances that are put into food either intentionally or unintentionally. An additive may be dirt or hair (unintentional) or artificial food coloring preservatives, or vitamins (intentional).

There has been much discussion of late concerning whether or not additives are dangerous. Some recent, though inconclusive, research relates certain food additives to hyperactivity in children and other problems. However, one can generally state that food additives are subjected to considerable evaluation before they are permitted to be used. The FDA is continually doing research in this area, and if there are any doubts concerning an additive, it is immediately withdrawn from use.

ORGANIC FOODS

Organic foods have always been available, but they have proliferated in recent years. The early 1970s witnessed the introduction of a large number of organic food stores and products. An organic food is a product grown without the use of herbicides and pesticides. No additives are used in these foods.

The misconception that applies to many so-called organic food is that they are not really organic. Many health food stores are selling nonorganic foods at high prices. Other studies have revealed that there is no nutritional advantage to buying the higher-priced organic foods even if they are organically

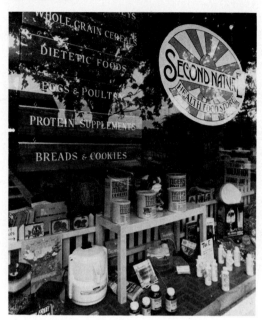

Health foods: fact or fallacy?

grown. Many states are presently looking into possible fraud by organic and health food retailers.

FOOD MYTHS

There are so many food-related myths that it would be impossible to list them all. An example of such a myth would be: fish is brain food. This is false as no one food goes to develop a particular part of the body. Other myths include: avoid pickles and milk; starve a fever, feed a cold; and do not drink water with your meals. Do you have any favorite food myths? Share them with the class. It is both funny and interesting to hear these myths and find out how they began.

THINKING IT OVER

1. Why is good nutrition essential to total good health?
2. Why is food necessary in humans and other animals?
3. Explain the word "calorie." What is the relationship between calories and the food we eat?

4. Define the word "nutrient" and list the basic nutrients.
5. Discuss the functions of proteins and carbohydrates.
6. Discuss the functions of fats and minerals.
7. What is a vitamin and why are excess vitamins usually not necessary?
8. Discuss the functions of water and roughage in the human body.
9. What is meant by a balanced diet? Write a balanced diet for one day.
10. Discuss some of the factors that affect your selection of foods.
11. Discuss the nutritional needs during pregnancy and lactation.
12. How do infants, children, and teenagers differ in their nutritional needs?
13. Discuss the nutritional needs of adults and senior citizens.
14. Discuss additives and organic food products and some misconceptions about them.

KEY WORDS

Additives. Substances added intentionally or unintentionally to food.

Amino acid. Compounds of proteins, often called the building blocks of the body.

Anemia. A condition characterized by a reduction in red blood cells or in hemoglobin quality.

Atherosclerosis. The narrowing of artery walls by fatty deposits.

Basic food groups. Food groups essential to nutrition including milk, meat, cereal and bread, and fruits and vegetables.

Calorie. Units of food energy that provide energy for activity and heat.

Cholesterol. A fatty alcohol found in animal and dairy fats, egg yolks, and other substances; also produced in the body and essential to body functioning.

Edema. Accumulation of excess fluid in the body tissues.

Lactation. The act of breast-feeding an infant.

Nutrients. Substances needed by the body for adequate functioning: (1) proteins, (2) carbohydrates, (3) fats, (4) minerals, (5) vitamins, (6) water, and (7) roughage.

Nutrition. The science of food, its utilization, and necessity for body function.

Organic foods. Foods that are grown without herbicides or pesticides and do not contain additives.

Rickets. Poor bone formation in children caused by a deficiency of calcium, phosphorus, and vitamin D.

Vitamins. Compounds necessary (in small amounts) for normal growth, development, and tissue maintenance.

GETTING INVOLVED

Books and Periodicals

Ewald, Ellen B. *Recipes for a Small Planet.* New York: Ballentine, 1973. Well-balanced vegetarian recipes.

Lappe, Frances M. *Diet for a Small Planet.* New York: Ballentine, n.d. The case for vegetarianism.

Movies

Vitamins — and Some Deficiency Diseases. A documentary about what happens if you don't take your vitamins. Distributed by Lederle.

The Vegetarian Gourmet, with Alan Hooker. A food authority shows how to cook with vegetables. Distributed by Association-Sterling Films.

Food for a Modern World. About food sources and requirements. Distributed by Association-Sterling Films.

13
WEIGHT CONTROL AND DIETING

Weight control and dieting is a subject of great interest to many people. A high percentage of Americans are overweight and this chapter will give you some insight into the reasons for this situation. You will learn why overweight and obesity are considered serious health hazards.

Is there a difference between overweight and obesity? The answer is "yes." You will learn how to tell if you fall into either of these categories. You will also read about the different types of obesity and their causes. There are physical, social, and psychological causes of obesity that many people tend to overlook. Some of these causes are explored in this chapter.

The chapter also concerns itself with the process of weight gain and loss and how these processes are linked to caloric intake and expenditure. You will also learn how to figure your daily caloric needs based on your present body weight. The importance of exercise in any program of weight loss is stressed in this chapter.

If you have ever dieted, you will be interested in the reasons why people diet and some of the fad diets they go on. The elements of a proper diet are also stressed. Some of the help available for dieters is discussed, including diet pills, surgical techniques, fat farms, and weight-reduction groups. The fat person who wants to remain fat is also discussed and the point of view that fat people are discriminated against is explored. After reading this chapter, you will have examined the basics of diet and weight control and some of the interesting topics that are related to this subject.

While reading this chapter, think about the following concepts:

■ Overweight, once a sign of prosperity, is now considered a health hazard.

■ Obesity has physical, psychological, and social causes.

■ Most people diet for aesthetic rather than health reasons.

■ Most fad diets provide quick but temporary weight loss.

■ Effective dieting must be gradual and must include a balanced diet, fewer calories, and increased exercise.

■ Some fat people want to be fat and feel that they should be left alone.

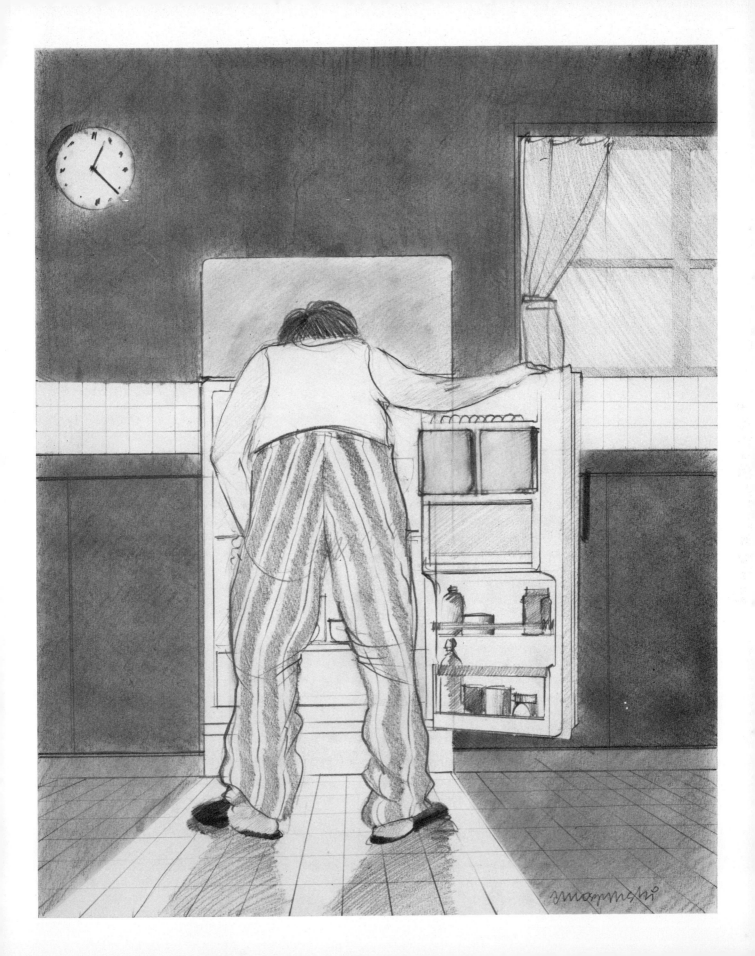

Do you have difficulty in controlling your weight? If so, you are certainly not alone. According to life insurance statistics, which are keyed to life expectancy, an estimated 6.7 million people are overweight. This is about 5 percent of the adult United States population.

If you have difficulty in controlling your weight, the problem may be life style and not diet. In a recent interview Dr. Van Itallie, a professor at Columbia University's Institute of Human Nutrition, emphasized that the answer to obesity may be found by focusing on the individual and his environment rather than his diet alone. One's approach to food and the factors in the environment that encourage certain eating habits often are the key to an overweight condition. This and other factors concerning weight control are discussed in detail in this chapter.

overweight and obesity

At one time people who were overweight were looked upon as being prosperous. It was a sign of having enough money to afford the "good life." However, overweight is no longer considered an admirable characteristic. It is a health menace and considered unattractive by many individuals. Excess body fat has been shown to be associated with diabetes, hypertension, and heart disease. It is also linked to respiratory problems, digestive disorders, arthritis of the bones, varicose veins, and many other disorders. The relationship between overweight and health is discussed in detail in a later section of this chapter.

Millions of Americans are overweight and the problem is much greater than many of us think it is. For many people it means the aggravation of a serious disease and not just the gain of a few unwanted pounds. In addition to the physical problems there are concurrent emotional problems. Emotional problems are frequently the reason why people tend to overeat while other emotional problems result from being overweight. The emotional aspect of weight gain and loss

will also be discussed in a later section of this chapter.

THE DIFFERENCE BETWEEN OVERWEIGHT AND OBESITY

Overweight may be defined as weighing more than one should for his or her body, structure, sex, and height. Some people are slightly overweight; others are significantly overweight. If one has too much fat tissue or body fat then he or she can be called obese.

Some people are overweight because their work calls for extra poundage. Examples of this would be a football lineman or a weight lifter. Many individuals who do work that requires a high degree of muscular development weigh more than what might be considered an "ideal" weight for their height, sex, and body structure. On the other hand, some people weigh less than their ideal weight because of their work. A model or an actress or actor might be an example of this situation. Can you think of any other examples?

How can you tell if you are overweight or obese? There are many methods that are used to determine this factor. One method is to compare one's weight to the weight he or she was at the age of 22. Of course, one can only use this method of comparison if he or she were thin at 22. A more accurate method of determining obesity is by pinching the skin at certain points. The skin under the shoulder bones of the back and on the upper arm reveal the extent of fat tissue stored in these areas. Try this test on yourself. What does it reveal?

Another more accurate method of determining obesity is the use of height–weight tables. These tables are frequently used by insurance companies in determining a person's health for insurance purposes.

There are two types of tables generally used. One type is the average weight chart. This type of chart gives the weights and heights of a nationwide sampling of individuals. The charts also indicate body build by small, average, or large frame. These charts allow a person to compare his weight to the so-called average in the country. These charts are not that accurate and may not give a good indication of comparative weights.

A better type of chart is the ideal or desirable weight chart, which is based upon weight and longevity, or how long a person will live (see Table 13-1). These charts are constructed by insurance companies and indicate the weight at which statistically a person is most likely to live the longest. These charts are based on height, sex, and body frame, but not on age. When referring to these charts, persons 25 years of age or older are usually grouped together. Those younger than 25 years are usually instructed to subtract one pound for each year under 25. One method of determining obesity by using the

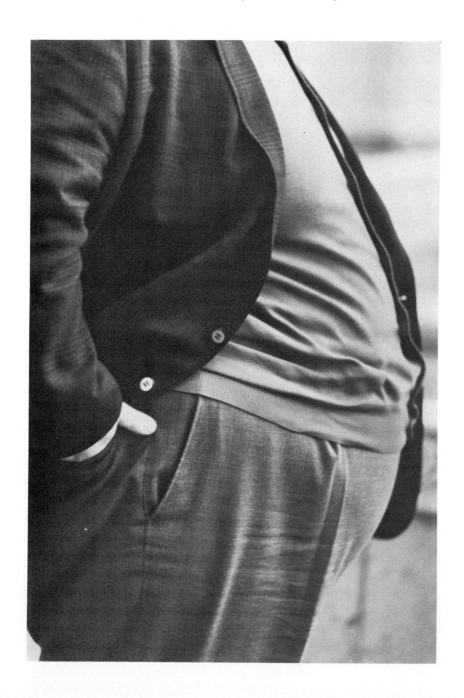

ideal weight charts is to figure that if one weighs 30 percent more than his or her ideal weight one is considered obese.

Table 13-1
DESIRABLE WEIGHTS—AGES 25 AND OVER
Weight in Pounds According to Frame
(In Indoor Clothing)

MEN			
Height (with shoes on) 1-inch heels Feet Inches	Small Frame	Medium Frame	Large Frame
5 2	112—120	118—129	126—141
5 3	115—123	121—133	129—144
5 4	118—126	124—136	132—148
5 5	121—129	127—139	135—152
5 6	124—133	130—143	138—156
5 7	128—137	134—147	142—161
5 8	132—141	138—152	147—166
5 9	136—145	142—156	151—170
5 10	140—150	146—160	155—174
5 11	144—154	150—165	159—179
6 0	148—158	154—170	164—184
6 1	152—162	158—175	168—189
6 2	156—167	162—180	173—194
6 3	160—171	167—185	178—199
6 4	164—175	172—190	182—204

WOMEN			
Height (with shoes on) 2-inch heels Feet Inches	Small Frame	Medium Frame	Large Frame
4 10	92— 98	96—107	104—119
4 11	94—101	98—110	106—122
5 0	96—104	101—113	109—125
5 1	99—107	104—116	112—128
5 2	102—110	107—119	115—131
5 3	105—113	110—122	118—134
5 4	108—116	113—126	121—138
5 5	111—119	116—130	125—142
5 6	114—123	120—135	129—146
5 7	118—127	124—139	133—150
5 8	122—131	128—143	137—154
5 9	126—135	132—147	141—158
5 10	130—140	136—151	145—163
5 11	134—144	140—155	149—168
6 0	138—148	144—159	153—173

For girls between 18 and 25, subtract 1 pound for each year under 25. Courtesy, Metropolitan Life Insurance Company.

Charts and other methods of finding one's ideal weight should only be used as a guide. Many of us are quite familiar with what a good weight is for us. One can tell if he is overweight by how he looks and how clothing fits. When we put on too many pounds, it becomes obvious rather quickly. For the person who is truly obese, the way he or she looks is enough of an indication that he or she weighs too much. The charts can further emphasize that factor, but in most cases it is already understood.

Think about the following statement: "People who are overweight are not necessarily obese, but most obese people are overweight." Do you agree with this statement? It is true! There are many people who weigh too much but do not have much excess body fat. You might not even think of them as being overweight. They wear clothes well and look attractive even though they may weigh more than the charts say they should for their height. However, it would be difficult to find an obese person who was not overweight. Some physical conditions may make a person look obese—but this is a rarity.

There are usually two types of obese individuals. One type of obese person has what is called regulatory obesity. This individual has lost the ability to voluntarily control his or her food intake. In simple terms, this person eats too much food. A second type of obesity is the metabolic type. This is an inborn or acquired disorder that involves the body's metabolism. However, many more people are obese because they eat too much than because they have a metabolic disorder.

Research seems to indicate that there are two types of regulatory obesity. One type is called juvenile-onset obesity and the other type is called adult-onset obesity. Juvenile obesity can begin at a very early age and there is evidence of a genetic factor in this type of obesity. It has been found that children of obese parents are more likely to be obese than children of normal weight parents. Part of this may be linked to heredity but part may be a reflection of parental eating patterns.

Research has also indicated that the old saying "the plumper the child the healthier he is," is not true. Children fed excessively during certain periods of their growth may develop larger fat cells than normal-weight children. They also develop more fat cells that may make it very difficult for them to lose weight at a later age. These critical years in a child's fat cell development are thought to be prior to the age of two and between the ages of 10 and 16. From your own experience, have you found this to be true? If you are overweight now, were you also an overweight baby and child?

Is obesity a disease? It can be called a disease because it can be a serious physical handicap, it can aggravate existing physical conditions, and it may indicate an abnormal distribution of fat. A person does not have to be "fat all over" in order to be considered obese. Many individuals have problem "fat" areas where diet and overweight are not necessarily involved. Are you one of these people?

OBESITY AND HEALTH

There are many dangers in prolonged obesity. Most physicians and experts in the area of nutrition would agree that the life expectancy of very obese individuals is significantly reduced. Obesity may precipitate diabetes in some obese individuals and may aggravate hypertension, or high blood pressure. Obese individuals, especially men in their middle age, may show a rise in triglycerides in the bloodstream. The fat stored in the body is almost entirely composed of triglycerides. Refer to Chapter 12 for a review of triglycerides and cholesterol.

From the present scientific research, there seems to be a correlation between heart disease and obesity. However, it is not entirely clear whether this is so because the obese individual tends to be sedentary and does little exercise or because of the more direct effect of excess calories as a cause of heart disease.

Diet and proper exercise are essential to total good health which includes "normal" weight. In order to lose weight and maintain a "normal" weight, one must change his or her life style so that a balanced diet and exercise becomes a part of one's life. Many people go up and down in weight because they diet and exercise *only* until they reach their ideal weight. Then they go back to their old way of living and soon gain all of the weight back. Losing pounds and maintaining a low weight requires constant vigilance and a complete change in eating and exercise habits.

PSYCHOLOGICAL FACTORS AND OBESITY

There are many psychological factors involved in why some people overeat and become obese. One of the most common reasons given for obesity is tension. Many people say they eat as soon as they become nervous or upset. It is the same type of tension that causes people to smoke excessively or take pills. These people feel a certain amount of relief from eating, smoking, or taking tranquilizers. They may feel guilty about the habit but the sense of sedation overcomes the sense of guilt.

Others eat to get back at someone. Children may choose to eat too much in order to anger their parents. Some children will not eat in order to accomplish the same effect. Some obese individuals think that they are punishing those closest to them while others enjoy punishing themselves. By being fat they may feel that less is expected of them and they can, in a sense, hide behind their fat.

The individual who remains obese may do so to stay unattractive. An unattractive man or woman avoids confrontation with the opposite sex. This is one method of trying to avoid a situation they are afraid to cope with.

Other psychological reasons often given for obesity include boredom, loneliness, anger, guilt, need for a reward, and fatigue. Can you think of any other reason? If you are overweight or have ever been overweight, did you use any of these reasons for your obesity? It is interesting to note that many of the same psychological reasons given for overeating are also given for eating too little. Why do you think this is so? Why do you think we tend to recognize these reasons for overeating but not for the opposite condition?

Does the overweight person feel differently about himself than the normal-weight person? It all depends upon how the obese person views himself. Fat people and thin people share the same range of emotions. A fat person who is very unhappy with himself will carry this attitude into his daily life. However, the stereotype of the fat, jolly person is not true. Fat people of course can be jolly, but certainly not all fat people are jolly—in fact, the opposite seems to be closer to the truth.

Is the fat person neurotic? Not necessarily. One is only neurotic if the obese condition affects the way he acts. If one denies that he or she is obese then this would be a neurotic reaction. If one always eats alone or hides food to fool people then he is acting in a neurotic manner. In order to determine neuroticism one may ask himself if he is

facing the problem realistically and if he is changing his life style because of the obesity. If answers to one or both of these questions is "yes" then the individual is probably reacting with some degree of neurosis.

SOCIOLOGICAL FACTORS AND OBESITY

There are many social patterns that result in obesity. Children of obese parents often become obese because of the eating habits that they are exposed to. Food is often pushed on people in certain families, and in some ethnic groups eating is a ritual. If one grows up in a family where eating frequently and in large amounts is expected, he or she may very well have a weight problem.

The type of food prepared, size of meals, and type and frequency of snacks are all patterns that people become accustomed to. In some homes diet snacks and drinks are commonplace while in other homes sweetened soft drinks and candy are eaten as snacks. What type of home did you come from? How was your weight affected by the eating patterns of your household?

Dieting can be difficult.

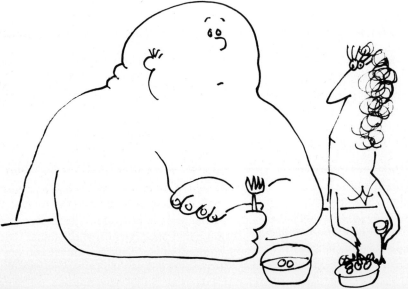

Another sociological factor is the peer group. Young people are especially affected by this type of influence. If one's friends are going out for pizza or sodas, the overweight person finds it hard to refuse to go or to abstain once he does go. The same is true for the adult who may eat large business lunches or consume too much alcohol. Alcohol is a significant source of calories. For example, an ounce and a half of gin is about 100 calories. If one is on a restricted calorie intake, this is a great deal of calories to consume in one drink. One drink may only be the beginning of a many drink, calorie binge.

Food is all around us most of the time. Many people feel that it is not polite to refuse an offer of something to eat by a host or hostess. These are some of the problems that the obese person who wants to lose weight must learn to cope with. Losing weight involves much more than restricting one's diet. There are social and psychological problems that must be dealt with "up front" so that a person can successfully diet and keep those pounds off.

the process of weight gain and weight loss

Weight gain and weight loss are primarily concerned with food intake and energy expenditure. This may be measured by calories, which are energy-producing units of food. Refer to Chapter 12 for a discussion of calories.

There are three body processes concerned with energy output. Body metabolism is one such process and may be defined as all the chemical changes that take place in the tissues of the body. Basal metabolism is the minimum amount of energy required to maintain the life processes.

You may have heard of the basal metabolic rate (BMR) that determines one's own basal metabolism. This rate gives one an idea of how many calories are needed just to continue the life processes. The BMR can be calculated by multiplying 1 calorie per hour (24) times your body weight in kilograms or

$$1 \times 24 \times \text{kg of body weight}$$

In order to determine your body weight by kilograms, devide your weight in pounds by 2.2. For example, if one weighs 154 pounds his weight in kilograms would be 70 kg. Then following the previous formula his BMR would be:

$$1 \times 24 \times 70 = 1,680$$

This number will be referred to later in this section when basic calorie needs for an individual are explained.

The second process involved in energy output is specific dynamic action (SDA). This is action of food on the body and it can be looked at as a 10 percent tax on the food you eat. For example, if you were to eat 100 calories, 10 percent or 10 calories would be taken up by SDA, leaving 90 calories for body use.

A third process involved in energy output is the amount of exercise one does and the number of calories used in this exercise. It has been estimated that the average sedentary individual burns up about 500 calories in carrying out his daily routine. Any additional exercise will burn up more calories.

In order to determine the approximate number of calories that one needs in order to maintain his present weight, one can take his BMR, add to it the calories needed for daily activities plus the 10 percent SDA. The following example is based on the weight of a 154 pound sedentary man.

BMR	1680
Daily activity	500
	2,180
SDA (10 percent)	218
Number of calories needed to maintain present weight	2,398

Very few of us are completely sedentary; therefore, more calories would be needed if more exercise was performed.

WEIGHT GAIN AND LOSS

In order to gain weight one must consume more calories than he expends. Therefore one should either eat more or exercise less. However, it is important to remember that since exercise is essential to total body fitness, less exercise is probably not the best of the two choices. Though overweight is a more common condition than underweight, this is a problem for many people. Do you have a problem of weighing too little? If so, how do you cope with this situation?

In order to lose weight one must consume fewer calories and/or exercise more. Usually a combination of both practices is the healthiest approach to losing weight. Exercise is an important factor in weight loss that many people tend to ignore. This is discussed in the next section of this chapter.

Different types of work demand varying calorie expenditure. For example, 2,400 calories is usually the amount needed by an individual employed in a sedentary occupation (teacher, student, secretary). A carpenter might require 3,200 calories, while a stone mason would require 4,400 calories. These are only calorie estimates for a certain occupation; only additional exercise would require more calories in order to maintain body weight. What would you estimate your calorie requirements to be based on your occupation and additional activities? Do you estimate that you are eating more or less than your required caloric intake?

exercise and weight control

As you learned in Chapter 11, exercise is very crucial to any weight control program. Exercise is a determining factor in daily caloric needs and is beneficial for total health and fitness. Many people tend to be unconcerned about exercise when they go on a diet. Are you one of these people? Some of the reasons that they are unconcerned are: (1) they are not aware of the importance of exercise in weight control; (2) they are not accustomed to exercising in a regular manner; and (3) they find exercise to be tedious while they are dieting. Can you think of any other reasons why people avoid exercise in weight control programs?

There are some interesting facts concerning exercise that you may not be familiar with. Many calories can be burned by exercise. The "cost" of these calories can be seen in Figure 13-1. In one experiment, a group of university students increased their daily calorie intake from 3,000 to 6,000 calories and did not gain weight because they increased their exercise at the same time.

Figure 13-1
Energy Expenditure for Different Activities

Number of Calories expended in 1 hour by a woman weighing 120 pounds:

Calories per hour

Awake—lying still (basal rate)	56
Sitting quietly	72
Walking slowly (2.6 mph)	145
Walking moderately fast (3.75 mph)	217
Swimming	362
Dishwashing	104
Typing rapidly	102
Sweeping the floor	122

Number of Calories expended in 1 hour by a man weighing 154 pounds:

Calories per hour

Awake—lying still (basal rate)	77
Sitting quietly	100
Walking slowly (2.6 mph)	200
Walking moderately fast (3.75 mph)	300
Swimming	500
Dishwashing	144
Carpentry or painting	240
Active exercise	290

Energy expenditure is affected by body weight. A heavier person will burn more calories doing the same exercise as a lighter-weight individual. This is so because more calories are burned when the individual has to move his own weight while doing the exercise. The heavier the person, the more

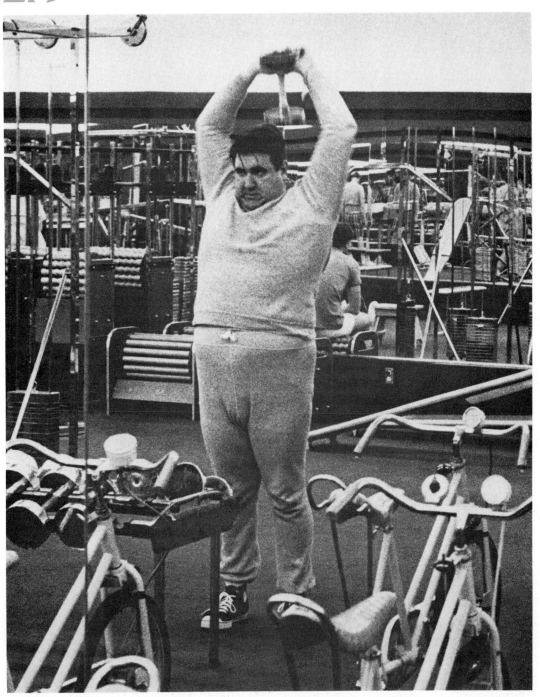

The high cost of food.

calories are burned in moving his body weight. For example, a 100-pound person who walks 3 mph will burn about 50 calories in 15 minutes. A 200-pound person would use up about 80 calories in the same amount of time.

Contrary to public opinion, increased physical exercise will *not* increase appetite significantly. The thin person may eat more following strenuous exercise, but the exercise will burn up the additional calories. However, an obese individual does not respond this way to exercise. The obese person's large fat deposits supply the calories burned during exercise. He will not feel a need to immediately replace these calories by eating.

It has also been shown that a decline in activity usually triggers an increase in weight. In one study of overweight adults, their obesity corresponded directly to a decline in exercise. This can often be seen in adults who were active as teenagers and became less active after they started working. Their inactivity usually precipitated a gradual weight gain. A lack of exercise coupled with unchanged caloric intake can result in weight gain. Most adults, especially those who do not exercise, need less calories than they consumed as teenagers. Even a gradual weight gain begins to add up. If one gains only two pounds a year, he could weigh ten pounds more after five years. Most people can easily gain more than two pounds a year if they do not try to control their weight.

What are the benefits of exercise in weight control? Exercise not only helps to burn calories but it also strengthens muscles and reduces flabbiness. Sagging skin is prevented by proper exercise. Inches can be taken off as well as pounds. Exercise helps one to overcome the feeling of fatigue and sluggishness and replaces these feelings with alertness and energy. In addition, one is often able to sleep better following exercise.

Exercise also allows for needed social relationships where the overweight person can seek companionship and concentrate on something other than his diet. Exercise is an excellent outlet for tension and anxiety that is often a reason why a person overeats. The person who exercises will be healthier physically and emotionally, will keep active longer, and is less apt to suffer from diseases of the heart and blood vessels in later life. Exercise is one of the most important elements in losing pounds and maintaining weight when one has lost those pounds.

dieting

It is difficult to go through one day without encountering someone who is on a diet. This makes sense because of the large number of persons in the population who are overweight or obese. Dieting means different things to different people. Some people diet by eating only one type of food for days; others go on near-starvation diets to accomplish their goal quickly. Some of these "diets" are discussed later in this section.

Why do people diet? Most people diet for health and aesthetic reasons. However, more people diet to be fashionable than to be healthy. Many people who one might consider thin are constantly dieting in order to be able to wear the newest fashions. The expression "thin is in" is true in today's American society and has been true for a number of years. Fashions are geared to the youth market and this is considered to be the "thin market." If you have dieted, why did you do so? Which health reasons entered into the picture?

FAD DIETS

You are probably familiar with one or more fad diets. These are the diets that "everyone" is on for a while and then no one hears about them again. These diets often add interest to those people who are constantly looking for a new approach to weight loss. Many of these diets are scientifically based and include nutritionally balanced meals. Other diets can be dangerous if the person suffers from certain physical disorders or stays on the diet too long. Some of the most popular fad diets of recent years are discussed here.

Dr. Irwin Stillman's Quick Inches Off Diet. The Stillman diet has been made popular by a book by the same name as the diet and by the author himself who routinely appears on radio and television talk shows. Dr. Stillman's diet requires one to keep within a 500 calorie a day allotment. It consists of eating large amounts of vegetables and fruits and avoiding protein entirely. The diet claims that low-protein eating helps one to burn up fat layers between the muscles— reducing bulges. The AMA's Department of Food and Nutrition disagrees. They feel the diet is hazardous to one's health because it is dangerously low in protein and may cause the dieter to become listless and depressed.

Dr. Atkin's Superdiet. The Atkin's diet was outlined in his book, *Dr. Atkin's Diet Revolution.* This diet includes a list of permitted foods that are low in carbohydrates and high in protein. A variety of food is allowed and there is no limitation on foods high in cholesterol. There has been much criticism of this diet because of the lack of carbohydrates and excess cholesterol. The Council on Foods and Nutrition of the American Medical Association has issued a critique of this diet. The report expresses concern with the unrestricted use of fats and cholesterol in the diet. This may not be that much of a problem while the person is losing weight but if the dieter stays on this diet after his weight is stabilized, the chances are that the blood cholesterol will be elevated.

The Drinking Man's Diet. This diet is taken from Robert W. Cameron's (Ed.) *The Drinking Man's Diet Cookbook.* It limits one's intake of carbohydrates and relies chiefly on high-protein foods such as meat, fish, and

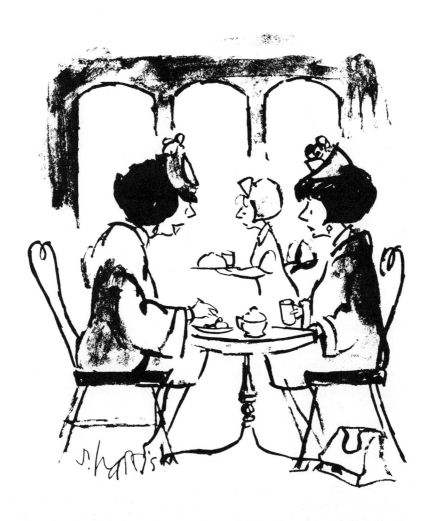

" I JUST LOVE THESE FAD DIETS. I'M ON FOUR OF THEM RIGHT NOW."

eggs. The diet works by burning the body's fat reserve because of the low carbohydrate regimen. Alcoholic beverages are allowed on this diet.

These are only a few of the different diets that have appeared in recent years. There are many others that appeal to every possible taste. Other diets include the "eat-anything diet," "the ice cream diet," "the nibblers' diet," and "the only diet that works diet." Have you tried any of these diets? If not, what type of diet is your favorite one?

Most fad diets seem to be successful because the weight loss may be somewhat quicker than a conventional diet that a doctor might prescribe. However, in most cases the weight loss by the fad diet is temporary, and, as we have seen, these diets can be nutritionally unsound. The reason why weight loss on these diets is often temporary is because one has not changed his or her eating habits. Very few people will stay on these "special" diets for longer than it takes to lose the desired number of pounds. Once the weight is lost, one will begin to eat the foods he did before he went on the diet. One may eat moderately at first, but will soon return to his old patterns. These people are sometimes called "yo-yo's" because their weight is constantly going up and down. Are you a "yo-yo" or do you know someone who is?

One of the latest fads in weight loss is the ear staple or "staplepuncture." This procedure consists of placing a surgical staple in a person's ear in order to reduce hunger pangs. The theory behind staplepuncture is related to Chinese acupuncture, where stimulation of a certain part of the body affects certain bodily processes. Ear stimulation is thought to be related to reducing hunger pangs. The staplepuncture is combined with a highly restricted diet. In some cases the diet has been under 400 calories. Some physicians who use this technique are careful to avoid any chance of infection by the use of the staple and prescribe a balanced diet to their patients. Some persons using this technique are not physicians and their patients are put on low-calorie, nutritionally poor diets and receive little or no follow-up

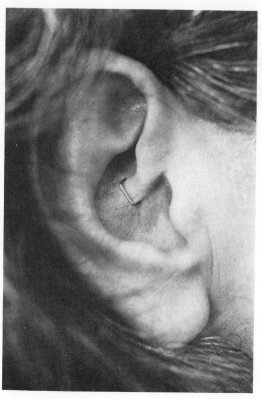

Staplepuncture.

care. The AMA has noted that there is no scientific evidence that this procedure helps to reduce hunger. They have warned the public to be on the lookout for unscrupulous people who practice this technique and make false claims as to its success. Do you know anyone who has had staplepuncture? How successful was it?

Weight loss is big business in the United States today. It is estimated that more than 10 billion dollars is spent annually on diet groups, special foods, and exercise clubs. For example, there are presently more than 70 books in print under the general category of "diet." Other books pertaining to this subject also appear under different headings. The next time you are in your local library, check the number of titles in the diet category.

Why do people never seem to tire of new fads where dieting is concerned? There seems to be a willingness on the part of the overweight or obese person to look for the least painful method of shedding those extra pounds. A new diet gives some people a topic of conversation for a while and helps to relieve boredom. Many obese people refuse to seek medical treatment and if they do it usually does not last long. Different types of diets make these individuals feel they are trying everything and they often conclude that nothing is going to work.

THE PROPER DIET

There probably is no one "proper" diet that would be suitable to everyone. But there are some guidelines that should be followed if one decides to lose weight. Every serious attempt to lose weight should be preceded by a medical examination. This examination will reveal any physical reasons for obesity and any conditions where certain types of diets should be avoided. Many people never bother to get medical advice before starting a diet. Many problems could be avoided by seeing one's doctor first and not taking dieting into one's own hands.

The most effective dieting program should include a balanced diet, fewer calories, and increased exercise. One should concentrate on low-calorie, nutritious food and think about meal planning. Weight loss should be gradual and over a long period of time if it is to be permanent. For the average person, the loss of about two pounds a week is considered desirable. This loss of weight is loss of body fat not water. When you hear about people who lose many pounds in the first week of a diet, they are losing water weight not body fat. This is not a good way to lose weight and it could be harmful to one's health.

In a gradual weight-loss program, one may lose weight more slowly as the program continues. Frequently, the body begins to resist further weight loss and some individuals find that they are at a standstill. The individual who keeps to the diet and does not get discouraged will continue to loose pounds, although at a slower rate than at the beginning of the diet program. If one's caloric intake is less than what he needs for

daily living, one will continue to lose weight. Have you ever gone on a "crash" diet? These diets may result in weight loss but one's physical condition and quick weight gain after the diet usually defeat the purpose of this approach to losing weight. The author has a friend who goes on a crash diet every January 1st. The dieter loses between 15 and 20 pounds in a month of agony. However, this type of starvation diet results in a short temper, headaches, stomach pains, sluggishness, and general discomfort. In case you are interested, this dieter gains back all of the weight lost by January 1 of the next year so that he must undergo this "crash" diet once again. What would be a more sensible approach to losing this weight?

HELP FOR DIETERS

Help for the dieter is available in many different forms. Some dieters take diet pills which are amphetamines. (Refer to Chapter 7 for information about these drugs.) Amphetamines can produce serious side effects and possible dependency. If used under a doctor's supervision, they may be helpful for a limited time to a person who is beginning to diet. They serve as a temporary "crutch" for this individual until he becomes accustomed to the diet regimen.

If one chooses to go to a so-called "diet doctor," one should be sure that this person has legitimate medical credentials. There are physicians who only treat obesity, but there are others who pass themselves off as doctors. These "doctors" often use a combination of amphetamines and vitamins in injection form. Some of these practitioners inject their patients with useless substances; others restrict caloric intake drastically without appropriate medical supervision.

There are also some surgical techniques to help obese patients who have had difficulty losing weight in other ways. One technique involves the removal of a large segment of the intestines, so that less fat is absorbed into the body. This treatment has been successful with some patients but there are uncomfortable side effects. The operation is recommended only for those who are extremely obese and have failed with other more conventional dieting methods.

Another type of surgical procedure is wiring the jaws shut. The patient cannot open his or her mouth wide enough to consume anything but liquids. Only a few obese patients have had this procedure done and it is one that is thought to be a last resort to help take off weight.

Help is also available through "fat farms" and health spas that concentrate on weight reduction through diet and exercise. Some fat farms are very exclusive and expensive. Diets may be greatly restricted or in some cases a liquid diet is promoted. Here, the patient will drink only liquids for a few days. Weight is lost and some people say the system is flushed of all impurities. For some people this is a relaxing way to take off extra pounds; however, such places are too expensive for the majority of individuals.

Many people who need help to lose weight turn to weight reduction groups. Here they find other people who share a common problem. If you have a weight problem, you can easily understand how difficult it is to communicate that problem to a thin person. Thin people think that all it takes is a little will power to take off weight. But, as you have learned from this chapter, there are many social and emotional reasons why people gain weight and find it difficult to lose.

There are many types of weight reduction groups. Most of them charge a minimal fee for a meeting and the group is based on a common goal: reaching and staying at one's ideal weight. Some of the groups that you may be familiar with include Weight Watchers, TOPS (Take Off Pounds Sensibly), Lean Line, and Overeaters Anonymous (O.A.). All of these groups operate differently, but precise, nutritionally sound diets and group pressure and acceptance are essential elements of most groups.

Let us take a look at two of these groups in order to find out more about how they operate. Weight Watchers was started in 1962 by Jean Nidetch. Mrs. Nidetch had been overweight all of her life; she weighed 214 pounds before she began to lose weight. In 1961 she began to go to the New York City Department of Health Obesity Clinic. She lost 72 pounds on their diet and started

Lean Line is a weight-reducing organization that uses a psychological regime developed at Rutgers University. The program includes special menus and daily weigh-ins, exercises, and lectures. There are also group meals that are policed by the members themselves. But it's not all work — the group also sponsors social events, including weight-loss cruises.

Weight watchers listening after a week of watching.

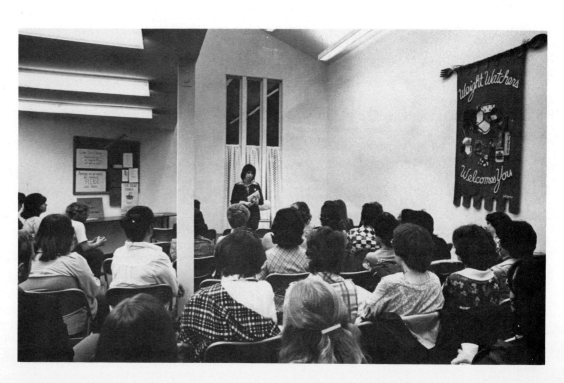

285

TOPS (Take Off Pounds Sensibly) is a pioneer among reducing groups. It was founded in 1948 as a nonprofit organization. Its methods, like those of Alcoholics Anonymous, include self-confession and group encouragement. Weekly meetings begin with a public weigh-in; members who have lost weight are rewarded, and those who haven't must tell why. Then the members relax with discussions, songs, and games.

Weight Watchers the following year. The Weight Watchers diet is not as unusual as its method of involving other overweight people in the weight-loss process. At Weight Watchers, people talk about their weight problems, exchange ideas, and recognize that they are overweight and must face the reality of it. Obesity is looked at as a battle that must be waged daily. The overweight person has to live with this problem every day in order to lose weight and then maintain an ideal weight.

The Weight Watchers Diet allows one to select food from various categories in carefully measured quantities. The dieter is supposed to eat everything on the menu and to eat three meals a day. At weekly meetings, a leader charts each member's progress and discusses problems. The diet is well-rounded, nutritionally sound, and combines calorie reduction with high-protein, low-fat food. Starches are used in moderation. The average weight loss is about two pounds a week. The advantage of this type of diet is it provides for the psychological need of the dieter through group interaction. The diet itself is satisfying and contains a variety of foods. The only disadvantage is that some people become confused with figuring out their daily and weekly food allotments. However, most people who stay with this diet are successful and keep their weight down.

Overeater's Anonymous (O.A.) was established in California in 1961, but it has only recently become popular throughout the country. O.A. is patterned after Alcoholics Anonymous (A.A.) (see Chapter 5). It follows the 12 steps of A.A. and teaches its members to take each day as it comes and not worry about the next day. The basis to this program is giving members the strength to say "no" to foods that are fattening. The program has sponsors and babies. Sponsors are people who have been in the program for 30 days while babies are new members. Each "baby" has a sponsor. O.A. provides a place for people to talk about their weight problems and people can be called upon at other times to help them cope with staying on their diets. In some areas O-Anon

is being formed to help family members of overweight people to better understand their problems. O-Anon is patterned after Al-Anon.

For those of you who are of normal weight, it may be difficult to understand the need for such groups. It might be interesting to invite a representative of a diet group to speak to your class.

CAN DIETING GO TOO FAR?

For some people dieting can get completely out of control. A bizarre affliction known as anorexia nervosa is an emotional disorder that affects thousands of young women. Most anoretics are in their high school or college years. The individual who becomes a victim of this disease is usually slightly overweight, but after losing weight she continues to diet, insisting that she is still too heavy. Some patients have lost so much weight that they die of starvation. Weights of below 65 pounds are not uncommon.

Psychiatrists seem to agree that the illness stems from an intense feeling of inadequacy about meeting the demands imposed by growing up or facing new situations. Many of these girls demand too much of themselves and are never satisfied with what they are doing and how they look. This was discussed in Chapter 1 in the "I'm OK—You're OK" section.

Behavioral modification therapy and hospitalization has helped some victims of the disease. In behavior modification, the patient negotiates a contract with the therapist so that she is rewarded with family contact, privileges, and material items if she continues to eat and gain weight. The patient is also under a doctor's supervision and receives psychotherapy while involved in the behavior modification program.

WHAT ABOUT THE FAT PERSON?

There is a saying that "inside of every fat person there is a skinny person just waiting to get out." Is it true that all fat people really want to be thin or do they feel that "fat is where it's at?" A recent book called *Fat Power* by Llewellyn Lauderback points out that many Americans are brainwashed to think that fat is more of a problem than it really is. The book contends that the fat person's major problem is not his obesity but the view that society takes of it. Fat people are a minority group that is subject to prejudice in relationships, jobs, and general public attitude. The author of this book feels that the majority of overweight adults are doing themselves a distinct disservice by dieting. If they are otherwise healthy, they should stop making themselves miserable by trying to attain a weight that may not be right for them. They should stay at a weight that is most comfortable for themselves. Do you think a "fat" person can be healthy?

An organization that supports the philosophy of *Fat Power* is the National Association to Aid Fat Americans, a nonprofit organization for fat people that is not built around the concept of losing weight. Have you ever thought about the possibility that many fat people would not mind being fat if everyone just let them alone? Many of us tend to look at a person's fat without trying to find out about the real person. People should lose weight because they want to not because they feel they have to because of family or public pressure.

THINKING IT OVER

1. Why is obesity considered dangerous to one's health?
2. Define overweight and obesity. How do they differ from each other?
3. Discuss some of the ways that one can tell if he or she is obese.
4. What types of height–weight tables are there? Which type do you think is more accurate? Why do many people object to the use of these tables?
5. Discuss the two types of obesity. How do they differ?
6. What are the two types of regulatory obesity? Which type do you think is more common?
7. What are the three body processes concerned with energy output?
8. How can one compute his or her BMR?

9. Determine your own daily caloric needs based on the formula presented in the text. Do you think your actual caloric intake is close to what it should be based on this calculation?
10. Discuss the relationship between calories and weight gain or loss.
11. Discuss the value of exercise in a weight control program.
12. What are some of the reasons for dieting?
13. Discuss some "fad" diets and practices. What do you think about this method of weight reduction?
14. What are some of the essential elements in proper dieting?
15. What help is available to dieters? Discuss the value of a diet group such as Weight Watchers or Overeaters Anonymous.
16. How do you feel about the premise of the book *Fat Power*?

KEY WORDS

Adult-onset obesity. Obesity that begins later in life and is usually caused by excessive caloric intake and lack of exercise.

Anorexia nervosa. A disease characterized by a gradual weight loss until the patient is extremely underweight. The cause is thought to be emotional.

Basal metabolism. Minimum amount of energy required to maintain the life processes.

Basal metabolic rate (BMR). Amount of energy necessary to keep an individual's life processes going; calculated according to body weight.

Body metabolism. All the chemical changes that go on in the tissues of the body.

Childhood-onset obesity. Obesity that begins in childhood with early formation of fat cells, making it more difficult to lose weight later in life.

Metabolic obesity. Inborn or acquired difficulties with the body metabolism that cause obesity.

Obesity. Having too much body fat, which is determined by measuring adipose tissues and referring to height and weight charts.

Overweight. Weighing more than one should for his body structure, sex, and height.

Regulatory obesity. A lack of control over the amount of food eaten.

Specific dynamic action. Action of the food on the body that represents a 10 percent tax on the food you eat.

GETTING INVOLVED

Books and Periodicals

Danowski, T.S. *Sustained Weight Control: The Individual Approach.* Philadelphia: F.A. Davis, 1973. A doctor discusses overweight.

Lauderback, Llewellyn. *Fat Power.* New York: Hawthorn Books, 1970. Points out the prejudice that exists against fat people and the right that the fat person has to remain fat.

Marotta, Antonia S., and Wurtzel, Lorraine F. *Diet Cybernetics for Lean Lines.* New York: Pyramid, 1973. The Lean Lines method of losing weight.

Wilkinson, Charles B. *Bud Wilkinson's Guide to Modern Physical Fitness.* New York: Barnes & Noble, 1969. How to improve general health and sports performance through diet and exercise.

Movies

La Grande Bouffe, with Marcello Mastroianni, 1973. The people in this movie are so gluttonous that they eat until they die. Distributed by Abkco Industries, Inc.

PART V
DISEASES

14
HEART DISEASE

Heart disease claimed about 700,000 lives in 1974 and though there has been a recent decline in numbers of cases, it is still considered the number 1 killer and crippler of Americans — mostly men in their younger years.

In this chapter, you will learn about all aspects of heart disease. The structure and function of the heart is briefly discussed so that you will understand the organ and blood vessels that are affected in heart disease. What physically happens during a heart attack is explained.

The factors that increase the risk of heart disease are explored in some detail. These factors include: sex, age, heredity, smoking, diet, lack of exercise, high blood pressure, and stress. All of these factors should be controlled so that one can prevent a heart attack or the recurrence of one. If these factors are multiplied, the risk of heart attack is much greater.

Symptoms and emergency treatment for heart attack are discussed. Emergency treatment involves resuscitation and cardiac massage. In addition, various forms of heart disease are examined. These forms of heart disease include: angina pectoris, congenital heart disease, rheumatic heart disease, high blood pressure, and stroke.

Treatment for heart disease is also discussed. Treatment includes a control of the risk factors associated with the disease and various surgical procedures. After reading this chapter, you will have a better understanding of heart disease and how to prevent it.

While reading this chapter, think about the following concepts:

■ Exercise is as important to the heart muscle as it is to other muscles.

■ There are numerous, proven risk factors associated with heart disease.

■ The risk of heart disease is multiplied by the number of risk factors that one has.

■ There are various forms of heart disease other than heart attack.

■ Heart disease affects the young as well as the old.

■ Treatment of heart disease requires physical as well as behavioral change.

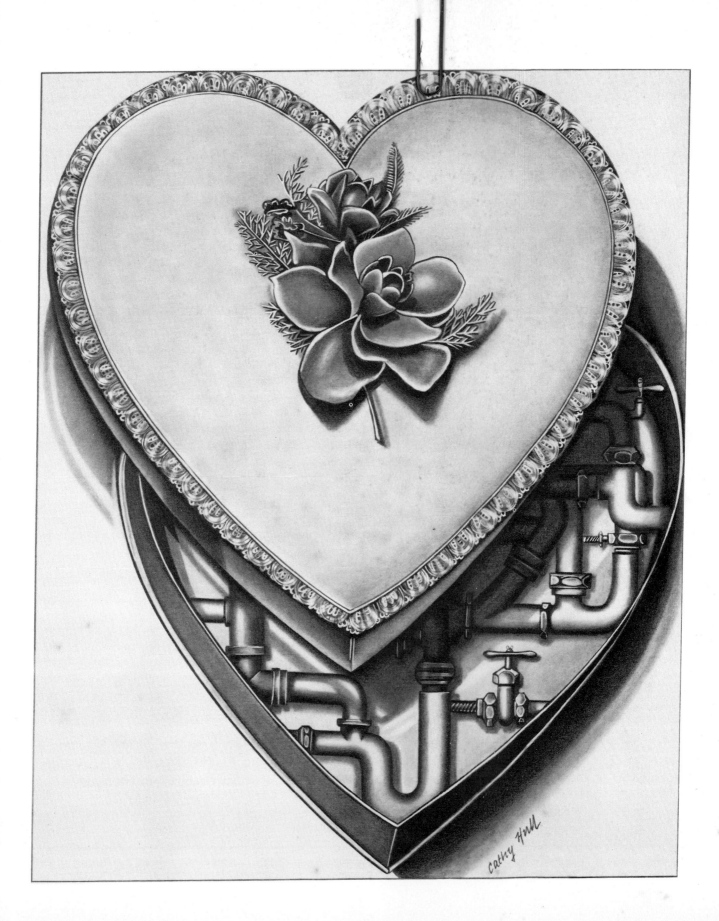

cathy Hill

The subject of this chapter is heart disease; two words with which you are probably somewhat familiar. When you think about heart disease, do you think that it only affects people over the age of 40? Do you also think that it is a disease that primarily affects males? These are two rather common misunderstandings concerning heart disease.

Autopsies of American soldiers killed in Vietnam revealed that many young men had advanced heart disease at the time of their death. These men had passed rigorous physical examinations and training programs and were considered to be healthy and physically fit. Advanced heart disease at the age of 19 or 20 indicates the onset of the disease years before.

There are many types of heart disease and until recently the most common type associated with younger people was a rheumatic heart. This disease results from childhood rheumatic fever. Other forms of heart disease that occur between the ages of 15 and 35 are bacterial infection of the heart's inner lining, viral infection that affects the heart muscle, and congenital heart defects. Blockage of the coronary arteries may also exist to some extent. All of these conditions are discussed in detail in this chapter.

The other common misunderstanding mentioned was that women are not susceptible to heart disease. Although it is true that young women generally exhibit a greater resistance to heart disease (particularly coronary heart disease), they do catch up to the men after the age of 40. Although authorities in the area of heart disease do not fully understand what happens, they believe that women are in part protected by the female sex hormone, estrogen. They also conclude that, in general, women tend to watch their weight and are more active physically than men.

Perhaps, some of your questions concerning heart disease have already been answered. But there are many other misunderstandings that remain to be explained. The first section of this chapter is concerned with the heart's structure and function. These "basics" will help you to better understand what is happening when one suffers from a form of heart disease.

the heart — its structure and function

What does the heart look like? It does not look like the valentine that may come to mind. Actually, the heart is about the size of a fist and is located near the center of the chest, slightly more to the left side than to the right. An adult heart weighs about 11 ounces.

The heart is made up of *cardiac muscle*. It is the largest involuntary muscle in the human body. An involuntary muscle is one over which we have no control, unlike the muscles in an arm or a leg. Though it is involuntary, it does respond to anger, fear, and rage as well as other emotions. It also responds to exercise, sleep, and other conditions to which the body is exposed. As you read about the structure of the heart, refer to Figure 14-1.

A thin layer of cells called the endocardium lines all of the internal surfaces of the heart. A double membrane called the pericardium covers the outside of the heart. The pericardium is a protective sac that is filled with a watery fluid that provides movement without friction and also provides protection for the heart.

Heart tissue has the ability to contract rhythmically or beat without any nerve stimulation. For example, if one placed a piece of animal heart tissue in a nutrient solution it would continue to beat. The heart beat is thought to be transmitted by muscle fibers that are similar in structure to nerve fibers. These heart fibers are called Purkinje fibers.

Contractions begin in a part of the heart muscle called the sinoatrial node (S-A node). This structure is also referred to as the *pacemaker*. It is located on the upper right side of the heart. The beating impulse travels to the central part of the heart where the atrioventricular node is located (A-V node). The

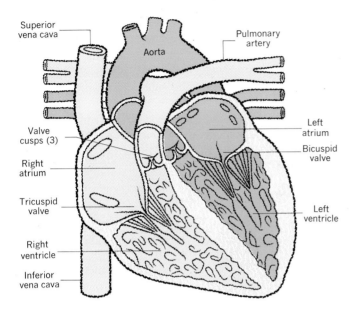
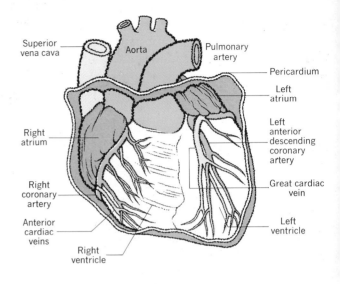

Figure 14-1
The heart.

impulse then radiates from the A-V node throughout the heart muscle, producing the contractive heart beat.

The rate of the heartbeat is controlled by impulses from the autonomic nervous system. The heart of a normal adult beats between 70 to 80 times per minute. There is a decrease in number of beats per minute from the child to the adult. For example, a three-year-old child will have an average heart rate of about 100 beats per minute. Many factors affect heart beat rate, including changes in temperature, drugs, and a change in the carbon dioxide level of the atmosphere.

The heart is divided into four chambers. There are two pumping chambers or ven-tricles (right and left). The two ventricles are closely joined in their muscular structure but are separated by a muscular tissue or septum. The atria forms the other two heart chambers. The right and left atria are thin-walled muscular cavities. The right atrium receives "blue" blood (not oxygenated) from the heart, arms, abdomen, and legs via two large veins. The left atrium receives

oxygenated or "red" blood from the lungs via the pulmonary veins.

There are four heart valves. Two valves separate the two atria from the two ventricles. This prevents a return of blood to the atria when the ventricles contract. The valve on the left side is called the mitral valve. The valve on the right side is called the tricuspid valve. The aortic valve prevents the return of blood into the aorta (large artery that carries blood away from the heart). The pulmonic valve prevents the return of blood from the pulmonary artery. Be sure to refer to Figure 14-1 to help you better understand the structure of the heart.

As circulation of blood through the body is the major function of the heart, a brief review of this process is in order. Blood enters the right atrium of the heart via the *superior vena cava* and the *inferior vena cava*. This blood has come from the upper and lower body regions. It then passes through the right A-V valve into the right ventricle. When the right ventricle contracts, blood is pushed through a set of valves into the pulmonary artery. The blood is then carried to the lungs. The oxygenated blood is then returned to the heart via the pulmonary veins. These veins open into the left atrium through the left A-V valve into the left ventricle. The blood is then pumped through the aorta and is distributed to all parts of the body. Figure 14-2 shows the flow of blood through the heart.

CORONARY CIRCULATION

A vital function of the heart is served by the network of coronary arteries and veins that cover the surface of the base of the heart. There are two main arterial trunks connected to the aorta. They bring oxygenated blood to the heart muscle. The coronary veins collect the blood that has provided the heart muscle with nourishment and oxygen and return it to the right atrium where other "blue" blood enters from the two large body veins.

There is a considerable interlacing of coronary arteries that provide for the circulation of the heart. It is these arteries that become blocked in certain forms of heart disease. If there is partial or complete blockage of a coronary artery, the existing arteries may form collateral arteries to bypass the obstructed areas and provide for continued circulation. Many individuals who suffer heart attacks as a result of severe coronary artery blockage are able to lead relatively normal lives because of the formation of these "extra" or collateral arteries.

One cannot expect to learn all about the heart's function and structure in a brief description of the subject. It is sufficient to know the basic structure, the function of heart muscle in beating and circulating the blood, and the function of the coronary arteries. If you wish to know more about this subject there are a number of books available in the library that detail the structure and function of the heart and its relationship to the rest of the body.

You have probably heard the expression "coronary" in reference to someone who has suffered a heart attack. The word is taken from the *coronary arteries*. When the blood supply is blocked by an obstructed artery, a *coronary* or heart attack occurs. The severity of the heart attack depends on how much

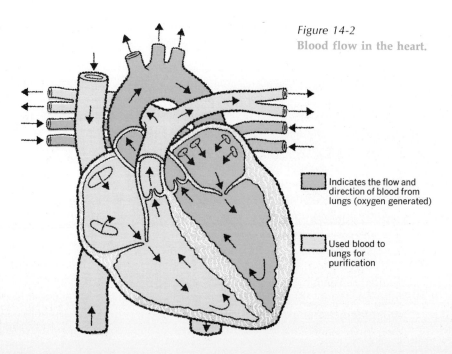

Figure 14-2
Blood flow in the heart.

Indicates the flow and direction of blood from lungs (oxygen generated)

Used blood to lungs for purification

Denton A. Cooley
(1920-   ), surgeon-in-
chief of the Texas Heart
Institute in Houston, is
one of the pioneers of
open-heart surgery. In
this type of operation, a
machine temporarily
takes over the heart's
functions so that the
surgeon can correct prob-
lems within the heart
itself. Among Dr.
Cooley's recent innova-
tions is a new type of
artificial heart valve.

of the heart muscle was deprived of blood. This deprivation of blood (and the oxygen it carries) results in damage to an area of the heart muscle. If there is great damage, the muscle will lose some of its contractual ability. As you can see, it is essential that the heart muscle have a constant supply of blood.

Exercise is as essential to the heart muscle as it is to other muscles. During exercise the heart develops the collateral coronary arteries that were previously mentioned. If a major vessel of the heart becomes obstruct-ed, these arteries can take over and keep the heart functioning. Dr. Denton Cooley, a renowned heart specialist, has said in refer-ence to the heart and exercise, "The question of exercise isn't just to keep the weight down. It keeps all the muscles including the heart muscle in tone and this is a very important safeguard. . . . You don't have to go into a vigorous time-consuming program like some men have of jogging thirty minutes a day." Dr. Cooley goes on to say that hopping on each foot 50 times twice a day or running in place twice a day for five minutes will provide as much exercise as a singles game of tennis. Refer to Chapter 11 for a complete discussion of exercise and fitness.

risk factors of heart disease

You have probably heard the term "risk factor." In health this term applies to certain conditions that can influence the onset of heart disease. There are certain factors that do exist to a greater degree in those who have heart disease. However, a *risk* factor is only that—a risk or chance of becoming ill and not a definite fact that one will suffer from heart disease. Not all of the research into certain risk factors and heart disease has been completed. Some of these factors are examined in the following sections of this chapter.

SEX

As discussed in an earlier section, males have a higher incidence of heart disease

than do premenopausal women. There seems to be a relationship between the female hormones released prior to menopause and the lower incidence of heart disease. Women who stay at home often get sufficient exer-cise through housework and child care to make them nonsedentary. If women work, they often carry the double responsibility of the home and the job and this too keeps them very active. Women, in general, tend to take their weight more seriously than men and weight is an important factor in heart disease.

However, women should not feel that they are completely protected from this disease, especially past the age of menopause. At this point in life, incidence of heart disease among women increases, although it does not equal the male incidence for the disease. Women who smoke heavily add to the risk of the disease. In addition, women who have high blood pressure or are obese increase their risk of suffering from heart disease. Women should follow the general good health requirements related to smoking, diet, and exercise in order to keep their "risk factors" down.

AGE

Although more and more Americans are having heart attacks at earlier ages, it is true that the older the person is the higher the risk. The older one becomes the greater the amount of coronary artery obstruction. Fig-ures reported from the National Center for Health Statistics indicate that coronary deaths among white American males between the ages of 35 and 64 dropped by 8.7 percent between 1968 and 1972. This decline was estimated at saving about 10,000 lives per year. The rate was also somewhat reduced for black men and for all women.

Why this sudden downturn in deaths from heart disease among younger people? Dr. Jeremiah Stamler, chairman of the depart-ment of community health and preventive medicine at Northwestern University Med-ical School suggested the following factors as contributing to the decline: (1) a decrease in cigarette smoking, especially among men over 25; (2) a shift from smoking cigarettes that are high in tar and nicotine content; (3) better screening for high blood pressure and increased use of drugs to control it; (4) increased use of unsaturated vegetable fat replacing animal fats high in cholesterol; and (5) increased availability and use of coronary-care units and emergency services.

Dr. Stamler feels that "the United States may, at long last, be 'over the hump' in regard to the epidemic of premature heart attacks, the No. 1 killer and crippler of Americans—particularly American men—in the prime of life." He made this statement at a recent annual forum of the American Heart Association. Evidence is mounting that medical science has turned the corner in the battle against heart disease. However, one can readily see that the individual has had much to do with this, specifically in his control of smoking and cholesterol intake.

HEREDITY

What part does heredity play in the onset of heart disease? This is a question that authorities are still researching. However, there are some forms of heart disease that are inherited (high cholesterol level in hyper-cholesterolemia) and other diseases where there *seems to be* certain familial trends. In hypercholesterolemia, cells keep on pro-

ducing cholesterol even when their cholesterol level is high enough for all body needs. This disease affects at least one out of 20 patients suffering from coronary heart disease.

Research is presently being conducted to find a biochemical that will "turn off" cholesterol synthesis at the cellular level. In addition, adult patients with a family history of heart attacks should be suspected of having the disease and their cholesterol levels should be measured.

SMOKING

The heart attack rate among men is 50 to 100 percent higher for cigarette smokers than it is for nonsmokers, depending on the age and amount smoked. For those who stop smoking, the death rate declines to that of people who have never smoked. Refer to the findings illustrated in Figure 14-3. These findings were adopted from data gathered by the National Heart and Lung Institue. As you can see, the rate of first heart attacks per 1,000 of the male population is greatly elevated for those who smoke more than one pack of cigarettes a day. Review Chapter 6 for more information on the effects of smoking on one's health.

DIET

How much one weighs and what he eats is extremely imporatnt to cardiac health.

Figure 14-3
Factors leading to heart trouble.

[1]Reprinted from "U.S. News & World Report." Copyright 1975 U.S. News & World Report, Inc.

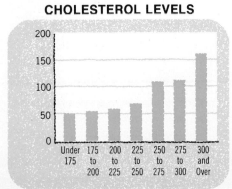

CHOLESTEROL LEVELS

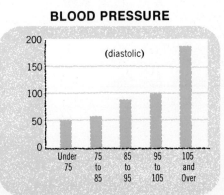

BLOOD PRESSURE

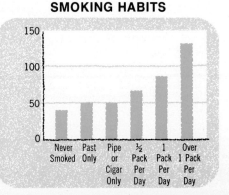

SMOKING HABITS

The heavier a person is, the greater the demand on his heart. The heart will, in time, compensate for additional weight, but obese individuals often suffer from complications related to the circulation and heart disease. Refer to Chapter 13 for methods of finding and achieving one's most ideal weight.

Cholesterol was discussed in Chapter 12 concerning nutrition. It is an important factor in any discussion of heart disease. Most studies have shown that high levels of blood cholesterol contribute to changes in the blood levels that can lead to coronary disease. Fats should not be eliminated entirely from the diet as they are a principal source of energy. However, certain fats that contain high levels of cholesterol can be replaced and limited. Animal fats should be avoided as much as possible. Substitutes include fish, fowl, vegetable oils, margarine, and low-fat milk. In general, a combination of exercise and a somewhat restricted diet will help to keep cholesterol at normal levels.

We have spoken about the problem of blood or serum cholesterol, but how exactly does it affect the coronary arteries? *Atherosclerosis* is the term given to the gradual narrowing and hardening of the arteries. This occurs when fatty deposits build up on the inside of arteries. This build-up may occur in arteries throughout the body and is not limited to the coronary arteries. However, when the deposits obstruct a coronary artery, blood may clot and cause a heart attack.

What is the relationship between cholesterol and this build-up in the arteries? Cholesterol is a fatty substance carried in the blood. If the conditions are right, an excess of this substance will be deposited in the arteries as the blood flows through the vessels. Conditions have to be right in that the level of cholesterol is excessive, the individual does not break down excess cholesterol through exercise; and other factors such as smoking and stress are elevated. Figure 14-4 illustrates how an atherosclerotic artery appears and shows how a blood clot may be formed in the narrowed vessel.

Most people suffer from some degree of atherosclerosis. This is expected, especially in an older person. After many years, the arteries will have become somewhat constricted by fatty deposits. Other factors, however, are involved in the rapidity of the deposit build-up; these factors as we have learned are both external and internal. Research is far from completed into the "whys" of atherosclerosis.

LACK OF EXERCISE

We have already discussed the importance of exercise in this chapter and in Chapter 11. Refer to Chapter 11 for a review of the value of exercise to cardiac health. Let it suffice to state here that exercise is a component of total good health which, of course, includes a healthy heart and circulatory system.

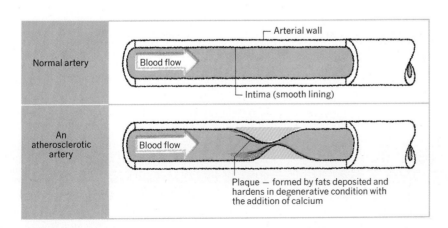

Figure 14-4
(a) A normal artery; (b) an atherosclerotic artery.

Normal artery

Arterial wall

Blood flow

Intima (smooth lining)

An atherosclerotic artery

Blood flow

Plaque — formed by fats deposited and hardens in degenerative condition with the addition of calcium

HYPERTENSION

Hypertension is better known as high blood pressure. Blood pressure is the force with which the blood pushes against the walls of the blood vessel. The blood pressure device used by your doctor determines this reading. The higher number is the systolic pressure which tells the level of pressure at the moment of the heart beat. The lower number or diastolic pressure is the pressure upon relaxation of the heart. A pressure of 120 over 70, for example, illustrates the pressure the heart exerts at work (120) and at rest (70).

Why is high blood pressure dangerous and a contributing factor in heart disease? If the blood pressure is too high, the arteries may "wear out" prematurely. In other words, years of high blood pressure may cause the arteries to lose their elasticity and become scarred. The fat deposits, previously discussed, accumulate more readily on the damaged walls of the arteries. Hypertension causes the heart to work harder and can result in an enlarged heart. This condition can lead to heart failure, the inability of the heart muscle to function.

What are the causes of hypertension? This question has only been partially answered. Some hypertension can be traced to a blockage of certain blood vessels, infections, or tumors. Often this type of hypertension can be treated and cured. This type of hypertension, however, only accounts for about 5 percent of all cases.

Heredity has been considered a possibility by some researchers. Others feel that diet is involved, especially a high intake of salt. Others combine both theories to conclude that there may be an hereditary predisposition toward a high degree of salt intake. Obesity has also been found to be related to high blood pressure.

Who gets high blood pressure? It affects people of all ages, races, and socioeconomic groups. It is more common among men than women, until about the age of 50. After 50, the reverse is more the rule. More older than younger people are affected; however, the disease does occur in children and teenagers. In fact, most people will first discover that they are hypertensive around the age of 30. The disease affects about 23 million Americans or about one out of seven, making hypertension the most common chronic disease in the United States.

It is interesting to note that high blood pressure is the leading cause of death among blacks and is the major reason why the life expectancy of blacks is shorter than that of the white population. It develops earlier among blacks, is often more severe, and results in a greater number of deaths at an earlier age. Some authorities in the field think that the high incidence of hypertension among blacks is related to the degree of stress to which they are exposed.

In many cases, high blood pressure can be successfully treated. A physician's regimen might include dieting, cutting salt intake, and exercise. If drug therapy is indicated, there are a number of drugs that can control high blood pressure. The important thing is to catch the disease before too much damage has been done.

In order to accomplish this, one must have his blood pressure taken. Many people do not go for routine examinations and may not know that they have this disease. In general, especially in the early stages, there are no symptoms. Only after 15 or 20 years of the disease do symptoms begin to appear. These symptoms may include headaches, dizziness, shortness of breath, and heart palpitations. However, after this many years, serious damage has already been done to the blood vessels.

Recently there has been a nationwide campaign to get people to have a simple blood pressure test. The National Heart and Lung Institute acted as a coordinating agency for the government's National High Blood Pressure Program. This program was aimed at mobilizing the medical community, the pharmaceutical industry, and the American public. Its purpose was education concerning high blood pressure and screening tests on a large scale. Hospitals, clinics, organizations, and mobile units sponsored free blood pressure testing. Dentists and other members of the medical profession were encouraged to take blood pressure readings as a part of their normal routine. Early discovery will go a long way to help control the disease and its complications. Have you had your blood pressure taken recently?

STRESS

Are you familiar with the terms *Type A* and *Type B?* No, they do not refer to blood types, but to personality types that are more or less prone to heart disease. Consider the following questions: (1) Are you highly competitive? (2) Do you become easily irritated? (3) Are you always trying to do too much in

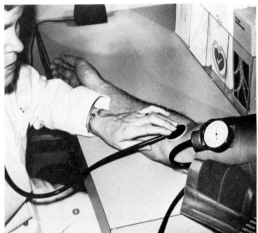

Free blood-pressure check-up at a local shopping center.

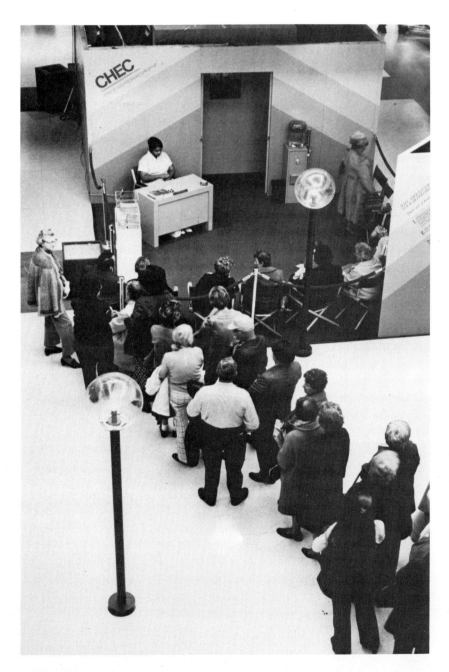

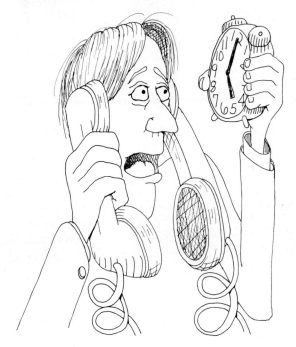
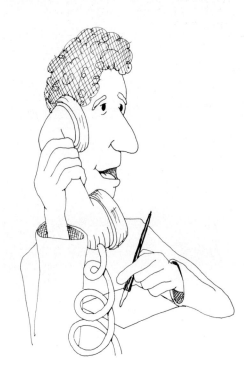

Type A and
Type B behavior.

too little time? If you answered "yes" to all of these questions, then there is a good chance that you may have a "Type A" personality.

Drs. Meyer Friedman and Ray Rosenman of Mount Zion Hospital, San Francisco, have done extensive studies of the relationships between personality and heart attacks. They have concluded that certain personality traits are a major factor in the occurrence of heart attack. Those who have high risk personality traits are called "Type A," while those with low risk personality traits are called "Type B." They have found that at least 90 percent of all the patients they have treated for heart attacks (under the age of 60) exhibited a Type A behavior pattern.

What is meant by these two personality classifications? Type A's tend to have a faster-paced life style. They are less able to cope with stress than Type B's. They are characterized by extremes of competitiveness, striving for achievement, aggressiveness, and briskness. They move quickly, are impatient, constantly under stress and pressure, and they always feel that the day is not quite long enough. Type A's tend to be truck

drivers, salesmen, auto racers, trial lawyers, television personalities, reporters, and high-level executives.

Type B's are basically opposite to Type A's. Though most people are a combination of both types of personalities, often one set of traits is more dominant than the other. Type B's know their capabilities and limitations. They do not rush into decisions and are generally more cautious than Type A's. They are better able to take one task at a time and complete it to their satisfaction. Type B's are generally "lower keyed" and are more apt to be patent lawyers, accountants, government clerks, or teachers.

Research at Mount Zion Hospital indicated that twice as many Type A's as Type B's suffered heart attacks. In addition, a Type A's heart attack was twice as likely to be fatal. An interesting factor that came to light was that Type A's who never smoked had nearly the same heart attack rate as Type B's who smoked. However, leading cardiologists are not in total agreement concerning this theory. Some authorities feel that the Type A-B approach is simplistic and puts too much weight on the personality theory.

301

They argue that it is dangerous to give that factor precedence over other established internal and external risks (cholesterol, high blood pressure, obesity, smoking, and exercise). The authorities do agree that stress is significant; however, they have yet to agree on the *degree* of significance.

MULTIPLYING THE RISKS OF HEART DISEASE

A number of risk factors have been discussed in relation to heart disease. A variety of the risks combined make the possibility of a heart attack that much greater. Heart disease is not caused by an isolated factor, but by many factors that vary in significance according to the individual's makeup (see Table 14-1). In most cases of heart disease, the individual exhibits a combination of risk factors that together have given rise to the onset of the disease.

heart attack—symptoms and emergency treatment

Symptoms of a heart attack vary with different people and the severity of the attack. Sweating and a feeling of weakness are usually present in a heart attack. There may be severe squeezing or burning pain in the area of the breastbone and frequently in the left arm and shoulder. Sometimes there is a feeling of heartburn or indigestion. There may be vomiting and loss of consciousness. Shortness of breath may also be experienced.

Immediate attention is urgently needed by the heart attack victim. If any of these symptoms persist, don't delay. Call an ambulance in order to get the individual to the hospital emergency room as quickly as possible.

EMERGENCY TREATMENT

Is there any emergency treatment that can

An emergency unit of a hospital is pressed into immediate service to treat a heart-attack victim.

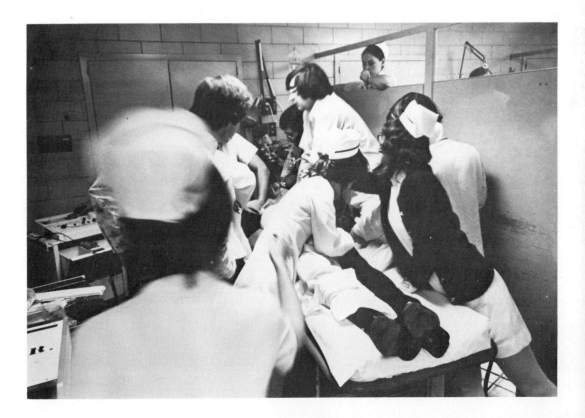

be administered while waiting for the ambulance to arrive? Loosen any restrictive clothing and have the patient rest quietly in a comfortable, semireclining position with his head and chest higher than the rest of the body. Try to talk to the person and help him to relax.

Two forms of emergency treatment can often save the life of a heart attack victim. These emergency treatments are resuscitation and cardiac massage. If a person has stopped breathing and the heart beat is weakening, mouth-to-mouth resuscitation can restore respiration and strengthen the weakened heart beat. If there is a lack of oxygen to the brain (for as few as four or five minutes), permanent brain damage can occur.

In order to accomplish mouth-to-mouth resuscitation, follow these procedures:

1. Lay the victim on his back, turn his head to one side, and remove any mucus, vomit, or gum from his mouth. Then turn the head forward.

2. Place one hand under the victim's neck and the other on top of his head. Tilt his head back so that the chin is pointing up.

3. Take a deep breath, open your mouth wide, and place it over the victim's mouth. Pinch the victim's nostrils closed as you do this. Exhale into the victim's mouth. Remove your mouth and listen for a return of air from the victim. Repeat this pro-

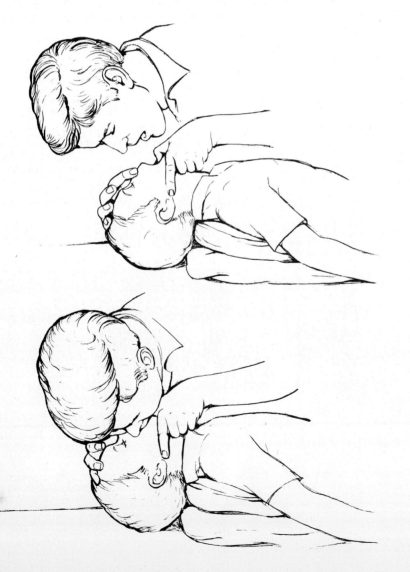

Mouth-to-mouth resuscitation.
a) Pull up jaw and pinch nostrils closed.

b) Press mouth firmly over victim's mouth and blow.

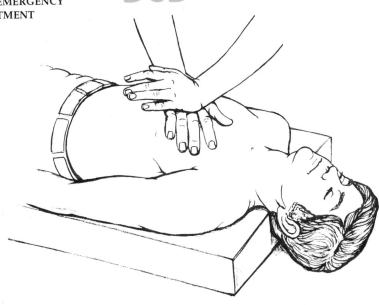

External cardiac massage.

cedure again, listening for a return of air. If there is no return, check for possible blockage of the respiratory tract.

4. Continue this breathing at a regular rate of approximately 12 breaths per minute.
5. If the victim begins to breathe on his own, time your breathing with his to allow for exhaling. Once breathing has returned and is sufficiently strong, resuscitation can be stopped.

The other emergency procedure, external cardiac massage, is only used in combination with mouth-to-mouth resuscitation.

1. The victim should be placed on his back. The surface should be rigid—not soft.
2. Before starting massage, have the person doing resuscitation breathe three times into the victim's mouth. Then hit the victim's chest once (upper chest—left of the center) with a closed fist. If this does not start the heartbeat then start immediately with cardiac massage.
3. Place the back of your hand on the victim's breastbone and put your left hand across your right hand. With your elbows straight, lean forward and press on the victim's chest. Do not hold the pressure but release it and then do again.

4. This should be continued at a regular rate of about once a second. Check for a pulse; but continue the massage until the victim is breathing on his own.

PREVENTIVE TREATMENT

Preventive treatment has been discussed in relationship to risk factors. Controlling these factors is a form of preventive treatment. A regular checkup is another way of detecting heart and circulatory disease in its early stage.

There is also a Cardiac Stress Test that helps to find those people who test normally with certain other routine heart testing. This type of testing involves performance on a stationary bicycle or treadmill, while a cardiologist continuously monitors the heart. This gives the cardiologist an indirect image of the extent of narrowing in a patient's coronary arteries. It can also detect the danger of stroke in cases where a patient exhibits extremely high blood pressure during exercise. It is also valuable in ruling out suspected coronary artery disease.

The American Heart Association recommends stress testing for adults with one or more of the following risk factors: a history of heart

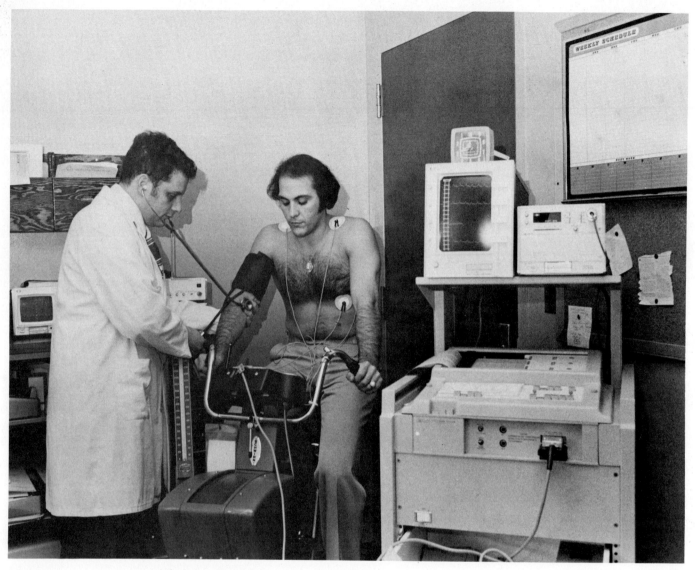

Administration of the cardiac stress test.

disease, high blood pressure, diabetes, high cholesterol, overweight, smoking, and highly pressured life style. Stress testing is available in most medical centers and large hospitals.

various forms of heart disease

Though heart attack may be the best known heart ailment, there are various forms of heart disease. Some of the more common diseases are discussed here.

ANGINA PECTORIS

The most common symptom of angina is a squeezing or burning pain that may radiate to the left arm or shoulder. This disease results from a brief lack of blood flow which deprives the oxygen supply to the heart. Some angina pain is an early warning of a heart attack. Individuals who have suffered heart attacks and those who have not suffered heart attacks may experience angina pectoris.

Anyone suffering this type of pain should seek medical treatment. Medication and rest will help to alleviate the condition. If symptoms other than chest pain occur, a heart attack should not be ruled out. Generally speaking, most angina attacks give no symptoms except chest pain.

CONGENITAL HEART DISEASE

Volumes have been written on the subject of congenital heart defects. A congenital defect is one with which a baby is born. Some defects can be corrected by cardiac surgery; others may be too severe for surgery procedures.

There are three general classifications of congenital heart disease. They include: (1) an imperfect separation between the right and left sides of the heart so that the oxygenated and deoxygenated blood mix; (2) a narrowing in the path of the flow of blood causing an obstruction; and (3) a combination of these defects.

More than 10,000 babies are born each year with congenital heart defects. If not corrected by surgery, these babies will die. Until recently, such surgery was considered a high risk and involved a high mortality rate. A new type of surgery employed at Children's Hospital Medical Center in Boston has met with a high success rate.

The child is anesthetized, then packed in ice until his temperature is below 77 degrees Fahrenheit. The child is then taken out of the ice pack and hooked up to a heart-lung machine, which further cools the heart and blood until circulation and heart beat stop. "The use of the ice pack has opened up a new era in the treatment of congenital heart defects" says Dr. A. Castaneda, head of the Boston surgical team.

RHEUMATIC HEART DISEASE

Rheumatic fever is much less common today than it was 20 or 30 years ago. Rheumatic heart disease is an inflammation of the valves and muscle of the heart that occurs during rheumatic fever. Scar tissue may be formed that may prevent the heart valves from functioning adequately and may also reduce the strength of the heart muscle.

Rheumatic fever is caused by a streptococcal infection. These "strep" bacteria usually attack the nose and throat. A "strep" throat is a fairly common infection, especially among children. Rheumatic fever often begins two to three weeks after the onset of a streptococcal infection. The patient may have a fever and sore throat for days, become well, and then have an attack of rheumatic fever. Symptoms of rheumatic fever include: (1) painful and inflamed joints; (2) high fever; (3) fatigue; and (4) aching of the arms and legs.

The onset of rheumatic fever can be prevented if streptococcal bacteria are destroyed in the early stages of "strep" throat. Throat cultures can be taken to determine if "strep" is present. If it is, penicillin and other antibiotics will destroy these bacteria. Any sore throat, particularly those accompanied by fever, should be examined and cultured if the doctor thinks it might be a "strep" infection.

Once one has had an attack of rheumatic fever, bed rest and quiet are prescribed. Aspirin, cortisone, and ACTH may help to suppress the inflammation of the heart. A course of penicillin treatment is also given to destroy any remaining streptococci. It is important that rheumatic fever patients do not get additional "strep" attacks. All sore throats should be cultured and penicillin therapy prescribed, if "strep" exists.

HIGH BLOOD PRESSURE

This subject was discussed in detail in the section concerning risk factors. Refer to this section for information concerning high blood pressure and heart disease.

306

STROKE

The medical term for a stroke is cerebro-vascular accident (CVA). A stroke is an interference with the circulation to the brain or part of the brain. It results from a disorder of the blood vessels rather than the heart.

Most stroke victims have had previous circulatory problems. High-risk individuals are often those with known heart or vascular disorders, high blood pressure, diabetes, high blood cholesterol, and obesity.

Strokes are caused by hardening of the arteries. This condition may be due to *atherosclerosis* or *arteriosclerosis*. Both conditions involve the blood vessels and may result in blood clots and disruption of circulation. Atherosclerosis is the hardening of the arteries and the accumulation of fat deposits in the inside walls. Arteriosclerosis is part of the aging process and involves a hardening of the outside walls of the blood vessels. Strokes are often a result of arteriosclerosis, as the arteries of the head harden and a blood clot may be formed.

The symptoms of a stroke may differ depending on the part of the brain that is affected. Symptoms may include: severe headache; difficulty in speech; impaired vision; and weakness, paralysis, or numbness of the body or of one side of the body. If you think that someone has suffered a stroke, be sure to get him to the hospital as quickly as possible.

treatment for heart disease

Rest, medication, and usually a change in life style are encouraged in the treatment of heart disease. Patients are urged to control the risk factors that were discussed at the beginning of this chapter. In addition to physical risk factors, one must also change his behavioral patterns.

Many cardiologists believe that the Type A individual must attempt to adjust his behavioral reactions. In order to help these people cope with stress, programs of Cardiac Stress Management Training are being conducted.

Christiaan Neethling Barnard (1922-   ), a South African surgeon, performed the world's first human heart transplant operation in 1967. However, heart transplant patients didn't survive very long, because their bodies developed a reaction against the "foreign" tissue of the new heart. So in 1974, Dr. Barnard introduced another new technique: the "twin heart" operation. He connected a second heart to the patient's own heart. It was hoped that the second heart would lessen the strain on the diseased heart by taking over some of its functions.

One such program at Colorado State University teaches patients to tense and relax muscles, to identify stress situations, to develop self-control, and be able to relax in a short period of time. Patients in the original program experienced lower blood cholesterol levels. The program will also be opened to Type A's who have not suffered a heart attack. This will be a preventive approach.

There are various forms of heart surgery that are a possibility for some patients with heart disease. Bypass surgery, valve replacement, and transplants are only a few of the procedures being used today. Dr. Christiaan Barnard made history in 1967 when he performed the first human heart transplant. Dr. Barnard made history again in 1974 when he performed a new transplant technique by implanting a second heart into a terminally ill cardiac patient. The second heart acts as a backup heart to the patient's own diseased heart. Barnard believes that the twin-heart operation may overcome some of the difficulties of the total heart transplant. The problem of rejection (the body's failure to accept another individual's heart) is controlled to the degree that if the transplanted heart is rejected, it can be removed and the patient still has his own heart.

Great strides have been made in the treatment of heart disease, but many problems are yet to be solved. Controversy exists in medical circles as to procedures to be used in diagnosis and treatment of these diseases. What is definitely known, however, is that the risk factors to some degree do affect the chance of cardiac disease. These risk factors should be controlled for one's cardiac health as well as one's total health.

THINKING IT OVER

1. Briefly explain the basic structure of the heart.
2. Discuss the circulation of blood through the heart.
3. Discuss the importance of the coronary arteries and what happens when the circulation to these arteries is cut off.
4. Explain the importance of exercise to the heart muscle.

5. Discuss the risk factor of sex in relation to heart disease.
6. Explain the role that heredity may play in heart disease.
7. Discuss nutrition and obesity in relation to heart disease.
8. What is hypertension? How does it relate to heart disease?
9. Discuss the characteristics of "Type A" and "Type B" personalities. How do these personality types relate to heart disease?
10. Discuss the symptoms of heart attack.
11. Briefly describe the two methods of emergency treatment for heart attack.
12. What is angina pectoris?
13. What are the common classifications of congenital heart disease?
14. What is a stroke and how does it affect its victims?
15. Describe the types of treatment available to victims of heart disease.

KEY WORDS

Angina pectoris. Pain in the heart and chest area caused by oxygen deprivation to the heart muscle.

Arteriosclerosis. Hardening of the outer walls of the arteries.

Atherosclerosis. Hardening of the arteries accompanied by the laying down of fat deposits on the inside walls of the arteries.

Congenital heart disease. Defects in the heart at birth; can often be corrected by surgery.

Coronary arteries. The circulatory system of the heart.

Heart attack. Formation of a blood clot within a coronary artery.

Hypercholesteremia. An inherited condition that causes elevated blood cholesterol levels.

Hypertension. High or elevated blood pressure.

Rheumatic heart disease. An inflammation of the heart muscle and valves caused by rheumatic fever.

Stroke. A blood clot in an artery of the brain due to atherosclerosis or arteriosclerosis; blood is cut off to a part of the brain.

"Type A." Personality type associated with heart disease and characterized by aggressiveness, competitiveness, and striving for achievement.

"Type B." Personality type not associated with heart disease and characterized by an even temper, thoughtful decision making, and a controlled personality.

GETTING INVOLVED

Books and Periodicals

Barnard, Christiaan. *Heart Attack.* New York: Dell, 1973. The transplant surgeon's suggestions for coping with heart attacks.

Friedman, Meyer and Ray Rosenman. *Type A Behavior and Your Heart.* New York: Knopf, 1974. Examines the kind of behavior that seems to work with other risk factors to increase coronary artery disease.

"Latest in Fight Against Heart Attack," *U.S. News and World Report,* February 3, 1975. Among other things, the latest techniques in preventing heart attacks.

Lesher, Stephan. "There Comes a Will to Live," *New York Times Magazine,* January 27, 1974. One man's experiences after having a heart attack.

Young, Patrick, "Your Personality May Be Killing You," *Reader's Digest,* August 1974. Heart disease and how it may be affected by the "Type A" personality.

Movies

Highway to Healthy Hearts, 1969. Research shows what keeps the heart going. Distributed by the American Heart Association.

The Human Body: Circulatory System, 1956. The workings of the heart—with a side look at the lungs and kidneys. Distributed by the American Heart Association.

Pulse of Life, 1962. Life-saving methods for victims of heart attacks and other disasters. Distributed by the American Heart Association.

Strokes, 1957. What happens when a stroke occurs, shown in animated cartoons. Distributed by the American Heart Association.

15
PULMONARY AND OTHER SYSTEMIC DISEASES

In this chapter you will learn about some of the diseases that frequently affect the respiratory system and other body systems. You have probably heard of most of these diseases, but you may not be familiar with their symptoms, causes, or treatment.

The first section of this chapter examines diseases that are related to the respiratory system. These diseases include the common cold, influenza, bronchitis, pneumonia, tuberculosis, asthma, and emphysema.

Diseases of the gastro-intestinal system are discussed in the next section of this chapter. Stomach upset, ulcers, colitis, ileitis, and appendicitis are examined. Diseases of other body systems are also examined. Diseases of the kidneys, liver, and nervous system are discussed.

In addition, arthritis and diabetes are examined. It is hoped that this chapter will provide you with a better understanding of some of these diseases. You may wish to study one or more of these diseases in greater detail by doing individual research.

While reading this chapter, think about the following concepts:

■ Disorders of the lungs result in many respiratory ailments.

■ The common cold is not really one disease, but a composite of ailments.

■ Many lung diseases are associated with smoking and air pollution.

■ Ulcers have been found to be closely related to stress situations.

■ Many people fear certain diseases of the nervous system because they do not understand their causes or symptoms.

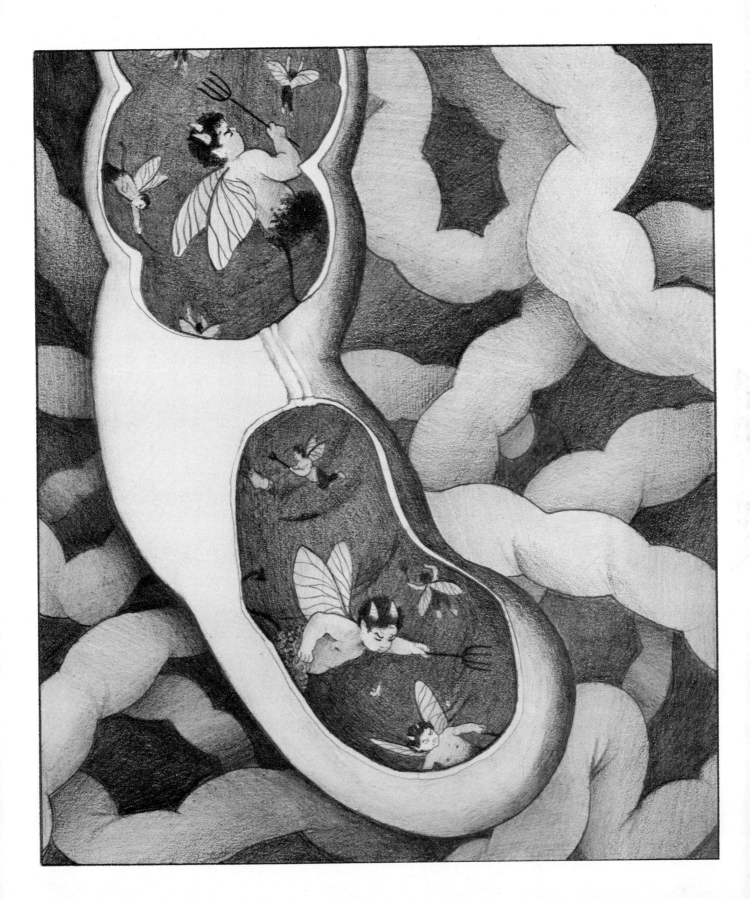

The title of this chapter, "Pulmonary and Other Systemic Diseases," may sound somewhat technical, but you are probably familiar with the diseases discussed in this chapter.

One disease, the common cold, is probably very familiar to you. How many colds have you had this year? According to a recent article in the *Journal of the American Medical Association,* persons in the 20 to 24 age group have approximately 2.8 colds a year. This study indicated a decrease in the number of colds as one got older, except for a slight increase in the 20 to 24 age group.

Other findings in this study were quite surprising. It was found that people with higher levels of education tended to suffer from a greater number of respiratory infections. Researchers concluded that perhaps better educated people were able to recognize the early symptoms of their illness. Another finding of this study was that more people became ill with colds on Monday than any other day of the week. This was particularly striking in the 5 to 19 or school-age population. The "blue Monday" or "back to school or work" syndrome seemed to be operating here. Have you found this to be true? The next time you get a cold, take note if it happens to be on a Monday!

Colds are just one of the diseases that you will learn about in this chapter. New treatment methods and research into these diseases are also discussed. Many people are unaware of the origin and treatment of many diseases. This chapter will give you an opportunity to become more familiar with both the common and uncommon diseases that afflict many people.

respiratory system — its structure and function

The structure of the respiratory system is often compared to the branching of a tree. Refer to Figure 15-1 as you read this section of the chapter. The windpipe, through which air passes, is called the trachea. This tube extends from the larynx (voice box) through the neck and into the chest cavity. At its lower end, it divides into two tubes, the bronchi. Each bronchus extends into a lung.

In the lungs, each bronchus divides into small branches called bronchioles. These bronchioles continue to branch into smaller passageways where their walls become very thin. Each bronchiole ends in a cluster of small air sacs or alveoli. Here the gases are exchanged between the circulatory system and the air. The exchange takes place between the thin walls of the alveoli and the capillary walls, where oxygen can easily pass into the bloodstream, while

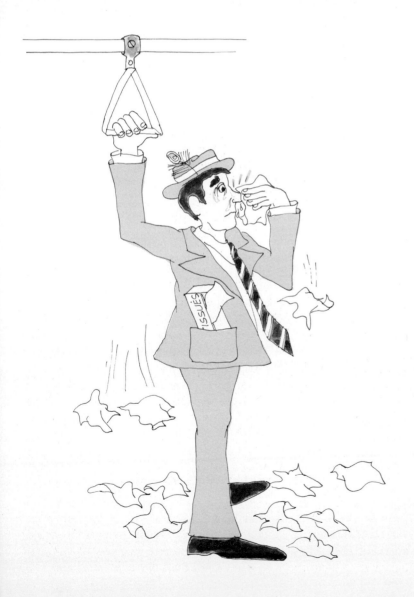

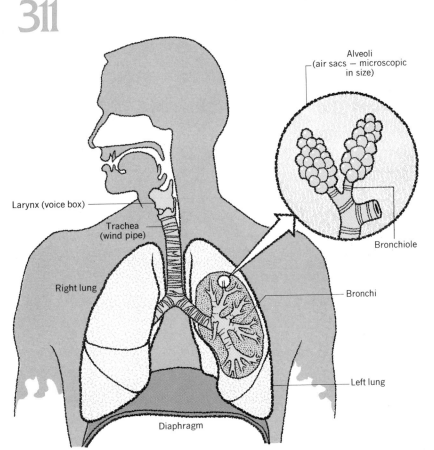

Figure 15-1
The respiratory tract.

Alveoli
(air sacs — microscopic in size)

Bronchiole

Bronchi

Larynx (voice box)

Trachea (wind pipe)

Right lung

Left lung

Diaphragm

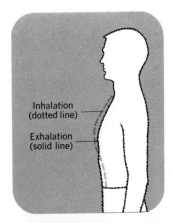

Inhalation (dotted line)

Exhalation (solid line)

Figure 15-2
Changes in the chest cavity caused by inhalation and exhalation.

carbon dioxide can pass out through the lungs into the air.

The lungs are surrounded by a double <u>pleural membrane</u> that protects them from the friction of the breathing movements. The two plueral membranes are separated by a fluid that prevents them from rubbing against each other during breathing.

How do you breathe? Breathing, as most body processes, is very complex. Here it will be described in a simplified way so that you will have a general idea of what is happening each time you breathe. During the breathing process, there are marked changes in the size of the chest cavity. See Figure 15-2. When you inhale, the chest cavity expands to allow the air to flow into the lungs. When you exhale, the chest cavity contracts to force the air from the lungs. This is accomplished by the <u>diaphragm</u>, a muscle that divides the chest and abdominal cavities and the muscles attached to the rib

cage. The abdominal muscles also play a role in breathing.

The heart and lungs work together to efficiently supply the body with oxygenated blood and remove the carbon dioxide from the bloodstream. These two systems (circulo-respiratory) are closely involved in physical fitness. Circulo-respiratory (C-R) endurance (as you may recall from Chapter 11) referred to the combined training effect of both these systems after a successful, long-term exercise program. Review sections of Chapter 11 for more information in this area.

diseases of the pulmonary system

Few people escape some diseases of the pulmonary system. The most common disease of the respiratory system is the cold. A cold is not really a disease, but rather a composite of ailments that usually affect the lungs and respiration. Colds are caused by several different viruses. Cold-causing organisms are usually present in the respiratory system. However, depending on one's resistance, one may be able to avoid a cold. Rest, proper diet, and total good health may help in preventing the onset of a cold.

Much has been written recently about the role of vitamin C in preventing colds. Linus Pauling (a renowned scientist) has proclaimed that vitamin C (taken in large doses) will prevent most colds from occurring and will lessen the symptoms of those that do occur.

A recent study by Canadian scientists (*U.S. News and World Report,* December 23, 1974) indicated that vitamin C does relieve the chest pains, fever, and general discomfort of the common cold. This study also indicated that small doses worked as well as massive doses. Studies done in the United States have warned that massive doses of vitamin C destroy substantial amounts of vitamin B-12. A lack of vitamin B-12 can cause a form of anemia, which can be fatal.

Researchers have been looking for a "cure" to the common cold for many years. This

may be a reality soon according to a report from the University of Illinois. The drug, *propanediamine,* is currently being tested. This drug is said to stimulate the production of *interferon.* This is a chemical agent produced by the body that is a natural defense against colds and other viruses.

INFLUENZA

Influenza or the "flu" is another common disease of the respiratory system. It is caused by many different viruses and often affects both the respiratory and digestive systems. Symptoms often include fever, chills, head-ache, prolonged cough, weakness, and sore throat. If the digestive system is involved nausea, vomiting, and diarrhea may ensue. In most cases, recovery will occur in two to seven days.

There are many varities of "flu" that often make the headlines each year. The "Asian flu," "Hong Kong flu," and a newly rec-ognized strain, the "Port Chalmers flu" (from New Zealand) are a few of the strains that have been recognized in recent years. During the 1968–1969 epidemic of the

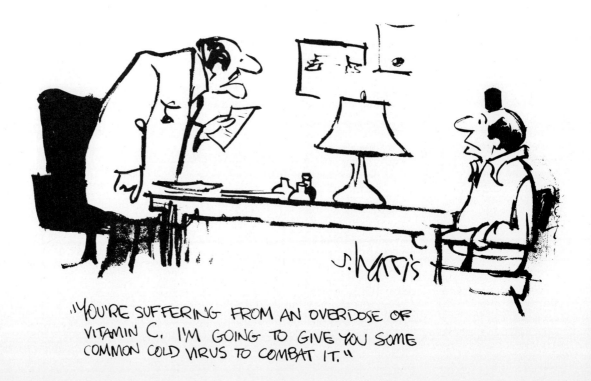

"YOU'RE SUFFERING FROM AN OVERDOSE OF VITAMIN C. I'M GOING TO GIVE YOU SOME COMMON COLD VIRUS TO COMBAT IT."

"Hong Kong flu" approximately 28,000 people died from influenza and the complication of related pneumonia.

Immunization is available for influenza and is encouraged for those who are extremely susceptible to respiratory infections and for the elderly. However, most flu vaccines are only moderately effective. Personal hygiene and the avoidance of large crowds during an epidemic are helpful in avoiding these diseases.

BRONCHITIS

There are two types of bronchitis: acute and chronic. The acute condition usually involves the bronchi and the lower trachea and accompanies a virus infection of the respiratory tract. Bronchitis causes an excessive secretion of the mucous glands and a cough that may last for many weeks. In both types of bronchitis, there is an inflammation of the bronchial tubes.

There are several antibiotic drugs that are effective in certain cases of bronchitis. Individuals with chronic bronchitis should avoid smoking, inhaling irritating gases, and areas of heavy air pollution.

Chronic bronchitis is similar to acute bronchitis except that the cough is more severe and long-lasting. In addition, there is a greater accumulation of thick mucus or sputum. There may be an accompanying shortness of breath and wheezing. This type of bronchitis usually occurs each year and may last from one to three months. Most people who suffer from chronic bronchitis are heavy smokers, hence the term "smoker's cough."

PNEUMONIA

Pneumonia is a common lung infection that may be caused by a bacteria or a virus. Bacterial pneumonia may affect the bronchioles (bronchial pneumonia) or the bronchioles and the alveoli (lobar pneumonia— affects one or more lobes of one or both lungs). The lungs are divided into lobes by deep fissures that are easily observable if one were to look at the lung.

Bacterial pneumonia is usually characterized by fever, chills, chest pain, coughing, and difficulty in breathing. In pneumonia, the bronchioles and alveoli become filled with fluid and pus and there may be a thick discharge from the lungs. There are varying degrees of severity. In most cases, antibiotics are effective in the treatment of pneumonia, if they are given in the early stages of the disease.

Virus pneumonia, as its name implies, is caused by a virus rather than a bacterial agent. It often follows a cold or other viral infection. The symptoms may be less severe than those of bacterial pneumonia and in some cases the symptoms are mild or nonexistent.

TUBERCULOSIS

Tuberculosis is a disease that is nearly eradicated in the U.S. today. However, it was once a leading cause of death in the United States and other countries. It still is an important cause of death in many parts of the world. Tuberculosis still kills about three million persons each year in Asia, South America, and Africa.

Tuberculosis is a bacterial disease that causes lesions in the lungs called tubercles. These lesions may be cut off from circulation and the tissues within the area will die. If there are many lesions, an entire lobe of a lung or the whole lung may be involved and the tissue destroyed.

In the early stages of tuberculosis, there may be no symptoms or pain. Months may pass before some of the symptoms become evident. Symptoms include fever, sweats, and loss of weight. Months later, a cough or blood-stained sputum may be noticed. At this stage, the disease is well-advanced.

If treated in its early stages, tuberculosis can be cured. Antibiotics and complete rest are effective in curing this disease. There are also methods of control that are valuable in identifying the disease at an early stage.

Skin tests, such as the tine test, can identify the presence of the tubercle bacteria. Chest X-rays will show up tuberculosis lesions. Routine X-ray examinations and/or skin tests are urged for certain segments of the population that are most susceptible to the disease (long-term hospital or institution patients or people who live in overcrowded conditions).

People who have public contact, especially those who are in contact with children, should be tested as a routine precaution. Have you been tested for tuberculosis recently? It is a simple procedure that should be given or requested as a part of a routine physical examination.

ASTHMA

Asthma is a condition that causes the constriction of the bronchial tubes resulting in breathing difficulty, wheezing, choking, and a shortness of breath. It is the leading respiratory condition of children under the age of 16, but occurs in adults as well as children.

There are two types of asthma, *extrinsic* and *intrinsic*. The extrinsic type is caused by a reaction to substances called allergens; these substances include pollen, dust, animal hair, and a variety of foods. Some individuals will not exhibit any symptoms until they have been exposed to the offending allergen for many years. Asthma may also come on suddenly and disappear just as suddenly. Intrinsic asthma is diagnosed when no allergen can be found that is causing the asthma attack. This type of asthma is thought to be related to a respiratory tract infection.

What causes asthma? It is currently thought that asthma is related to a chemical deficiency that causes the air passages to become clogged, swelling of the mucous membranes, and muscle spasms in this area. This leads to the wheezing and coughing associated with an asthma attack. Heredity is thought to be an important factor, especially in extrinsic asthma. Emotional and psycho-

logical pressures can aggravate an asthmatic condition.

There are many treatments available to asthmatics. Skin tests are given to determine the allergens responsible for the attack. If the allergen or allergens are identified, then injections of small amounts of these materials are gradually increased until the body builds up a tolerance to the substance or substances.

Drugs such as *aminophylline* are often prescribed to relax the muscles and open the air passages. Adrenalin is also injected to keep open the air passages. A new drug, called *cromalyn,* helps to prevent asthma attacks in some individuals. Individuals who suffer from asthma should avoid self-medication. Many over-the-counter drugs can be harmful to the asthmatic. This is particularly true of medications containing aspirin. They can cause a serious asthma attack, especially in the intrinsic form of the disease.

EMPHYSEMA

Emphysema is a serious disease of the lungs that has been increasing in recent years. Incidence of the disease has tripled in a recent 11-year period. More than 20,000 Americans die from emphysema each year.

Emphysema usually afflicts individuals who are between 50 and 70 years of age. More men than women are victims of this disease. A very high percentage of emphysema patients are heavy cigarette smokers and have smoked for many years. Air pollution is another factor in the incidence of the disease. Some individuals have a certain chemical deficiency that makes them more likely than others to get the disease at an earlier age.

Emphysema is caused by a chronic irritation of the bronchi, bronchioles, and the alveoli. The walls of the alveoli may tear or be stretched resulting in the entrapment of air and impairment of the air exchange process and circulation in the lungs. If the irritation continues, the entire lung may become enlarged and there is a marked decrease in gaseous exchange. The name *emphysema*

comes from the Greek word meaning
"to inflate."

The symptoms of emphysema in its early
stages may be difficulty in breathing following
mild exercise. As the disease progresses,
breathlessness may occur following normal,
routine activities. Some people have difficulty
in breathing when they walk or climb stairs.
Some patients need a constant flow of oxygen
to help them to breathe.

As the alveoli deteriorate, the passage of
blood through the lungs is affected. The
heart must work harder in order to pump
the blood. Heart failure, due to enlargement
of the heart, often results from emphysema.

Individuals with emphysema can be treated
by medication, oxygen, breathing retraining,
exercise, and by learning to use to its fullest
advantage what breathing capacity is left.
In order to prevent emphysema, one should
not smoke and one should avoid polluted
air whenever possible. If one is a heavy
smoker and emphysema is diagnosed, one
should immediately quit smoking.

OTHER INFECTIOUS DISEASES

Many of the diseases discussed so far in
this chapter could have been discussed in
Chapter 16, "Infectious Diseases." However,
because of their relationship to each other,
it was decided to include them in this chapter.
If you want to find out more about any of
these diseases, you may want to write to
the local chapters of the American Lung
Association, Heart Association, or the
National Interagency Council on Smoking
and Health, 419 Park Avenue South, New
York, N.Y. 10016. Lung cancer is discussed
in Chapter 17, where the entire subject
of cancer is examined.

diseases of other major body systems

In this section of Chapter 15, some of the
more common diseases of the body systems
other than the respiratory system are discussed. There are many other systemic
diseases, but this group was chosen because

a large percentage of the population is
afflicted by them.

THE GASTROINTESTINAL SYSTEM

Many organs and glands make up the
gastrointestinal system. These structures
include the mouth, salivary glands, esophagus,
stomach, small intestine, large intestine, gall
bladder, liver, and pancreas. These organs
and glands work together to break down
and absorb food substances and to pass
solid waste matter out of the body.

The function of the digestive system is
briefly described here so that you will better
understand some of the common diseases
that are related to this system. Refer to
Figure 15-3 as you read this section of
the chapter.

Digestion begins in the mouth by means
of chewing the food and mixing it with
saliva. The saliva is secreted by salivary
glands. There are three pairs of salivary
glands that produce between two and three
pints of saliva daily. The enzymes contained
in the saliva are active in beginning the
breakdown of carbohydrates. Other enzymes
in the digestive system complete this action
and break down other food nutrients.

The food is then swallowed and passes
through the esophagus into the stomach.
This occurs through peristaltic or squeezing
contractions of the esophagus. Once in the
stomach, the partially digested food or
bolus is further digested by the gastric juices
secreted by the inner lining of the stomach.
The stomach aids digestion by a continual
churning and mixing action. The bolus then
becomes a smooth paste called chyme.
The chyme then passes through the pyloric
sphincter, a muscle located at the end of
the stomach where it joins the small intestine
(see Figure 15-3).

Most of the digestive process takes place in
the small intestine and it is here that the
digested food is absorbed into the body.
Various secretions in the small intestine help
to further break down food nutrients. The food
is absorbed by millions of small, fingerlike

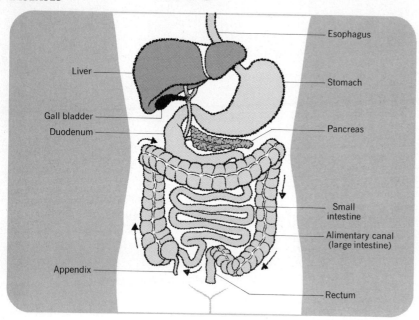

Figure 15-3
The digestive
tract.

Esophagus

Liver

Stomach

Gall bladder

Duodenum

Pancreas

Small
intestine

Alimentary canal
(large intestine)

Appendix

Rectum

structures called villi (see Figure 15-4). Each villus has a network of capillaries and a central tube called a lacteal. The lacteals contain lymph (a body fluid). Broken-down fatty substances pass through the villi capillaries into the lacteals and other substances pass into the villi and enter the bloodstream in this manner. At the completion of the digestive process, only water and undigested matter remain in the small intestine.

This remaining material is the substance of the solid wastes or feces. These materials are passed from the small intestine into the large intestine or colon. It is here that excess water and salts are absorbed into the body and the remaining waste materials are passed out of the colon through the rectum during a bowel movement.

There are many major and minor conditions that affect the digestive system. You are probably most familiar with two of them: *indigestion* and *heart burn*. These two conditions are commonly grouped under the general term, *upset stomach*. An upset stomach means different symptoms to different people. Some individuals have a feeling of discomfort or fullness, while others complain of gas or a burning sensation in the upper

portion of the stomach. Sometimes all of these symptoms are experienced at the same time.

What causes upset stomach? Some of the major causes are eating too rapidly or too much, drinking too much alcohol, smoking, certain medications, tight or restrictive clothing, or eating foods that one is not accustomed to consuming.

In addition, nervousness and tension are also related to stomach upset. They can cause the stomach to secrete excessive amounts of digestive juices that may irritate the stomach lining, which can be more harmful when there is no food in the stomach. Too much stomach acid can, in time, eat away a part of the stomach lining and result in a gastric ulcer. This is discussed in more detail in the next section.

What can one do to avoid an upset stomach? One of the most important factors is to make mealtimes relaxed occasions where there is little commotion or few highly emotional discussions. This will help to reduce nervous tension while eating. Food should be eaten slowly and thoroughly chewed before swallowing. Spicy foods should be avoided if they cause stomach

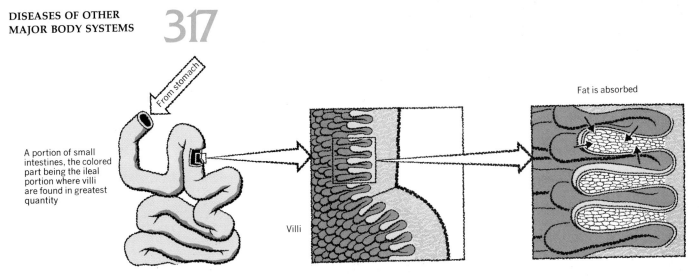

Figure 15-4
The villi.

discomfort. Drinking too much alcohol can also irritate the stomach lining. This effect can be reduced by consuming food prior to and along with the alcohol.

Are there any medications available to help relieve the symptoms of an upset stomach? There are numerous over-the-counter preparations that are widely advertised and well-known to the public. If the stomach upset is minor, these substances may be helpful in relieving some of the discomfort. However, if the pain recurs and is severe, one should seek medical attention. A family physician or gastroenterologist (a doctor who specializes in diseases of the gastrointestinal system) should be consulted. Prescribed medications are available to help reduce stomach acidity, and certain diets will help control ulcerative conditions.

There are two types of gastric or stomach ulcers: gastric ulcers, which occur in the lining of the stomach, and duodenal ulcers, which occur in the duodenum (the first portion of the small intestine). These ulcers result from prolonged irritation of the linings of these structures. The lining becomes irritated and, in time, open sores or ulcers are produced. The acid in the gastric juice is responsible for this action.

Symptoms of an ulcer include stomach pain that may be present before eating (in a gastric ulcer) and after eating (in a duodenal ulcer). The symptoms often come and go for weeks at a time and may then disappear for several months.

Most ulcer patients can be treated by diet and medication. The ulcer patient often needs to eat smaller meals more frequently during the day. It is beneficial, in many cases, to keep the stomach partially filled with food so that the excess gastric juice is absorbed. This prevents the acid contained in the juice from irritating the stomach lining. In severe cases, surgical procedures are used to reduce the flow of acid into the stomach.

In many cases, the cause of ulcers is thought to be excessive stress. Refer to Chapter 4 where stress was discussed in detail. Stress tends to stimulate the secretion of excess gastric juice into the stomach. Alcohol, tobacco, and a poor diet can further complicate the condition.

One should not self-medicate for ulcers. This could be a dangerous practice. Many people take over-the-counter antacids that tend to neutralize the gastric juices, but this is usually followed by a greater secretion of this substance.

Two diseases of the digestive system are less well-known but affect approximately two and one-half million people. These diseases are colitis and ileitis. Colitis is the more common of the two diseases. At one time, these diseases were difficult to detect and often thought of as the same disease. *Colitis* is an inflammation of the colon or large intestine while ileitis is an inflammation and scarring of the *ileum,* which is a portion of the small intestine. The symptoms are very similar and include abdominal cramps, chronic diarrhea, mild fever, anemia, and weitht loss. As ileitis progresses, the bowel often becomes obstructed. Surgery may be required to remove portions of the ileum and colon.

A new test has recently been reported that will aid in the diagnosis of ileitis. This test measures the level of an enzyme in the blood called *lysozyme.* Amounts of lysozyme were found to be significantly greater in patients suffering from ileitis than in normal patients or those with colitis. The test was found to be most reliable in patients with severe or moderate ileitis, rather than in milder forms of the disease.

The National Foundation for Ileitis and Colitis (NFIC) was founded in 1967 and has provided funds for research and disseminated information about these diseases. If you wish to find out more about these conditions, write to NFIC, 295 Madison Avenue, New York, N.Y. 10017.

The final condition to be discussed in this section is appendicitis. You may have suffered from this condition or known someone who has. The appendix is a projection of the caecum (see-cum), a structure in the area where the small intestine joins the colon or large intestine. Because the circulation in this area is poor, the appendix may become inflamed or infected, resulting in appendicitis.

Symptoms of appendicitis include a general stomach discomfort which may become localized in the lower right portion of the abdomen. A decrease or lack of appetite and nausea and vomiting are also common symptoms. If these symptoms are recognized, the patient should be taken to the hospital immediately. No laxative or enema should be given and no food or water should be consumed. It is important to get medical attention before the appendix ruptures and the infection is spread throughout the abdominal cavity. If appendicitis is diagnosed, the appendix will be surgically removed.

DISEASES OF THE KIDNEY

Kidney disease has come to the attention of the public in recent years as a result of the great strides made in research in this area. Some of these developments are discussed later in this section. Kidney disease is more widespread than most people think. It affects more than eight million people and more than 60,000 Americans die each year from a form of kidney disease.

The function of the kidneys is to filter out harmful substances from the blood and to help in the maintenance of the water and chemical balance of the body. Figure 15-5 shows the kidneys, ureters, bladder, and urethra. The bladder holds the urine or liquid body waste until it is excreted through the urethra.

Figure 15-5
The urinary tract.

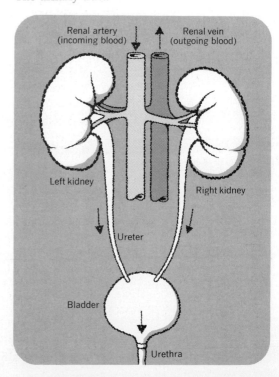

Kidney disease is not one disease but rather a group of diseases. More than 50 conditions that involve the kidneys have been identified. A few of the more common kidney diseases are discussed here.

Pyelonephritis is a common infectious disease of the kidneys. There may or may not be symptoms present. However, chills, fever, backache, and pain upon urinating are a few of the symptoms that may be recognized. If diagnosed in its early stages, this disease can be cured by antibiotics.

Glomerulonephritis, often referred to as *nephritis* or *Bright's disease,* is an inflammation of structures within the kidney called *glomeruli.* The urine is often red or rust-colored and there may be puffiness around the eyes. In most cases, the disease occurs as a result of a ''strep'' infection and will usually do no permanent damage to the kidneys. However, if the disease is chronic there may be no symptoms, but a high degree of kidney damage.

Nephrosis is a condition that causes water to accumulate around the ankles and feet, the abdomen, and under the eyes. This condition is called edema and it can often be treated by certain hormones. The disease is more common among children than adults, but it affects individuals of all ages.

Kidney stones are caused by the hardening of certain minerals and other substances into stone-like materials that collect in the kidney or obstruct the urinary tract. Infections, severe pain, and kidney damage may ensue. In some cases, symptoms are not apparent and small stones may be broken and passed without damage to the urinary system.

In general, symptoms of kidney disease in adults may include puffiness around the eyes; swollen abdomen, ankles, or feet; red or rust-colored urine; frequent, painful urination; and lower back pain. In children the symptoms often include fever; poor appetite and sleep patterns; poor growth; and discolored urine.

Hemodialysis: Everyday-life goes on with the life-saving "artificial kidney" that cleanses the blood.

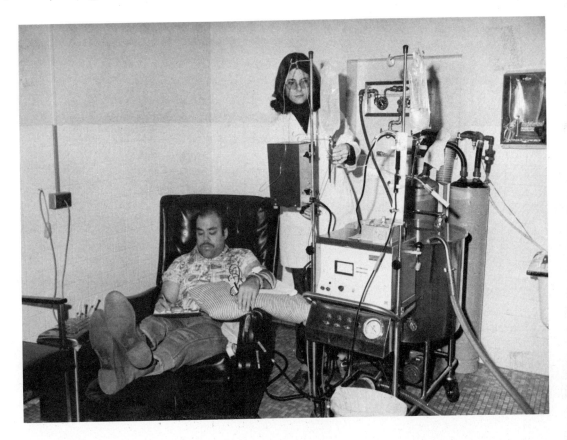

As mentioned earlier, there have been great strides in the treatment of kidney disease. There are X-ray tests that involve the use of radioactive solutions that illuminate the extent of kidney damage. Tissue can also be extracted through a needle that is injected directly into the kidney. Hormones, antibiotics, and diuretics (drugs that help to remove fluid that collects in the body) are also used in kidney disease.

You may have read about the artificial kidney, which is a machine that cleanses the impurities from the blood in those patients who have excessively damaged kidneys. This treatment is called hemodialysis and many patients would not be able to live without this treatment. The problem with dialysis is the expense and frequency of treatment needed to keep the patient alive. However, a recent amendment to the Social Security Act placed dialysis treatment under Medicaid so that patients needing this treatment could afford it.

A Hemodialyzer or Artificial kidney is used to do the kidneys' work when the kidneys cannot function properly. Like a normal kidney, the hemodialyzer filters certain harmful elements out of the blood.

Kidney transplants have also been used with success in many patients. Rejection is still a problem, but due to the use of certain drugs and techniques it is less of a problem than it was. However, there are certain side effects from the use of drugs that suppress rejection.

DISEASES OF THE LIVER

There are two commonly recognized diseases of the liver. One, infectious hepatitis, will be discussed in the following chapter where infectious diseases are examined. The second, cirrhosis, will be discussed in this section.

Cirrhosis of the liver is a disease commonly associated with alcoholism. According to the recent report on *Alcohol and Health* issued by the National Institute of Alcohol Abuse and Alcoholism (NIAAA), the death rate from cirrhosis has risen to the fourth leading cause of death of persons between the ages of 25 and 65. Cirrhosis is more common among heavy drinkers because poor nutrition is also a key factor in the development of

this disease. Alcoholics often neglect their diet and many are extremely malnourished.

The disease is characterized by destruction of the liver cells and replacement of these cells with scar tissue. Death may occur if treatment is begun at a late stage or if there is no treatment. Symptoms include fatigue, weakness, loss of appetite, jaundice, and enlargement of the liver. If treated early, the liver damage can often be reversed. Treatment includes rest, adequate nutrition, and avoidance of alcoholic beverages.

DISEASES OF THE NERVOUS SYSTEM

In this section of the chapter, diseases that affect the nervous system are discussed. You may be less aware of these diseases than those already discussed because they occur less frequently or are controlled by vaccines. Many people fear some of these diseases and the people who have them because they lack knowledge about the disease and what to expect from the patient. This section will help you to better understand these diseases and the individuals who suffer from them.

Neuritis is a disease of the nerve fibers and it affects more than seven million Americans. Generally speaking, neuritis includes any damage to the nerves and may result in inflammation, pain, and partial nerve degeneration. The symptoms and severity of the condition varies with the cause of the damage and the patient.

The causes of neuritis may be accidental injury to a nerve, a vitamin B deficiency (often related to excess intake of alcohol), and certain other conditions that cause nerve involvement and complications. Treatment varies depending on the cause of the condition.

There are a number of viral and bacterial infections that affect the nervous system. Some of these diseases are briefly discussed in this section.

Meningitis. There are two forms of meningitis.

One is caused by a virus and the other more commonly recognized disease is caused by a bacterium (Meningococcus). This disease is also known as *cerebrospinal meningitis* because it affects the membranes of the brain and spinal cord. Symptoms include fever, headache, backache, and a skin rash. Delirium and coma may occur. The disease can be cured if treated in its early stages.

Encephalitis. Encephalitis is a virus disease that affects the brain. It is often called "sleeping sickness" because it may result in headaches, sleepiness, and coma in severe cases. There are a number of viruses that may cause this condition.

Polio. This once dreaded disease is under control today as a result of successful immunization programs. Polio affects the central nervous system and can result in paralysis of the arms and legs and the respiratory system. The Salk and Sabin vaccines have saved countless lives. However, recent reports have indicated that many children are not being immunized and localized outbreaks of polio have appeared. People tend to become complacent about the disease because they think that it is under control. It is essential that all children be immunized in the early months of their lives and a booster dose be given at a later time.

Rabies. This disease is fatal if not treated. It is a viral disease, primarily of animals; that is, spread to man by an animal bite or through an open wound. The symptoms include depression, headache, and sensory changes. The disease then progresses to paralysis, muscle spasms, delirium, and convulsions. The most effective control of the disease is through the immunization of dogs with the rabies vaccine. If one is bitten, he should report the animal to the health authorities. The animal can be observed for seven to ten days to see if it has the disease. There is a vaccine available for humans who have rabies. However, it must be administered in the early stages of the disease.

Tetanus. This disease, often called lockjaw, is caused by a bacterium and is characterized by painful muscular contractions and muscular rigidity. The disease is fatal to one out of every two people who contract it. It is essential that one keep his immunization up to date. According to the United States Center for Disease Control, a tetanus booster is needed every ten years.

Botulism. Botulism is a rare bacterial disease that is often fatal. The toxin or poison of these bacteria are only produced in the absence of oxygen—in a can or other sealed container. In most cases, the bacteria are destroyed in the cooking and canning process. However, there are some warning signs that one should be aware of. If the can is bulging or swollen at one end or if the contents of a can spurt out of the can upon opening, do not eat the contents of the container. Most cases of botulism occur in the faulty home canning or processing of foods.

Multiple Sclerosis (MS) is a disease that affects the central nervous system. It affects most individuals between the ages of 25 and 40. The first attack usually strikes suddenly and then symptoms may disappear for several months. Some individuals never have a second attack and others may be in remission for as long as 25 years. The symptoms of the disease include impaired sensations, blurred vision, speech problems, stiffness of the limbs, and emotional instability. There is no known cause and most treatment methods have not proven to be successful.

Epilepsy is more of a condition than a disease. It is caused by a dysfunction of the electrical activity of the brain. In some cases, there is brain injury. However, in other cases, no injury can be found. The word *epilepsy* comes from the Greek word for seizure. There are three types of commonly recognized seizures that affect individuals with epilepsy. They are the grand mal, petit mal, and psychomotor seizures.

There are certain events that may cause epilepsy. These events may include: prenatal or birth injuries, congenital malformations, nutritional deficiencies, fever, diseases, brain tumors, and head injuries. There are many

Jonas Edward Salk (1914-), an American physician, in 1954 developed the first effective polio vaccine and thus put an end to the outbreaks of polio that had swept the nation almost every summer.

Dr. Salk is still interested in immunology. He is now doing research on the influenza virus at the Salk Institute for Biological Studies in California.

anticonvulscent drugs available to the more than four million people in this country who suffer from some form of the disease. Surgery is also utilized in certain forms of the disease.

Allergies are a reaction to a certain substance or substances called *allergens*. People may be allergic to many different allergens including foods, drugs, cosmetics, animal hair or feathers, pollens, and grasses. Skin testing can often point out the offending allergen or allergens.

The symptoms may vary according to the allergen. Symptoms may include skin reactions, itching, breathing problems, stuffed noses, coughs, cramping, and nausea. Treatment is available through the injection of small amounts of the allergen in order to build up a tolerance to that substance.

other common diseases

Arthritis is a disease that affects 17 million Americans. It is a disease that has a variety of forms, but it is primarily a disease of the joints that is especially common among older people. Because there are no cures and most people who are affected are older, arthritis patients are often victims of quackery. This is discussed in detail in Chapter 19.

However, there have been great strides in the treatment of the disease in recent years. New plastics and other materials have been used in operations on diseased joints. Artificial hips have also been used to replace the diseased joints. Drug therapy is widely used in the relief of joint inflammation and its pain. There is no permanent cure, but a variety of treatments can relieve some of the symptoms.

Diabetes is a nutritional and metabolic disease. True or sugar diabetes results from insufficient production of *insulin* by the islet cells of the pancreas. Insulin is the hormone that is involved in the storage and utilization of *glucose* (blood sugar). Individuals with this condition can have a fairly normal life if they watch their diet and receive regular dosages of insulin.

THINKING IT OVER

1. Briefly discuss the structure and function of the respiratory system.
2. What are some of the symptoms of the common cold and some of the interesting facts that have been discovered about it?
3. Discuss the symptoms and causes of two respiratory diseases. Do some research into these diseases and write a paragraph or two about each.
4. Discuss the relationship between smoking and emphysema.
5. What are the types of ulcers and what are some of the causes of this condition?
6. Discuss the "upset stomach syndrome," its symptoms and causes.
7. Discuss colitis and ileitis and some of the symptoms of these diseases.
8. What are some of the common types of kidney disease and the treatment available for individuals affected by kidney disease?
9. What is the cause of liver cirrhosis?
10. Discuss in detail (from research) any two viral or bacterial diseases that affect the nervous system.
11. What is epilepsy and what are some of the possible causes?
12. Do some research into new treatments available for people who suffer from arthritis.
13. What is the cause of sugar diabetes and how is it treated?

KEY WORDS

Air sacs. The *alveoli* where gases are exchanged in the lung.

Allergens. Substances that cause allergic reactions.

Alveoli. Air sacs where gases are exchanged in the lungs.

Appendicitis. Infection and inflammation of the appendix.

Asthma. An allergic reaction that results in an inflammation of bronchial tubes.

Bronchioles. Smaller branches of each bronchus in the lungs

323

Bronchitis. An inflammation of the bronchi.

Bronchus. Air passageways that branch into each lung from the trachea.

Cirrhosis. A disease of the liver that results in the hardening of the liver tissues.

Colitis. Inflammation of the colon or large intestine.

Diaphragm. A muscular partition that divides the chest cavity from the abdominal cavity.

Emphysema. A stretching and tearing of the alveoli of the lungs.

Gastroenterologist. A specialist in the disorders of the intestinal tract.

Ileitis. An inflammation and scarring of the ilium.

Influenza. A group of viral diseases of the respiratory tract.

Nephritis. Inflammation of the glomeruli of the kidneys.

Peristalsis. Squeezing contractions of the digestive organs.

Trachea. Windpipe where air passes from mouth into the lungs.

Tubercle. A lesion of the lung containing tuberculosis bacteria.

Tuberculosis. A bacterial infection of the lungs or other organs of the body.

Ulcer. A sore in the lining of the stomach or duodenum.

Villi. Fingerlike projections in the walls of the small intestine.

GETTING INVOLVED
Books and Periodicals

Bloom, Arnold. *Diabetes Explained.* Baltimore: University Park, 1971. Practical information about diabetes.

Crain, Darrell C. *The Arthritis Handbook: A Patient's Manual on Arthritis, Rheumatism and Gout.* New York: Arco, 1973. How to live with these diseases.

Morris, T. "Ileitis: The Disease People Won't Talk About in Public." *Today's Health,* June 1975. The causes and treatment of ileitis and colitis.

Petty, Thomas L. *For Those Who Live and Breathe: A Manual for Patients with Emphysema and Chronic Bronchitis.* Springfield, Ill.: Charles C. Thomas, 1972. Hygiene, therapy, and reconditioning.

Pool, James L. *Your Brain and Nerves.* New York: Scribner's, 1973. Various diseases simply explained.

Sands, Harry, and Caplan, Frances. *The Epilepsy Handbook.* Washington: The Epilepsy Foundation of America, in press. Epilepsy explained in layman's terms.

Serino, Girard S. *Your Ulcer: Prevention, Control, Cure.* Philadelphia: Lippincott, 1966. What to do about ulcers.

Movies

A Brief Vacation, with Florinda Bolkan, 1973. An Italian tuberculosis sanitorium is the setting for this drama of self-discovery. Distributed by Cinema International Corporation.

16
INFECTIOUS DISEASES

The subject of this chapter is infectious diseases. These diseases cover a wide range of ailments that include childhood diseases, mononucleosis, hepatitis, and the venereal diseases. Infectious diseases have an important effect on our general health, life style, and economy. For example, the cost of gonorrheal complications in females amounts to in excess of $200,000,000 each year according to the Center for Disease Control in Atlanta, Georgia. The same source reports that the hospitalization of the syphilitic insane costs taxpayers about $44,000,000 each year. Many people are unaware of the social and economic significance of these diseases.

In this chapter, you will learn about the organisms that cause infectious diseases and the diseases that they cause. You will read about some of the common childhood diseases, their symptoms, and treatment. Mononucleosis and hepatitis are discussed in detail. Immunity in general is discussed and specific immunization programs for certain diseases are stressed.

The last section of this chapter discusses venereal disease. You will read about how VD is transmitted, how it can be prevented, the main types of venereal disease, and what is being done to control these diseases. After reading this chapter, you will have a better understanding of infectious disease in general and some specific diseases.

While reading this chapter, think about the following concepts:

■ There is a difference between infectious disease and chronic disease.

■ Immunization programs are available for many infectious diseases, but they are being neglected in many cases.

■ Children should be routinely immunized for certain diseases in the early months of life.

■ In the majority of cases, permanent disability from mononucleosis is rare.

■ Anyone can get VD — it is a disease of "nice" people, too.

■ Venereal disease can be prevented; if contracted, it can be completely cured if medical attention is received when the disease is in its early stages.

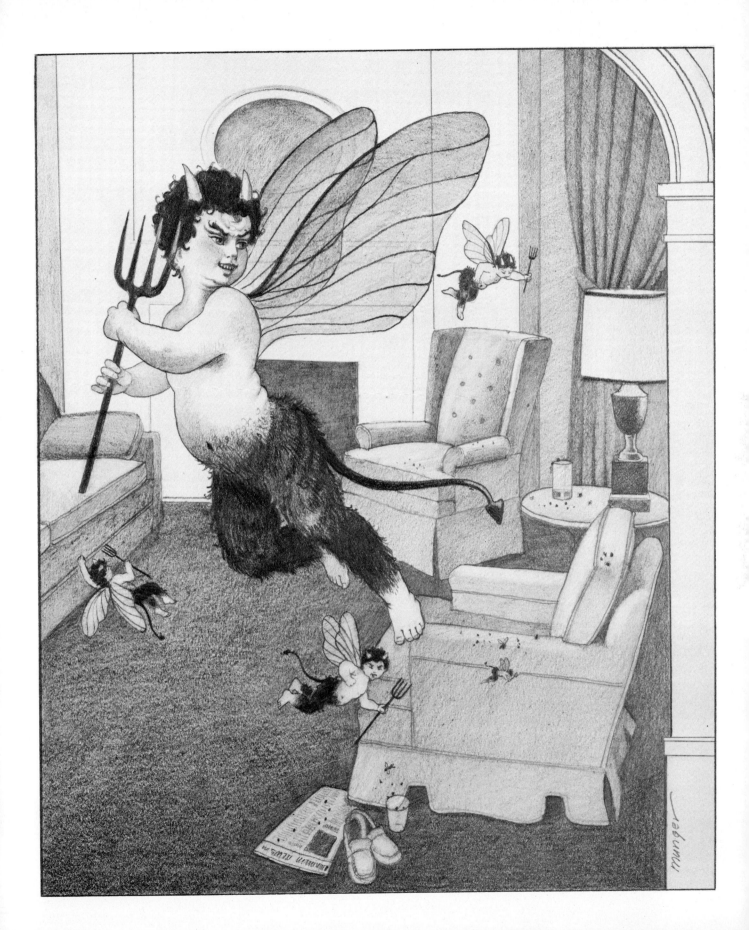

Have you ever heard of the term "city diseases?" In an article in *New York Magazine* (October 7, 1974), infectious and noninfectious diseases were examined. In the article entitled "City Diseases That Can Kill You," the disease cryptococcal meningitis was discussed. This is a disease caused by the cryptococcus fungi. It is a serious, often fatal disease that is called a "city disease" because the fungi often live and grow in pigeon droppings. Fortunately for New Yorkers and other city dwellers, it seems to affect a minority of individuals who have an immunity problem. However, pigeons are responsible for numerous other infectious diseases that affect man. These diseases include *histoplasmosis* (respiratory tract infection); *encephalitis* (virus infection of the nervous system); *salmonellasis* (bacterial food poisoning); and *pigeon ornithosis* (a mild viral disease).

Pigeons are only one way in which infectious disease organisms are transmitted to humans. In this chapter you will learn about a variety of infectious diseases, their symptoms, and immunity to these diseases. As you read this chapter, note any questions that may come to mind concerning a particular disease. These questions can then be researched and discussed in class.

what types of disease are infectious?

An infectious disease is one that is caused by microorganisms. If the disease can be transmitted from one person to another, directly or indirectly, then the disease is call communicable. Measles, mumps, chickenpox, and whooping cough are all communicable diseases. Can you think of any other? Due to immunization programs, many communicable diseases have been controlled and prevented from affecting large portions of the population.

A chronic disease differs from an infectious disease in that it is not caused by a microorganism. Chronic diseases are caused by metabolic, endocrine, or other organ and system disorders. In the case of some chronic diseases, the causes remain unknown. An example of such a disease would be certain forms of cancer. Other common chronic diseases include heart disease, diabetes, stroke, and certain nervous disorders. Most chronic diseases are longterm and progressively debilitating.

It is interesting to note that although there has been a decrease in the cases of infectious disease in recent years, there has been a marked increase in cases of chronic disease. Heart disease is the number one killer today, with cancer and stroke following closely behind. However, some people question whether chronic diseases are increasing or whether people are living long enough to suffer from these diseases. The life span has steadily increased and with these additional years come the problems of heart disease, stroke, cancer, and other chronic ailments, which tend to affect more older than younger people.

DISEASE-PRODUCING ORGANISMS

There are a number of disease-producing organisms that include the bacteria, viruses, fungi, protozoa, parasitic worms, and rickettsia. Each of these organisms and some of the diseases they cause will be briefly discussed in the following paragraphs.

Bacteria exist all around us in many different sizes and shapes. They are the most prevalent form of life on earth. However, most bacteria are not disease-causing organisms. Many bacteria are harmless and many others are beneficial to man. Those bacteria that cause disease are called pathogenic organisms.

Bacteria are often grouped by their shape. Refer to Figure 16-1 as you read this section. One type of bacteria is spherical in shape and called *coccus*. Coccus bacteria may form long chains, short chains, or appear in clusters. It is a coccus bacteria, streptococcus, that causes a "strep" throat. Rod-shaped bacteria are called *bacillus* and they may also join together in chain-like

Figure 16-1
The three types of bacteria: (a) *coccus*, (b) *bacillus*, (c) *spirillum*.

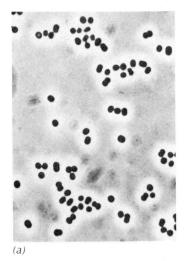

(a)

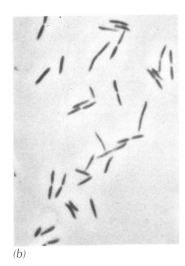

(b)

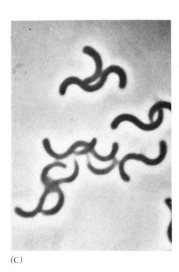

(c)

formations. Other bacteria resemble twisted rods and are called *spirillum*.

Bacteria are responsible for numerous diseases, some of which you have already read about in Chapter 15. Others include diphtheria, scarlet fever, typhoid fever, and whooping cough.

Viruses are the cause of a variety of diseases that affect humans. Many of the diseases with which you are most familiar are caused by viruses. In fact, many people now refer to a group of symptoms as a "virus." The word *virus* has become very much a part of our present-day vocabulary.

Viruses are extremely tiny organisms that require a living cell in order for them to be active. They tend to be *specific* organisms. This means that certain viruses tend to attack certain cells and tissues. Viruses are often classified according to the tissues they attack. Some viruses invade skin tissue and cause smallpox, chickenpox, or cold sores. Others are specific to the respiratory tract where they cause colds, influenza, and viral pneumonia. Polio, encephalitis, and rabies are caused by viruses that invade the central nervous system. The liver is affected in cases of infectious hepatitis (to be discussed later in this chapter). The glands are another site of viral infection. Examples include mumps (a disease that is controlled today by

immunization) and mononucleosis (a common disease of young people). "Mono," as it is called, is discussed in detail in a later section of this chapter.

Fungi are another type of disease-causing organism. Fungi were mentioned in the introduction to this chapter when cryptococcus was discussed (a fungi that thrives in pigeon droppings). Fungi are also responsible for ringworm, athlete's foot, and numerous other infections.

Protozoans are one-celled microorganisms that are larger than bacteria and more complex in structure. You may recall protozoans from your study of biology and the simple one-celled amoeba. The amoeba is a harmless protozoan but some of its "relatives" can cause disease. One type of protozoan causes dysentery, a disease of the intestinal tract common in certain tropical areas. Another protozoan causes malaria, a serious often fatal disease carried by a type of mosquito. A serious form of sleeping sickness is also caused by a protozoan.

Rickettsiae are microorganisms that are smaller than bacteria but larger than viruses. These organisms usually live and reproduce in ticks and are responsible for a serious disease called Rocky Mountain spotted fever. In about 20 percent of all cases of this disease, the infected individual dies. This disease is common in the Northwestern section of the United States and the affected individual has symptoms of a spotted rash, high fever, and painful joints. The organism is named after Dr. Howard T. Ricketts who had discovered that typhus fever was also caused by rickettsiae.

Parasitic worms are also disease-causing organisms. Up to this point in the chapter, the organisms discussed have been microscopic in size. However, parasitic worms are common causes of *infestation* in other countries as well as in parts of the United States. The tapeworm is one parasitic worm that many people refer to without thinking about disease. When someone eats too much, one may say "do you have a tapeworm?" However, tapeworms are no laughing matter and may go undetected while causing their hosts (man) to lose weight and strength.

Tapeworms are flat, ribbonlike worms that enter the human body through the meat of an infected animal. The meat of such an animal was improperly cooked so that the tapeworm cysts, as they are called, were not destroyed in the cooking process. Once the tapeworm passes through the human stomach into the intestine, the worm fastens itself onto the wall of the intestine where it will feed on the blood that it sucks.

Another parasitic worm is the trichina which is an extremely dangerous roundworm. Humans eat trichina cysts in infested pork that has been improperly cooked. The disease that results is a painful, serious disease known as trichinosis. The best way to prevent this and other parasitic worm infestations is to thoroughly cook all meat before eating it.

common infectious diseases

A number of childhood diseases are both common and highly infectious. Many of these diseases have been somewhat controlled by immunization programs. This will be discussed in a later section on immunity.

CHILDHOOD DISEASES

There are two types of measles. Rubeola is the more serious of the two types. It is a highly communicable viral disease that causes bronchitis, nasal discharge, and a blotchy-red rash. Children who are suffering from malnutrition have a greater chance of dying from the infection than do healthy children. Immunization is available and essential to the control of the disease.

Rubella or German measles is the other type of measles. The disease is milder than rubeola and has few symptoms in children other than a spread-out rash. Some cases do not result in a rash. Rubella is caused by a virus and is a highly communicable disease.

The serious problem of this disease is that if affects the unborn children of women infected in the first three months of pregnancy. Children born to these mothers may suffer from mental retardation, deafness, heart defects, eye cataracts, and several other birth defects. In some cases, fetal death results from the infection.

In 1963, an epidemic of rubella resulted in 30,000 stillbirths and approximately 20,000 serious birth defects. In order to prevent such epidemics, all young children should be immunized against this disease. Unfortunately, many parents and other adults who have young children in their care are neglecting measles and other routine immunizations. In a recent year, only 55.6 percent of all young children had been immunized against rubella. This lack of immunization in almost half the population of children this age can result in new major measle epidemics.

At one time children were very familiar with symptoms of mumps. This disease is caused by a virus and is characterized by fever and a swelling and soreness of one or more of the salivary glands. This often results in a large swelling on one or both sides of the face. This disease is more serious in adults than in children, as the testes in males and ovaries in females may be affected. This occurs more often in adult males than in adult females. Immunization is available and should be given at an early age.

Chickenpox is caused by a virus and is extremely communicable. It is not unusual to find half a class of young children absent from school at the same time because of this disease. The symptoms of the disease include a slight fever and a skin eruption that many cover parts of the body or most of its surface. Eruptions often appear on the scalp. There is no immunization; however, children who contract the disease should be kept at home for at least one week following the skin eruption. It is also important that the condition be accurately diagnosed to be sure that it is not smallpox.

Whooping cough (pertussis) is a serious bacterial disease that is characterized by a high-pitched, violent, or "whooping" cough. The symptoms of the disease include an irritating cough that worsens within a few weeks and may last for a few months. There is often an expulsion of thick mucus with the cough. Immunization is available and should be given to all children during infancy.

MONONUCLEOSIS

Mononucleosis or "mono" is a viral disease that is most prevalent among the 15 to 19 years old age group. Mono is not a serious disease and permanent disability is rare. However, the symptoms of the disease are extremely unpleasant and there is no preventive treatment.

Despite what you may have heard about the disease, the average person is completely well about two weeks after the onset of symptoms. In many high schools and colleges, stories abound concerning individuals who were sick for two years or had to drop out of school because of mononucleosis. In some cases, symptoms of fatigue and weakness may last about six weeks. In a few cases, students may fall so behind in their studies that they are forced to "drop out" for a semester—but these are the rare cases!

The usual symptoms of mono include a low-grade fever, a feeling of weakness and fatigue, swollen and sore lymph glands, and sometimes a fine, red rash. There is a blood test for mono that is extremely conclusive for the disease.

Mono has been called the "kissing" disease because this is one method of transmission. However, the disease can also be transmitted by the common use of drinking and eating utensils. It is interesting to note that mononucleosis is more common among college students, especially students in Ivy League colleges and those from the upper-middle classes. The reason for this is thought to be that young people from smaller families and less overcrowded conditions have a lesser immunity to the virus that causes mononucleosis than other young people. These students, therefore, have a greater susceptibility to the disease.

Most experts in this area agree that one cannot get the disease twice. There is a myth among many students that the disease can appear and disappear over many months. This is not the case. Another viral infection, with similar symptoms, may appear and the patient may assume that it is mono. The eventual control of the disease lies in the development of an effective immunization program. However, this is still in the future. An interesting article about this disease is "The *Kissing Disease* That Isn't So Romantic" (*Today's Health,* December 1974).

HEPATITIS

This disease was briefly mentioned in Chapter 15 under diseases of the liver. Infectious hepatitis (formerly known as "yellow jaundice") is caused by a viral infection of the liver. The virus causes destruction of liver cells that results in *bile* (a brownish fluid secreted by the liver) to enter the bloodstream causing a jaundiced or yellowish skin coloration.

Symptoms of infectious hepatitis include fever, general discomfort, loss of appetite, and abdominal pain. The disease may be mild or may last for many weeks. The liver may remain enlarged and sore for many weeks following the infection. Outbreaks of this disease are often related to contaminated water and food.

Another form of hepatitis is serum hepatitis. It is often difficult to distinguish between both forms of this disease. However, serum hepatitis results from the injection of human blood that has been contaminated. This may occur following a blood transfusion from a donor who had the virus in his bloodstream. This is still a problem today, especially in blood banks that operate in poor areas and pay their donors for their services. An interesting article entitled "Blood Farming" appears in the May 18, 1975 *New York Magazine*. The author of this article began researching the "blood-for-profit" business after the death of a friend from serum hepatitis contracted from a routine blood transfusion. Many individuals think that this type of situation no longer exists today, but the article points out that it does exist and is not that unusual.

Hepatitis is a frequent complication of heroin addiction. Heroin users tend to share needles and neglect routine sterilization procedures. They may also prepare their drugs and fill their needles in an unsanitary manner. Many addicts are hospitalized as a result of hepatitis.

IMMUNITY

Throughout this chapter, reference has been made to immunity to certain diseases and the fact that immunization is available to protect individuals from certain diseases (measles, mumps, whooping cough, polio, and others). Immunization has saved many people from death and incapacitating conditions.

Immunity may be defined as a condition where one cannot contract a certain disease. Even if the infectious agent is present, the individual is *immune* or protected from that disease. There are different types of immunity. Natural immunity is the immunity one has to certain infectious agents that are unable

to grow in the human body. Acquired immunity is that immunity gained by an individual either by developing one's own antibodies (that destroy the disease-producing organism) or through the injection of a serum that makes one immune to these organisms.

You may have heard the terms active and passive immunity. Active immunity is the immunity that individuals establish to a disease after having already had it. This occurs when antibodies are produced against the organism during the infectious period. These antibodies keep the individual from getting the disease again. Passive immunity is achieved by the injection of a vaccine made from the weakened disease-causing organisms. This vaccine causes the body to produce antibodies to the infectious organism and gives the individual immunity to the disease.

This is the basis of immune therapy programs designed to protect individuals from certain diseases. However, in order for individuals to build up this immunity, they must receive the serum at an early stage of life. Recent reports indicate that many children are *not* being routinely immunized in infancy and during the first years of life. Many adults mistakenly assume that children are protected from certain diseases in their early years. There may be some natural immunity from the mother in the early months of life, but not to all diseases and to varying degrees to certain diseases. Many parents wait until a child begins school to have him immunized; by then it is often too late. Who do you think should have the responsibility for seeing that children are immunized?

National surveys, for example, have indicated that in 1963, 84.1 percent of children from one to four had been immunized against polio. However, when similar surveys were conducted in 1973, only 60.4 percent had been immunized. These statistics are the reason behind polio outbreaks in recent years. Too many people are becoming too complacent about immunization. The possibility of large-scale epidemics does exist if

Immunization Programs are usually a great success when a vaccine is first developed; later on, people forget the dangers of the disease, and they may neglect to have their shots. The Center for Disease Control (the federal agency responsible for preventing communicable diseases) recommends that children be immunized against polio, measles, German measles, mumps, whooping cough, diphtheria, and tetanus.

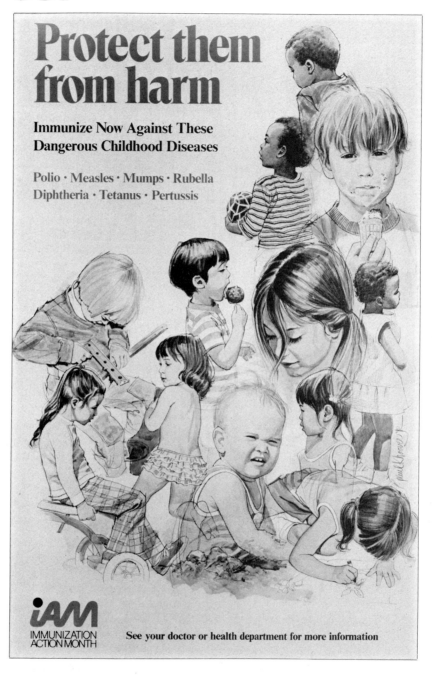

Protect them from harm

Immunize Now Against These Dangerous Childhood Diseases

Polio · Measles · Mumps · Rubella
Diphtheria · Tetanus · Pertussis

iAM
IMMUNIZATION
ACTION MONTH

See your doctor or health department for more information

people continue to neglect these routine immunizations. There are many free immunization programs at clinics and local health departments. If you wish to find out more about these programs, call your local public health department for immunization schedules.

the venereal diseases

The venereal diseases are a group of contagious diseases that are almost always transmitted during sexual activity, usually intercourse. There are a few exceptions, however, and they are very rare. Infants may be born with congenital syphilis. Infection occurs in the uterus and is caused by the syphilis germs of the mother. Gonorrhea can infect a baby during birth and cause a serious eye infection that can result in blindness. If the mother has gonorrhea, then the baby would come in contact with these germs as it passes through the birth canal. For this reason, the eyes of all newborn infants are treated with silver nitrate and other medications to destroy any gonorrhea germs that might be present. In a few isolated cases, young girls have contracted venereal disease from bed linens and towels. This is, however, a rare occurrence.

Sexual contact does not have to include intercourse, although this is the primary way of transmitting these diseases. Venereal disease may also be contracted through the mouth or rectum. If one has a syphilis sore on the mouth or fingers, someone who touches the sore could get the disease. One could, therefore, contract syphilis by kissing a person who has a syphilis sore on the lips or inside of the mouth. Syphilis germs can also enter the body through tiny breaks in the surface of the skin. Drug addicts have been known to spread the disease by sharing contaminated needles with one another. As you can see, there are many ways of contracting the disease; however, sexual intercourse is the most common source of infection.

You have probably read more about venereal disease in recent years than at any other time in history. Venereal disease has become a serious threat to the health of many thousands of people. Current statistics indicate that there are more than 800,000 reported cases of gonorrhea and 90,000 reported cases of syphilis. The Center for Disease Control, Atlanta, Georgia, estimates that there are 2,500,000 new cases of gonorrhea each year. That would mean a new case of gonorrhea every 14 seconds. It is also estimated that more than 500,000 persons in this country have syphilis.

You may be asking why there seems to be a discrepancy in the numbers of cases of these diseases. The reason is that the numbers 800,000 and 90,000 reflect *reported* cases. These are the cases reported to health authorities by physicians and clinics. However, many cases go unreported because physicians agree to keep the matter confidential at the request of the patient. This is an unfortunate practice because the disease control centers of the state boards of health are not able to follow up contacts and warn them about the possibility of having a venereal disease. It is important to note that state health boards are interested in protecting the public and they try to be discrete in questioning contacts that have been referred to them.

Venereal disease does not choose its victims. These diseases attack all people in all age

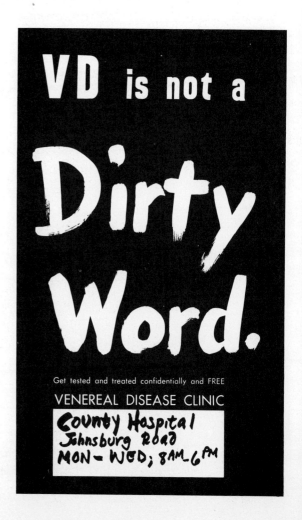

VD is not a Dirty Word.

Get tested and treated confidentially and FREE

VENEREAL DISEASE CLINIC

County Hospital
Johnsburg Road
MON - WED; 8AM-6PM

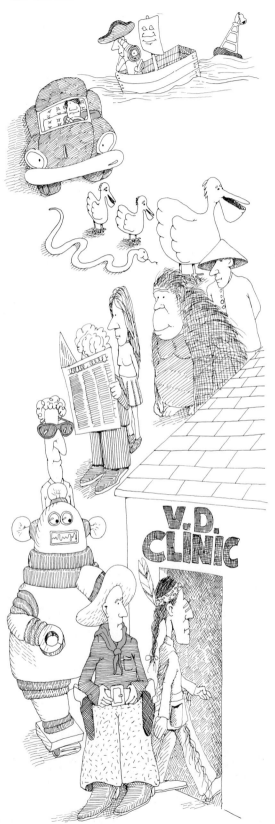

All kinds of people can get V.D.

groups. Because of the reporting problem, it is difficult to pinpoint the age group that has the greatest incidence of VD. However, statistics seem to indicate that about one-half of all cases of VD occur in persons under 24 years of age. A quarter of this group is between the ages of 13 and 19.

Is venereal disease really more prevalent in this country today or are we just hearing more about it? Venereal disease has definitely increased in recent years and there are many reasons suggested for this increase. One of the main reasons given is that many individuals have become complacent about VD because they assume that antibiotics has these diseases under control. This is certainly true to some extent, but an individual with VD must take the antibiotic in order to protect himself and his sexual contacts. To further complicate this situation, a number of gonorrhea strains have been found that are resistant to low dosages of penicillin. This means these germs cannot be killed by the usual dosage of the antibiotic.

Young people are tending to become sexually active at an earlier age and certain groups of individuals of all ages are having more sexual contacts than they did in past years. Some individuals may have several sexual contacts in a short period of time. This type of sexual activity increases the chances of contracting venereal disease. The birth control pill may also be in part responsible for the "new freedom" that many people have today in their sexual relationships.

Another reason for the increase of VD is that the world is smaller today than ever before. Sexual contacts may be widespread, thanks to our present-day mobility. This was found to be true when many servicemen returned from Southeast Asia with venereal disease. It is an impossible task to track down sexual contacts across the country or across the world.

PREVENTION OF VENEREAL DISEASE

At present there are no vaccines that are generally available for immunization against venereal disease. However, research is being done in this area. Once a person had VD it does not make him immune to the disease. One can get gonorrhea many times after having been cured of the disease. The same is true for syphilis. Many individuals become reinfected and think that they are protected by their previous antibiotic treatment. However, once the course of treatment is over and the person is told that he is cured, he is once again susceptible to the venereal disease bacteria.

There are certain things that one can do to prevent getting VD. The most effective method of prevention is the use of the condom. This birth control device was discussed in Chapter 9. The condom not only keeps the semen from entering the vagina, but is also keeps the penis from making direct contact with the vagina. This protects both partners from contracting the disease. The introduction of new birth control devices and pills resulted in many people not using condoms. This is another reason why VD has increased in recent years.

Other contraceptives in the form of foams, creams, and jellies may also be helpful in preventing VD. These products are available without a prescription. Although these products may be helpful, they will not necessarily prevent the disease. Cleanliness in the genital area is also helpful, but again it may not prevent VD. These products and cleanliness are good precautionary methods, but the use of a *condom* will provide protection.

THE MAIN
VENEREAL DISEASES

There are five main venereal diseases and a sixth that has become more well-known in recent years. The five major venereal diseases are chancroid (*shank*-royd), granuloma inguinale (*in*-gwih-nah-lee), lymphogranuloma venereum (vuh-*neer*-e-om), gonorrhea and syphilis. The sixth disease is called genital herpes (*her*-peez). In this section, all of the diseases except gonorrhea and syphilis will be briefly discussed. Gonorrhea and syphilis are discussed in separate sec-

tions because of their widespread incidence.

Chancroid is a venereal disease that causes a painful ulcer or sore in the genital area. This ulcer or chancroid begins as a small, reddened area and later becomes enlarged and infected. This disease can be treated if diagnosed in its early stages. If chancroid is not treated in time, permanent damage can result to the reproductive organs.

Granuloma inguinale is a bacterial venereal disease that causes small, hard eruptions that later become enlarged, infected sores or ulcers. The infection may then spread to other parts of the body. This disease may be spread without sexual contact.

Lymphogranuloma venereum or LGV for short, causes small ulcers to appear on the sex organs. These sores may appear about six weeks after exposure to the disease. A burning pain upon urination may also be experienced. The lymph nodes of the groin may become swollen and enlarged. Internal damage will result if the illness is not diagnosed and treated in its early stages.

Herpes is a venereal disease that has greatly increased in incidence in recent years. A recent article called it "the venereal disease of the new morality." According to Dr. Marcus A. Conant of the University of California Medical Center, San Francisco, the epidemic of herpes that we are experiencing today results of "changing sexual morals and practices rather than the development of a more aggressive virus."

Genital herpes is caused by the herpes simplex virus Type 2 that is similar to the virus that causes cold sores, fever blisters, and shingles (a nerve disorder). It has been estimated that at least 250,000 cases, and perhaps as many as one million cases, had been treated in 1975. The symptoms begin with itching or a rash in the genital area. A cluster of blisters may then form, break open, and ulcerate. The condition is extremely painful and may eventually involve the legs and urinary system. The condition has also been linked to cervical cancer in some research studies. There are some methods of treat-

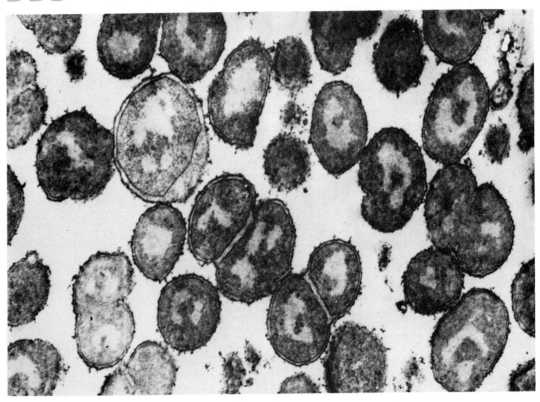

The gonococcus bacterium which causes gonorrhea.

ment, but they are not successful in all patients.

Gonorrhea. Gonorrhea (dose, clap, drip) is caused by the gonococcus bacterium. The incubation period is from three to ten days. As previously mentioned, gonorrhea may be indefinitely infectious if not treated. In a man, the main symptoms include burning upon urination and a discharge (a "drip") of pus from the penis. In some males, the disease is *asymptomatic* (there are no symptoms). In the female, there are usually no symptoms until the disease has progressed. If symptoms do exist, they may include swollen genitals and a vaginal discharge.

If treated in time with antibiotics, gonorrhea can be easily cured. However, if treated at a later stage, damage to the reproductive organs is often irreparable. The disease may cause scar tissue to form in the Fallopian tubes and vas deferens (refer to Chapter 9) and result in sterility. Untreated gonorrhea may result in gonorrheal arthritis (painful

joints) and may also affect other parts of the body.

Babies born to mothers infected with the disease may contract it during the birth process. As mentioned earlier in this chapter, all newborns are treated to prevent gonorrheal eye infection.

Syphilis. Syphilis is caused by a *spirochete*. The incubation period is between 10 and 90 days, with the average being about three weeks. Four stages of syphilis are usually recognized. The first or *primary* stage is when the chancre (*shank*-er) appears. This is a red sore that is often painless. The chancre contains the spirochetes and the disease is highly infectious at this time.

The *secondary* stage usually occurs when the chancre disappears. This will happen without any treatment. However, the disease is still present and highly infectious. Other symptoms may appear during this stage. Rash or skin lesions, headaches, fever, and

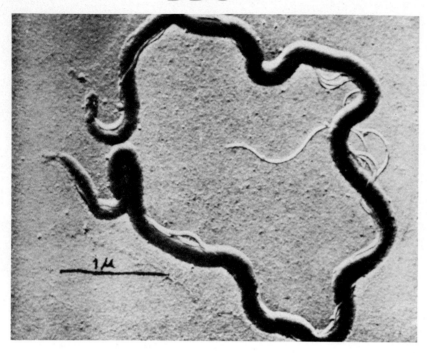

Treponema pallidum, the spirochete that causes syphilis.

sore throat are often misdiagnosed as another disease. During this stage, syphilis is often called "the great imitator."

The third or *latent* stage may last for 10 or 20 years. There are no symptoms of the disease during this period. The disease is hidden, but not gone. During this stage the syphilis spirochetes are infiltrating the body organs. The disease is usually not infectious during this stage. However, serious damage may result to the joints, liver, heart, eyes, and brain.

The *late* stage occurs where the damaging effects of the latent stage begin to appear. Heart disease, blindness, and mental deterioration often affect people during this stage.

Treatment of syphilis is the same as for gonorrhea—antibiotics. Syphilis can be cured in the first three stages and antibiotics can prevent further organ involvement in the latent and late stages of the disease.

Syphilis can affect the unborn child of a mother who has the disease. The spirochete is able to cross the placenta and attack the fetus. If the mother is treated and cured during the first three or four months, the fetus will not become infected. However, if the mother is not treated, the child will be born with syphilis and may be seriously deformed. Some babies are born dead from the infection.

CONTROL OF VENEREAL DISEASE

The control of VD can only be accomplished through widespread educational programs and contact tracing. Education is needed on all levels. The media has a responsibility to disseminate information regarding VD and to some extent this has been done. In addition, government at all levels have conducted campaigns to educate people concerning these diseases. There are a number of private groups that operate hot lines to answer questions about VD. One such group, Operation Venus, maintains a hot line operated by young people. The volunteers operate a toll-free number where people with questions about VD can call. Operation Venus is located in Philadelphia, Pennsylvania. Does your school or community have a VD education program? If not, find out about what can be done to start one.

CONTACT TRACING

This is the other factor involved in the control of VD. Contact tracing involves the tracking down of sexual contacts of an individual with venereal disease. One individual may be responsible for a number of cases of VD. Refer to Figure 16-2 to see how this may happen.

Contact tracing or case finding (as it is sometimes called) can only work if cases are reported to the state departments of health. Health investigators in this area are prohibited by law from revealing the name of the infected individual to his or her sexual contacts. Reporting one's contacts is essential to the health of these individuals and others who may become infected by the original contacts.

As you can see, venereal disease is a serious business. It can be easily cured *if* one seeks treatment as soon as he thinks he may have the disease. If you think you have been infected, do not wait for symptoms to appear—go for medical treatment immediately.

THINKING IT OVER

1. How would you define an infectious disease?
2. How do infectious diseases differ from chronic diseases? Give some examples of each.
3. What are some of the reasons given for the increase in chronic diseases in recent years?
4. What is a pathogenic organism? What are the three types of bacteria?
5. Discuss two disease-causing organisms other than bacteria.
6. Discuss two common childhood diseases, including symptoms and treatment.

Figure 16-2
The spread of venereal disease.

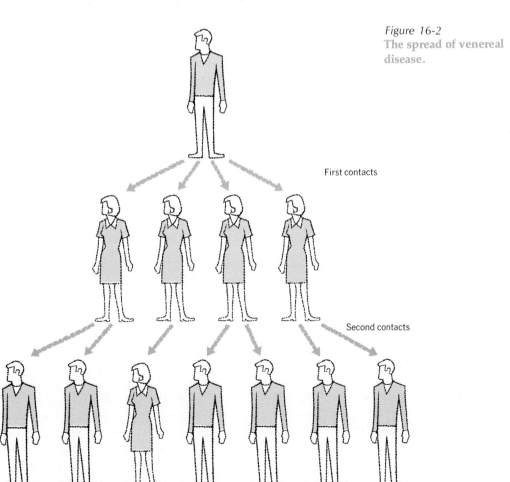

First contacts

Second contacts

7. Discuss mononucleosis, its mode of transmission, symptoms, and treatment. What are some of the myths associated with this disease?

8. How is infectious hapatitis transmitted? What are the effects of this disease?

9. What is immunity? Differentiate between *active* and *passive* immunity.

10. Why have there been many outbreaks of disease for which immunization is available? What can be done to change this situation?

11. What is venereal disease? Discuss ways in which these diseases are transmitted.

12. What are some of the reasons for the increase in venereal disease in recent years? Can you think of any additional reasons?

13. How can venereal disease be prevented?

14. Discuss one of the main venereal diseases (except gonorrhea and syphilis), its symptoms and treatment.

15. What are the symptoms of gonorrhea and syphilis? How are these diseases treated?

16. Discuss methods of venereal disease control.

KEY WORDS

Antibodies. Disease-fighting cells that are produced by the body.

Chancroid. A venereal disease that causes painful sores to appear in the genital area.

Chronic disease. A long-term, debilitating disease not caused by a microorganism.

Chickenpox. An infectious, viral, childhood disease.

Communicable disease. A disease that can be transmitted from one person to another by direct or indirect contact.

Congenital syphilis. Having syphilis at birth; syphilis passed from the mother to the unborn child.

Contact tracing. The finding of persons who have had sexual contact with individuals who have a venereal disease (also called case finding).

Gonorrhea. The most common venereal disease; caused by the gonococcus bacterium.

Granuloma inguinale. A disease that causes sores and infection throughout the body; may be spread in other ways than by sexual intercourse.

Hepatitis. A viral infection of the liver.

Herpes. A viral venereal disease that has become widespread in recent years.

Immunity. Protection against a disease naturally or by the injection of a serum (*active*—established after having had the disease; *passive*—established from a vaccine).

Infectious disease. A disease caused by a microorganism.

Lymphogranuloma venereum. A venereal disease that causes ulcers to appear on the sex organs and can result in internal damage if not treated.

Mononucleosis. A viral disease that is prevalent among young people.

Parasitic worms. Disease-causing worms that infest animals and humans.

Pathogenic organism. A disease-causing organism.

Protozoans. One-celled, disease-causing organisms.

Rickettsiae. Microorganisms that are smaller than bacteria and larger than viruses.

Rubella (German measles). A serious infectious disease that can cause stillbirth or deformity in newborns.

Syphilis. A common venereal disease; caused by a spirochete.

Trichinosis. A disease caused by the trichina worm.

Venereal disease. A disease transmitted through sexual intercourse.

Virus. A tiny organism that may cause disease.

Whooping cough (pertussis). A bacterial disease characterized by a high-pitched cough.

GETTING INVOLVED

Books and Periodicals

Bauer, Stuart, "Blood Farming," *New York Magazine,* May 19, 1975. The "blood-for-profit" business and how it affects us.

Brooks, Stewart M. *The V.D. Story.* Totowa, N.J.: Littlefield, Adams, 1972. The treatment and prevention of venereal disease.

Halberstram, Michael, "The Kissing Disease That Isn't So Romantic," *Today's Health,* December 1974. "Mono" and some of its symptoms and effects.

Karelitz, Samuel. *When Your Child Is Ill.* New York: Random House, 1969. About the common childhood diseases.

Levin, Arthur, "City Diseases That Can Kill You," *New York Magazine,* October 7, 1974. Urban diseases that are often misdiagnosed or remain undiagnosed.

Nicholas, Leslie. *How to Avoid Social Diseases: A Practical Handbook.* New York: Stein & Day, 1973. Questions and answers about VD.

Sharpe, Menell, "The Venereal Disease of the New Morality," *Today's Health,* March 1975. The herpes virus and how health investigators are attacking this recent epidemic.

Movies

Dr. Ehrlich's Magic Bullet, with Edward G. Robinson, 1940. Biography of the chemist who discovered a cure for syphilis. Distributed by United Artists 16.

17
CANCER

There are few diseases that cause more fear and misunderstanding than cancer. Many people would be less fearful if they understood more about the disease and the treatment that is presently available.

In this chapter, you will read about the steady progress that has been made in the treatment of different types of cancer. You will also learn about the warning signs of cancer and how early diagnosis and treatment can save many lives.

The answer to the question, "What is cancer?" is examined. You will learn how a cancerous cell differs from a noncancerous cell and how the cancer cells reproduce and spread without normal control. The causes of cancer are also examined. Cancer is caused by a variety of factors, many of which are known.

The last section of this chapter is concerned with the treatment of cancer. Early diagnosis is stressed. Methods of treatment are presented and examined. False "cures" for cancer, known as quackery, are also discussed. After reading this chapter, you will have a better understanding of what cancer is, the warning signals to look for, and how it is treated. Many of the misunderstandings and fears that you may have had will probably have changed after reading this chapter.

While reading this chapter, think about the following concepts:

■ Cancer is not a new disease.

■ Cancer has been on the rise in recent years because of a variety of factors that are indirectly related to the disease itself.

■ Although no "cure" is available, research and treatment methods have made steady progress.

■ Early diagnosis and treatment is essential to the control of certain types of cancer.

■ There are many successful methods of treatment available to cancer patients.

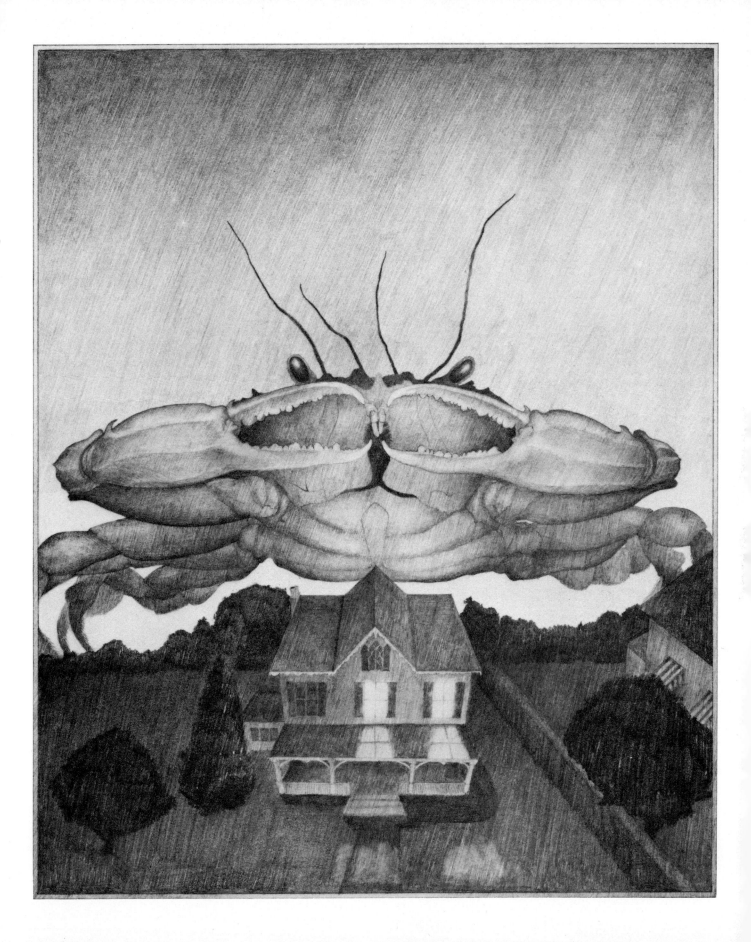

It is difficult to read a newspaper or magazine without coming across at least one article about some aspect of cancer. In late 1974, all the major magazines carried stories of Betty Ford and Happy Rockefeller and their mutual experience with breast cancer. For millions of American women, the publicity given these operations had a profound and beneficial influence on their lives. Many women called for breast examination appointments and clinics and screening programs were backed up for months. In New York City, for example, the Guttman Institute, which provides free breast examinations, was so backed up that one could not get through by telephone. Women without specific symptoms were advised to write for an appointment.

What does this tell us about cancer? One thing that becomes dramatically evident is that there is a great need for education on this subject. Women who had probably not planned to have a breast examination suddenly realized its importance after reading or hearing about it through the media. The importance of education, early diagnosis, and treatment are only a few of the topics that you will explore while reading this chapter.

cancer: past and present

Cancer is not a new disease. It is symbolized by the Greek name for "crab," which describes its "clawing," spreading characteristic. In recent times, the incidence of cancer has been increasing. There are two major reasons for this. One explanation is that there is earlier and more accurate diagnosis of the disease. In the past, many people may have died from cancer without knowing it. A second reason for the increase in cases of cancer is the longer life span. For example, in 1900, only about 6 percent of deaths were from cancer; in 1970, about 20 percent of deaths were from cancer.

According to recent statistics published by the American Cancer Society (ACS), approximately 53 million Americans now living will eventually have some form of cancer.

For the 1970s, there will be an estimated 3.5 million cancer deaths, 6.5 million new cases of cancer, and more than 10 million persons under treatment for cancer. In 1975, there were one million Americans under treatment for the disease.

How many will die as a result of cancer? About 365,000 persons died from cancer in 1975. If we break that number down, it comes to about 1,000 persons a day or a death from cancer about every minute and a half. The deaths from cancer have steadily risen in the twentieth century. Deaths per 100,000 persons have increased from 112 in 1930 to 125 in 1950 and reached 131 in 1971.

These statistics may sound depressing, but there are a large number of patients who have been "cured" of the disease. Today, there are approximately 1,500,000 Americans who have lived without evidence of the disease for five years following diagnosis and treatment. This is accepted as "cured" for most cancer patients.

THE IMPORTANCE OF EARLY DIAGNOSIS

Although no true "cure" is available, early diagnosis and treatment have resulted in about 222,000 Americans being saved in 1975. About one-third of all cancer victims do *not* die from this disease. Today, about 35 percent of cancer patients will live five years or longer after treatment. Although five years is the accepted "cure" time for most patients, some patients are discharged as being free of the disease after three years while others are "cured" after one year of treatment.

Why is early detection so important? The main reason is that about half of all cancers can be detected early enough to be curable. Certain types of cancer grow and spread very slowly, while other types grow and spread at a rapid rate. These types of cancer are incurable at the present time.

Most cancer originates on the surface of a particular tissue such as the mouth, intes-

The American Cancer Society is the nation's leading voluntary cancer organization, with chapters throughout the United States. Its programs are aimed both at finding a cure for cancer and at alerting the public about it. The society funds cancer research (by 1975 it had spent some $350 million in this way), sponsors training programs for physicians, supports antismoking legislation, and maintains breast cancer detection clinics.

tines, or bladder. This stage of the disease is localized or confined to one area. If cancer is detected during the early stages, it is much easier to control by various treatment methods.

One method of improving detection is by selective techniques of determining population groups more likely to have a particular type of cancer. These selected groups of people should be examined frequently for the presence of cancer. By identifying these high risk groups, many lives can be saved. Some of the major high risk groups are given here for your consideration.

Lung Cancer: Those who smoke cigarettes have a much greater risk of getting lung cancer than those who do not smoke. It is currently estimated that cigarette smoking is responsible for about 80 percent of all lung cancer. The heavy smoker also has a significantly higher risk of getting cancer of the larynx, bladder, and mouth.

Breast Cancer: The highest risk group includes: (1) women over the age of 35; (2)

women who have never had children; (3) women who bear their first child after the age of 25; (4) women whose mothers or sisters had breast cancer; and (5) women who menstruated at an early age and/or had a late menopause.

Stomach Cancer: Diet is considered to be a causative factor in stomach cancer. A high incidence of the disease occurs in people who consume large amounts of pickled vegetables and dried salted fish.

Colon-Rectum Cancer: A family tendency toward polyps (growths) in this area has been observed in cases of colon-rectum cancer.

Cancer of the Cervix: Women who come from a low-income background who have never had a Pap test (discussed in a later section) or regular checkups are more likely to have cervical cancer than other women. Other high risk factors include women who have borne children and had a history of early sexual intercourse with a number of partners.

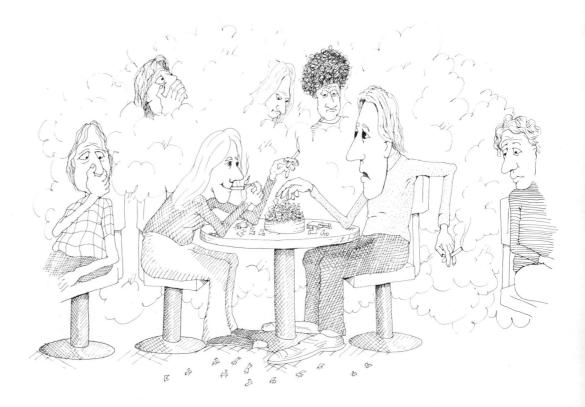

Any persons who fall into these high-risk groups should see a physician regularly and be checked for the possibility of cancer.

The American Cancer Society lists the follow-lowing safeguards for early detection of cancer:

1. Do not smoke cigarettes.
2. Avoid overexposure to the sun.
3. Monthly breast examination.
4. Regular examination of mouth by physician or dentist.
5. Uterine cancer test for women.
6. Rectal examination.
7. Annual complete physical.

Many lives could be saved if individuals followed these safeguards. How many of these seven points do you follow?

We hear so much about cancer and the importance of early diagnosis that it is surprising that more people do not avail themselves of these tests and checkups. However, many people allow fear to keep them from seeking diagnosis. These people are usually afraid of what they might find out. They do not realize that if they have cancer, the sooner they find out the better it is for them. Avoiding a medical examination will not cure the disease. Many people do not have annual examinations that might detect cancer. Cancer will not just "go away."

It is important to be aware of the seven warning signals of cancer: These signals include:

1. Unusual bleeding or discharge.
2. Lumps or thickening in the breast or elsewhere.
3. Sore that does not heal.
4. Change in bowel or bladder habits.
5. Hoarseness or cough.
6. Indigestion or difficulty in swallowing.
7. Change in a wart or mole.

If any of these symptoms lasts more than two weeks, one should seek a physical examination. It is important to remember that these symptoms do *not* mean that one

has cancer. They could be symptoms of many diseases and disorders, but one should be checked for the *possibility* of cancer being present. The warning signals are not a diagnosis of cancer, but rather a warning that a medical examination is necessary.

Pain is not a warning signal of cancer. Most cancers are not painful in the early stages. Pain only becomes a symptom after the disease has progressed. As mentioned previously, finding a lump or recognizing another symptom does not mean you have cancer. For example, only about 25 to 35 percent of all breast lumps are cancerous.

In order for more people to seek early detection, public education is necessary. As you recall from Chapter 6 on tobacco, public education concerning cancer and cigarettes has led to many people giving up the smoking habit. Education cannot start too early. Many school systems are showing films to young women about how to check themselves for breast cancer. If a girl begins to do this at a young age, she is likely to continue with it through her adult years.

Cancer education needs to be widespread so that the majority of people can learn about it. Television spots, magazine articles, and first-person books are all helpful in educating the public. The American Cancer Society is a very active organization which provides a multitude of services and publishes a voluminous literature about cancer. If you have any questions or problems concerning cancer, write or call your local chapter of the American Cancer Society.

Public awareness has increased because of the breast cancer of such women as Betty Ford and Happy Rockefeller. In fact, Betty Ford was the Honorary Chairman of the 1975 American Cancer Society Crusade.

In addition, public awareness has been benefited by programs on television that have dealt openly with the issue of cancer. Edith Bunker (played by actress Jean Stapleton) of *All in the Family* discovered a lump in her breast in one episode of this show. The lump was not cancerous which provided a double-learning experience for the viewer (self-examination and the fact that most breast lumps are not cancerous). Other television programs that have spot-lighted cancer have included *Not For Women Only, Medical Center,* and *Marcus Welby, M.D.* Another program entitled, *Why Me?,* told how the lives of ten women were affected by breast cancer.

Although much more remains to be done, it is encouraging that cancer has finally been brought into the public view. At one time, people so feared the disease that it was never discussed openly. In the past, television programs might have alluded to cancer, but never before has programming centered around this disease.

what is cancer?

Cancer may be defined as a group of living cells that grow and reproduce without normal controls. As was mentioned previously, cancer begins as a localized disease. At the start, one cell or a few cells undergo an abnormal change. These cells become malignant or cancerous. Each malignant cell will only reproduce malignant cells. This is how the disease begins to spread. Malignant or cancerous cells have an abnormal size and shape and do not form constructive body tissues. Refer to Figure 17-1 for a comparison of malignant and nonmalignant cells.

Masses of these cells cause a lump or swelling to develop. These swellings are called tumors. If the tumor is caused by cancerous cells, then it is called a malignant tumor. However, some tumors are caused by noncancerous cells; these tumors are benign. Most tumors are *not* malignant. If you notice a lump or swelling any place on your body, see a doctor immediately. In most cases, the tumor will be benign.

The most dangerous phases of cancer are the later ones. Masses of cancer cells may enter the blood vessels or lymph nodes and travel to other parts of the body. Colonies are formed and are called metastases. The process itself is known as *metastasis.* Sometimes, these cancer cells are trapped in a lymph node of the original organ of involvement. If this occurs, the disease is known as being regionally involved. This may retard the spread of the cancer for a while.

If cancer goes untreated, then the cells will eventually spread to other parts of the body. This is known as advanced cancer and death is almost inevitable. When cancer is in the metastatic or advanced stage it is extremely difficult to arrest. Early detection and treatment could "cure" most cancers that are in the early or localized stage of development.

There are many forms of cancer known to man. Although there are between 200 and

Figure 17-1
Cells of the cervix:
(a) malignant, (b) non-malignant.

(a)

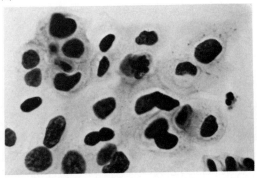

(b)

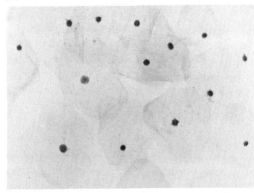

300 recognized kinds of cancer, there are about 30 common forms of the disease. Some of the most common forms include cancer of the: lung, breast, colon-rectum, uterus, cervix, pancreas, larynx, stomach, bladder, kidney, lip-tongue-mouth, brain, prostate, thyroid, skin, bone and connective tissue, as well as leukemia and Hodgkin's Disease.

One can see from this partial listing that with so many types of cancer it is difficult to find a "cure." As you will see in a later section of this chapter, different forms of cancer require different treatment or a combination of treatments.

causes of cancer

The abnormal cell growth that is characteristic of cancer may be initiated by a number of factors. Substances that are cancer-causing are called carcinogens. A carcinogenic substance includes smoke, tars, and certain chemicals and gases. Researchers are presently working to identify carcinogens and limit one's exposure to them. Some common carcinogens and their effects are discussed later in this chapter.

BIOLOGICAL CAUSES OF CANCER

A commonly asked question concerning cancer is whether or not it is inherited. A few very rare types of cancer have been traced to heredity. However, the most common types of cancer are not directly inherited. However, in some of these common types, there is a familial tendency. This means that a particular type of cancer occurs with greater frequency among members of a family. A family, in this sense, is not only the immediate family, as a tendency toward cancer may exist, for example, in parents, children, grandparents, aunts, uncles, and cousins. Familial tendencies have been found in cancer of the breast, colon, stomach, prostate, and lung, and in leukemia.

A familial tendency *does not* mean that one would get cancer if, for example, a parent had the disease. It *does* mean that there appears to be a tendency toward a greater

susceptibility to certain cancers among certain family members.

It is extremely important that high-risk individuals have frequent checkups for cancer. A study by cancer geneticist, Dr. David Anderson, indicated that relatives of patients who had cancer of both breasts were five times as likely to develop cancer as patients in a control group. Relatives of those patients who had cancer of the breast before the age of 40 were nine times as likely to get breast cancer as the control group. Dr. Anderson concluded that breast examinations should begin as soon as family members are identified, regardless of age, and should be conducted at regular, individualized schedules according to the risk-factor involved.

Another biological factor involved in cancer is age. Although cancer may occur at any age, it strikes with increasing frequency as one gets older. Certain types of cancer occur more frequently in children than in adults. Leukemia is the cancer most frequently found in children and is the single greatest cause of death in children.

Many of you may have heard about the virus theory of causing cancer. Viruses are presently under study, and there is some indication that a virus may be one cause of cancer. Presently, more than 100 viruses have been identified as capable of producing cancer in animals under special laboratory conditions. However, these viruses have not been found to be related to cancer in human beings.

A recent finding may, however, be significant to these virus studies. On January 8, 1975, the National Cancer Institute released the news that a virus has been discovered that is associated with a case of human leukemia. There is great interest in this discovery, as the isolation of this virus may help researchers develop new approaches to detection, diagnosis, and treatment of leukemia. The evidence is strong that this virus is a distinct virus; but whether or not it is a factor in causing human leukemia has not been conclusively shown. It should be noted that

The National Cancer Institute, one of the federal National Institutes of Health, is a research and planning agency. It also provides grants to private institutions' cancer research programs. The institute is planning a National Cancer Program that will put research findings into immediate use in the treatment or prevention of cancer.

the viruses under study are not infectious and are not passed from person to person.

Hormones are another biological factor that may cause cancer. There has been some indication that certain hormones either stimulate or inhibit the growth of cancer. However, no conclusive evidence exists concerning this theory.

ENVIRONMENTAL FACTORS

The World Health Organization (W.H.O.) and other agencies recently estimated that between 60 and 80 percent of human cancers are caused by environmental factors. There is a growing interest in the possibility that chemical carcinogens in the environment may activate viruses in the cell and cause a cell to grow abnormally.

There have been many occupational cancers linked to certain chemicals and gases. Bladder cancer has been found in dye and rubber workers. Lung cancer has been connected to asbestos and uranium miners and in coke oven and nitrogen mustard workers. Skin cancer has been associated with oil works; cancer of the pancreas has appeared in organic chemists; liver cancer has been observed in a number of polyvinyl chloride workers.

One of the problems with environmentally caused cancers is the long latency period. For certain chemicals, cancer becomes apparent 18 to 30 years after exposure to the carcinogen. In other substances, less than 10 years have been observed between exposure and malignancy.

The American Cancer Society recently released a geographic study that illustrates trends in cancer deaths for various parts of the country (see Table 17-1).[1] This study lends strong support to the theory that most cancers result from environmental causes. Some of the findings were not surprising. For example, the death rate from skin cancer was the highest in the southern United States. This finding is consistent with the belief that excessive exposure to the sun is related to skin cancer.

Deaths from cancer of the stomach were highest in the Southwest and certain northern states. These areas are populated by groups of people (Mexican and Scandinavian) whose diets are related to this type of cancer.

Deaths from lung and liver cancer were highest in smelt-industry communities. This fact suggests an air-pollution effect. However, deaths from lung cancer were also high in east coast cities and even higher along the Gulf Coast. Cigarette smoking and air pollution were considered causative factors; however, other factors may also be involved.

Food additives and pesticides have also been the subject of study as possible environmental causes of cancer. Recently two pesticides were prohibited from use because of their carcinogenic properties. And in early 1976, the FDA banned the use of a red dye that had been used for many years in thousands of food and drug products. There are many problems today involved with how to set up laws to protect the public from involuntary exposure to such carcinogens. More research has to be conducted in the area of consumer protection where carcinogenic substances are involved.

The highest mortality from bladder cancer was found among men in the highly industrialized Northeast. For example, of the 21 counties of New Jersey, 18 were in the top percentile for bladder cancer. Chemicals are thought to be a factor in this type of cancer.

The National Cancer Institute points out that these studies do not *prove* a cause and effect relationship in cancer; but they do identify areas where cancer is more likely to occur. Studies like this are extremely helpful in pinpointing areas of the country where specific population groups would benefit from screening programs for early detection of cancer.

[1]Reprinted by permission of the American Cancer Society, Inc.

348

TABLE 17.1

**CANCER DEATHS AND DEATH RATES
BY STATE, 1973**

State	Deaths	Rate per 100,000 Population	State	Deaths	Rate per 100,000 Population
Alabama	5,430	153.4	Montana	1,054	146.2
Alaska	202	61.2	Nebraska	2,628	170.4
Arizona	2,831	137.6	Nevada	805	146.9
Arkansas	3,647	179.0	New Hampshire	1,393	176.1
California	31,948	155.1	New Jersey	14,004	190.2
Colorado	2,849	116.9	New Mexico	1,192	107.8
Connecticut	5,457	177.4	New York	35,485	194.3
Delaware	928	161.1	North Carolina	7,400	140.3
District of Columbia	1,534	205.6	North Dakota	940	146.9
Florida	16,492	214.8	Ohio	18,463	172.1
Georgia	6,498	135.8	Oklahoma	4,730	177.6
Hawaii	901	108.3	Oregon	3,657	164.4
Idaho	1,009	131.0	Pennsylvania	22,651	190.3
Illinois	19,646	174.8	Rhode Island	1,939	199.3
Indiana	8,463	159.2	South Carolina	3,662	134.3
Iowa	5,212	179.5	South Dakota	1,141	166.6
Kansas	3,858	169.3	Tennessee	6,490	157.3
Kentucky	5,546	165.9	Texas	17,151	145.4
Louisiana	5,822	154.7	Utah	1,058	91.4
Maine	1,949	189.6	Vermont	816	175.9
Maryland	6,567	161.4	Virginia	7,245	150.6
Massachusetts	11,075	190.4	Washington	5,652	164.8
Michigan	14,129	156.2	West Virginia	3,254	181.4
Minnesota	6,172	158.4	Wisconsin	7,394	161.8
Mississippi	3,382	148.3	Wyoming	448	126.9
Missouri	8,856	186.2	Total United States	351,055	167.3

Source: Vital Statistics of the United States
Prepared by: Research Department, American Cancer Society, April 1975.

some common types of cancer

Throughout this chapter, different types of cancer have been mentioned. In this section, a few common types of cancer are discussed so that you will become more familiar with their causes, symptoms, and treatment (see Figure 17-2).

CANCER OF THE BREAST

In the United States, breast cancer occurs more often than any other form of cancer. It causes about 33,000 deaths in this country every year. It is found in women of all ages, but is more frequently found in women over the age of 35.

The cause of breast cancer is still unknown. However, an injury to the breast has *not* been found to be related to the development of breast tumors. Fortunately there is treatment for the disease. Breast cancer is often found by the woman (about 95 percent of all breast lumps) and most of these lumps are *not* cancerous. Early diagnosis is essential. Certain diagnostic methods are discussed in the next section of this chapter.

Treatment consists of surgery and radiation therapy. Some women require one method; others require both methods. Most women are treated by an operation called a mastectomy (removal of the breast, the muscles underneath the breast, and the lymph nodes of the armpit). This operation is designed to remove all cancerous tissue and prevent the recurrence and spread of the disease. The extent of the surgery is deterninded by the individual case. Hormones, certain chemicals, and operations to remove the ovaries, adrenal glands, or pituitary gland are sometimes helpful to certain breast-cancer patients.

CANCER OF THE COLON AND RECTUM

This cancer is often called "the cancer no one talks about." But more people should begin talking about it, because it results in about 47,000 deaths in the United States each year. There are about 100,000 new cases each year.

In about 75 percent of all cases, the patient can be saved. However, only about 40,000 patients are saved because not enough people

have regular physical checkups that include a proctoscopic examination. This test known as a "procto" is the visual examination of the lower colon and rectum through a lighted tube. "Procto" examinations can detect cancer in those areas at a very early stage.

Cancer of the colon or rectum usually causes an obstruction. The symptoms include constipation (sometimes diarrhea), gas pains, and rectal bleeding. In later stages, blood may appear in the bowel movement. Weakness, anemia, and shortness of breath may ensue. If rectal bleeding, blood in the stool, persistent change in bowel habits, and intestinal gas are observed, seek immediate medical attention. *Any* of these symptoms are important, though they may *not* mean cancer. All men and women, especially those past the age of 40, should have a rectal examination including a "procto."

CANCER OF THE LUNG

Lung cancer causes more deaths than any other type of cancer. Approximately 91,000 cases of lung cancer were cited in 1975 and about 81,000 deaths occurred from this form of cancer. Lung cancer is almost entirely caused by cigarette smoking. Therefore, it is largely preventable, if people would stop

Figure 17-2
Estimates for 1976:
(a) cancer incidence by
site and sex
(nonmelanoma skin
cancer and carcinoma in
situ of uterine cancer
are excluded); (b) cancer
deaths by site and sex.
(Reprinted by permission
of the American Cancer
Society, Inc. Copyright
© 1975 by the American
Cancer Society, Inc.)

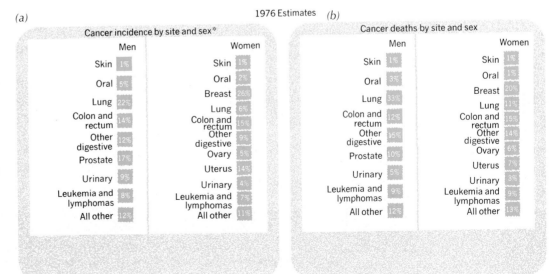

smoking or never start. Lung cancer is a difficult disease to diagnose in its early stages. For this reason, only about 10 percent of all lung cancer patients are presently being saved. Refer to Chapter 6 for more information about the relationship between cigarette smoking and lung cancer.

The symptoms of lung cancer vary depending on where the cancer occurs. If it starts in the air passage, it will cause partial obstruction and irritation and the symptoms may be a cough. The sputum, however, may contain blood. In its early stages, there may be no symptoms. All lingering coughs should be checked. Chest X-rays, especially for smokers, should be a part of every physical examination. A sputum examination may also indicate the presence of lung cancer cells. The bronchoscope allows for visual examination of the windpipe and lungs and a biopsy of lung tissue can be taken with this instrument.

Treatment involves surgery to remove the cancerous tissue. Under favorable conditions, many patients completely recover following surgery. The cure rate in lung cancer is low, however, because the operation is often performed in the later stages of the disease.

LEUKEMIA

Leukemia is often called "cancer of the blood," however, it is a cancer of the tissues where blood cells are formed. These tissues include the bone marrow, lymph nodes, and the spleen. The word leukemia means "white blood" and it is called this because one of the common symptoms is an oversupply of abnormal white blood cells.

The blood forming organs normally produce hundreds of millions of normal blood cells each day. When leukemia is present, a large portion of these cells are partially formed, abnormal white cells. In advanced leukemia, cancerous cells fill the bone marrow, crowding the production of red blood cells, normal white cells, and platelets (which clot

blood). Eventually this causes the symptoms of leukemia.

What causes leukemia? There is some evidence of inherited susceptibility, as in breast cancer and other forms of cancer. However, there is no evidence of the disease being transmitted directly from mother to child. A brother or sister of a child with leukemia has a 1 in 720 chance of developing the disease. In the general population under the age of 15, the risk of getting leukemia is only 1 in 2,880. If a child has leukemia, his brothers and sisters should be carefully watched.

There has been some evidence that overexposure to X-rays may be related to leukemia. Individuals who would be affected in this way include doctors and X-ray technicians.

The virus theory also exists for leukemia. Virus-like particles have been found in the cells of human leukemia patients. If viruses are discovered to be related to leukemia, then the possibility of an antileukemia vaccine does exist. Of course, research in this area is constantly being conducted.

There are few early signs of leukemia. If a case is discovered early, it is usually through a routine blood examination. During a later stage of leukemia, a person may experience fatigue, pallor, nosebleeds, hemorrhages, bone pain, and night sweats. Children may have symptoms similar to an infection. Advanced leukemia is often characterized by great fatigue, massive hemorrhages, pain, high fever, enlargement of internal organs and lymph nodes, swelling of the gums, and skin disorders.

Treatment usually involves chemotherapy (the use of drugs). A combination of drugs and certain antibiotics can put a patient in remission in about 90 percent of leukemias. Remission is the term used to describe the condition that stops and reverses the progress of the disease. However, some remissions are more temporary than others. In more serious leukemias, the rate of remission is about 40 to 50 percent. In many cases, patients with leukemia will go through periods of repeated remission and relapse, often extending from 10 to 20 years.

MOUTH CANCER

Mouth cancer is somewhat less common than the cancers that have been discussed, but it does occur in about 5 percent of the male population and 2 percent of the female population. It is very rare in children. It causes approximately 7,000 deaths per year.

There are a number of suspected causes of mouth cancer. It is thought that cancer of the lower lip might be caused by excessive exposure to sunlight. Constant irritation from a pipe, cigarette, or cigar may also cause a lip cancer. Any irritation by a denture or tooth may be a causative factor. Heavy drinkers have been found to have a greater incidence of mouth cancer than the general population. A combination of heavy drinking and smoking may also be involved in this type of cancer.

The best way to detect this disease is by having frequent dental or physical examinations. In addition, one can examine his own mouth for the presence of a sore; raised, irregular area; reddened area; or a lump or thickening of the cheek, gum, tongue or floor of the mouth. Mouth cancers are usually painless. Treatment usually consists of surgery and radiation. Either or both may be used. Radiation is often used to shrink large tumors so that they can be operated upon more easily.

SKIN CANCER

About 1 percent of the general population is affected by skin cancer. Approximately 120,000 new cases are reported each year, but estimates vary widely depending on whether or not the cancer is superficial. About 5,000 deaths from skin cancer occur each year. Who gets skin cancer? Studies indicate that overexposure to the sun is one of the major causes of the disease. "Sun worshippers" are more apt to get skin cancer than those who keep away from the sun's rays. Dark-skinned persons and those who tan easily are less susceptible than the general population.

If one does enjoy sunbathing, then common

medical sense should be used. Avoid the sun between the hours of 10:00 a.m. and 3:00 p.m. This is the time when the sun's rays are the strongest. If you do go out in these hours, use a protective lotion of a para-amino-benzoic acid (PABA) in alcohol. Many brand names utilize this formula. Start with 15 minutes of exposure and gradually increase the amount of sunbathing time.

Skin cancer is usually indicated by a reddened, ulcerated sore than does not heal in a reasonable amount of time. If detected early enough, most skin cancers can be cured. However, some are more malignant than others and are difficult to arrest. Treatment for skin cancer includes surgery, X rays, and chemotherapy. Some cancers can be removed in the doctor's office by the use of an *electric needle* while the patient is under a local anesthetic.

UTERINE CANCER

Cancer of the uterus occurs in about 14 percent of all women in this country. It causes about 12,000 deaths each year. This is one cancer that can be completely cured, if caught in time.

Cancer of the uterus includes cancer of two areas of this organ. The neck of the uterus, or *cervix* (the narrow area of the lower uterus which connects to the vagina) is one site of uterine cancer. The other site is the uterus itself. The growth of cancer cells in the cervix or body of the uterus can spread to other parts of the body if not treated.

Cancer of the uterus is most common in women past the age of 35. However, any woman old enough to bear a child can get uterine cancer. Younger women usually develop cancer of the cervix, while older women (during or after menopause) most frequently develop cancer in the body of the uterus.

As previously mentioned, there is a test for uterine cancer called the *Pap test.* It is named for its developer, Dr. George N. Papanicolau. The Pap test is a simple, painless procedure that is usually done during a routine pelvic examination. The doctor takes a sample of cells from the cervix and vagina for microscopic examination. The sample is taken on a cotton swab or flat stick. The test takes a minute or so and can save one's life. If you avoid going for a pelvic exam, why do you think you react in this way?

The Pap test will indicate if there are any suspicious cells in this area. If there are, further tests will be done to see if the patient has uterine cancer. A Pap test should be taken every year, more often in certain cases. A symptom of uterine cancer is often abnormal bleeding from the vagina. This is especially

true of cancer in postmenopausal women. However, all abnormal bleeding should be checked and in most cases it is related to another less serious condition. Treatment for uterine cancer usually involves surgery and radiation therapy.

treatment of cancer

Early diagnosis is imperative in the treatment of cancer. This fact cannot be stressed too often. Close to 100 percent of all breast and uterine cancers could be cured if diagnosed in time.

Figure 17-3
Breast self-examination. (Reprinted by permission of the American Cancer Society, Inc. Copyright © 1975 by the American Cancer Society, Inc.)

How to examine your breasts

In the shower:

Examine your breasts during bath or shower; hands glide easier over wet skin. Fingers flat, move gently over every part of each breast. Use right hand to examine left breast, left hand for right breast. Check for any lump, hard knot or thickening.

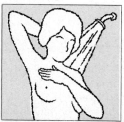

Before a mirror:

Inspect your breasts with arms at your sides. Next, raise your arms high overhead. Look for any changes in contour of each breast, a swelling, dimpling of skin or changes in the nipple.

Then, rest palms on hips and press down firmly to flex your chest muscles. Left and right breast will not exactly match—few women's breasts do.

Regular inspection shows what is normal for you and will give you confidence in your examination.

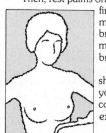

Lying down:

To examine your right breast, put a pillow or folded towel under your right shoulder. Place right hand behind your head—this distributes breast tissue more evenly on the chest. With left hand, fingers flat, press gently in small circular motions around an imaginary clock face. Begin at outermost top of your right breast for 12 o'clock, then move to 1 o'clock, and so on around the circle back to 12. A ridge of firm tissue in the lower curve of each breast is normal. Then move in an inch, toward the nipple, keep circling to examine *every part of your breast,* including nipple. This requires at least three more circles. Now slowly repeat procedure on your left breast with a pillow under your left shoulder and left hand behind head. Notice how your breast structure feels.

Finally, squeeze the nipple of each breast gently between thumb and index finger. Any discharge, clear or bloody, should be reported to your doctor immediately.

353

BREAST SELF-EXAMINATION

One method of diagnosing breast cancer is by a monthly breast self-examination, in addition to a physician's examination. The best time to do this is after one's menstrual period. Refer to Figure 17-3, as you read this section of the chapter.

The easiest time to do this is while bathing or showering, when your skin is still wet. (Figure 17-3a). Hold your fingers in a flat position and gently feel each breast for a lump or thickening. After this, do a more thorough check.

Lie down with one hand behind your head. With the flattened fingers of the other hand, gently feel your breast. Press lightly. Then examine the other breast in the same way. Begin where you see the A in Figure 17-3b and follow the direction of the arrows. Feel each breast for a lump or thickening. Repeat the same procedure while sitting up with one hand behind your head.

Another diagnostic technique used in screening patients for breast cancer is a mammogram. This is a low-dose X ray that can detect tumors before they are large enough to be felt. If a suspicious mass is found, then a biopsy is done to determine whether or not it is malignant. *Mammography* is particularly recommended for women over the age of 35, or those with a family history of breast cancer.

METHODS OF TREATMENT

The three most common methods of treatment for cancer include radiation therapy, chemotherapy, and surgery. Depending on the type of cancer, one or more of these

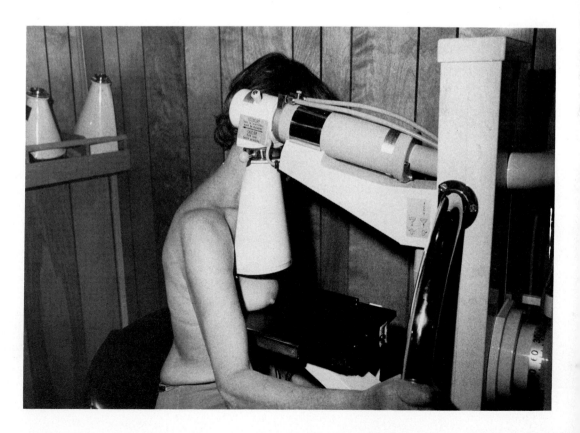

Administration of the mammogram.

methods may be used. Surgery is the most common and effective treatment method for most types of cancer.

Chemotherapy has led to many advances in the control of such cancers as leukemia and Hodgkin's Disease, which is a progressive cancer affecting the lymph and spleen. A new antibiotic, *adriamycin,* is proving to be effective against leukemia, bone cancer, and a wide range of malignant tumors. It is also useful in the treatment of lung cancer. Side effects do exist and at present the drug is very expensive.

Research in cancer is proceeding along many fronts and recent developments in the field are considered encouraging. It is an enormous job because of the wide variety of cancers that are known and those that still remain unknown.

CANCER QUACKERY

Cancer quacks prey on cancer victims by offering a variety of "cures." These so-called cures may include drugs, gadgets, special diet supplements, fad diets, and numerous other ploys. The cancer victim often goes

Radiation therapy.

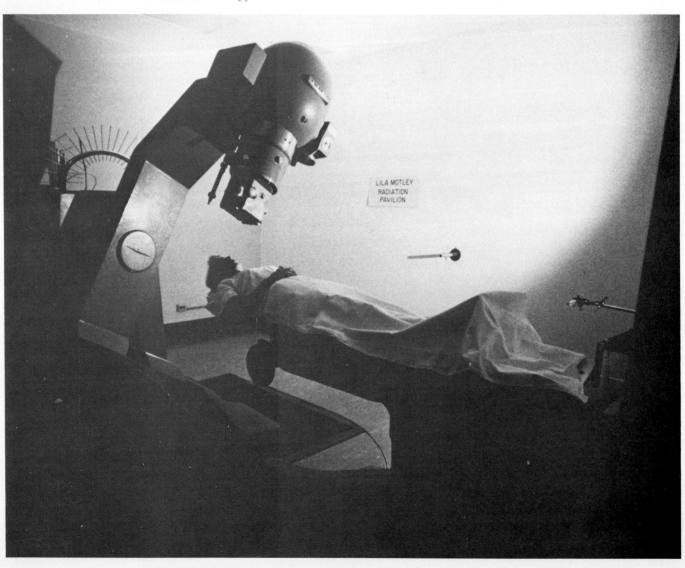

355

along with the quack because he feels "it is his last chance." Cancer quackery and other forms of quackery are a big business and attract many thousands of people each year. You will read about all types of quackery in detail in Chapter 19.

WHERE TO GET HELP

If you or a member of your family has cancer and needs help in coping with any related problems, there are agencies that you can contact. The American Cancer Society has offices in most major cities and the national office is located at 129 East 42 Street, New York, N. Y. 10017.

Most offices are able to provide service and rehabilitation programs as well as general information and patient assistance. In addition, certain units of the ACS provide for the "Reach to Recovery" program where women who have had mastectomies help those who have just undergone surgery adjust to this operation.

A number of services are also provided by Cancer Care, Inc., an arm of the National Cancer Foundation. This organization provides counseling and financial aid to the families of patients with advanced cancer.

THINKING IT OVER

1. Why has cancer been on the rise in recent years?
2. Discuss the need for education of the public through the media. Explain your answer.
3. Do you think adequate public information about cancer is presented by the media? Explain your answer.
4. Why are many cases diagnosed after cancer is in the advanced stage?
5. What are the seven safeguards against cancer?
6. What are the seven warning signals of cancer?
7. What is cancer? How does the disease spread to other parts of the body?
8. What is the difference between a *benign* and a *malignant* tumor?

9. What is the difference between *localized* and *regional* cancer?
10. What is a *carcinogen?*
11. Discuss the part that heredity may play in cancer.
12. What other biological factors may cause cancer?
13. Discuss some of the environmental factors that may cause cancer.
14. Why is early diagnosis so imperative in cases of cancer?
15. What is a *Pap test?*
16. What is a "procto?"
17. What methods can be used to detect breast cancer?
18. Discuss the three major methods of treatment for cancer.
19. What services are available to the cancer patient and his family?
20. What is cancer quackery? Why are many cancer patients open to quackery?

KEY WORDS

Advanced cancer. Cancer that has spread to various parts of the body.

Benign tumor. A noncancerous tumor.

Bronchoscope. An instrument used for the examination of the windpipe and lungs.

Carcinogen. An agent that causes cancer.

Chemotherapy. Use of drugs to treat disease.

Familial tendency. An inherited susceptibility to certain types of cancer.

Localized cancer. Cancer cells that remain at the site of the original cancer.

Malignant tumor. A cancerous tumor.

Mammogram. Low-dose X ray used to detect breast cancer.

Mastectomy. Removal of the breast, the muscles underneath the breast, and the lymph nodes.

Metastases. Groups of cancer cells that are carried in the bloodstream or lymph nodes to other parts of the body.

Pap test. Test for cancer of the uterus.

Proctoscopic examination. Examination of the rectum and colon to detect cancer.

Regional cancer. Cancer cells that have spread and are trapped in the lymph nodes in the region of the original site.

Reach to Recovery, sponsored by the American Cancer Society, is a rehabilitation program for women who have had breast surgery. It starts within a few days after surgery, when a trained volunteer (who has had breast surgery herself) visits the woman in the hospital, bringing information manuals, exercise equipment, and a temporary breast form. Consultation services are available after that; and in many areas Reach to Recovery hold discussion sessions for expatients. There is no charge for any of these services.

Remission. A condition that stops and reverses the progress of the disease.

Tumor. Masses of cells that form a lump or swelling (may be cancerous or non-cancerous).

GETTING INVOLVED

Books and Periodicals

American Cancer Society. *Answers to 101 Questions about Cancer.* A.C.S. Pub. No. 2025. Pamphlet answering the most commonly asked questions about cancer.

————. *Personal Memo for Today: Breast Self-Examination.* A.C.S. Pub. No. 2028. The recommended technique for examining one's own breasts.

Conniff, James, "Bask, Don't Burn," *The New York Times Magazine,* July 7, 1974. Sunbathing and the relationship between the sun's rays and skin cancer.

National Cancer Institute. *Cancer: What to Know, What to Do about It.* P.H.S. Pub. No. 375. Washington, D.C.: U.S. Government Printing Office, 1967. A government pamphlet about cancer.

Ross, W.S. *The Climate Is Hope: How They Triumphed over Cancer.* Englewood Cliffs, N.J.: Prentice-Hall, 1965. Cancer can sometimes be cured. . . .

Thomas, Lewis. *Lives of a Cell: Notes of a Biology Watcher.* New York: Viking, 1974. Well-written observations of life and biological processes.

Movies

Breast Self-Examination. Good visual presentation of this technique. Distributed by the American Cancer Society.

Man Alive. Cancer's warning signals. Distributed by the American Cancer Society.

Who Me? About the dangers of smoking. Distributed by the American Cancer Society.

PART VI
CONSUMER HEALTH

18
MEDICAL SERVICES

When you visit your dentist or doctor, do you think of yourself as a consumer who is purchasing health care? Most people do not use the term consumer when referring to health care. In this chapter, you will learn about the public as a consumer of health care, the status of health care today, and what one should look for when "buying" all types of health services.

You will also learn about the people who provide health care and the services that they provide. You will read about the different medical specialties and their place in providing medical services. Many health-related careers are also briefly discussed in this chapter. The nursing profession and a recent addition, the nurse practitioner, is examined.

An important aspect of health care is the hospital. Different types of hospitals and hospital services are discussed. In addition, nursing homes, rehabilitation centers, and clinics are examined.

Programs that aid in covering the cost of medical services are also discussed. There are private programs that include Blue Cross and Blue Shield, private insurance plans, and a more recent plan called the Health Maintenance Organization (H.M.O.). In addition, there are public programs that include Medicare, Medicaid, and the proposed National Health Insurance Plan. Each of these plans are discussed in this chapter. The cost of medical care and what this means to the consumer is also examined. The controversy over malpractice insurance and how this relates to health consumer costs is explored. After reading this chapter, you will be a better informed health consumer who will recognize the services performed by medical specialists and allied health personnel.

While reading this chapter, think about the following concepts:

■ We are all consumers of health services.

■ There are methods of determining the general competence of physicians and other medical personnel.

■ The cost of medical services is high, but there are programs that can help.

■ There are a number of allied health careers that are both interesting and rewarding.

■ Hospitals and other health care facilities vary in services offered as well as in level of treatment.

■ It is important to investigate all aspects of health care prior to "buying" any health service.

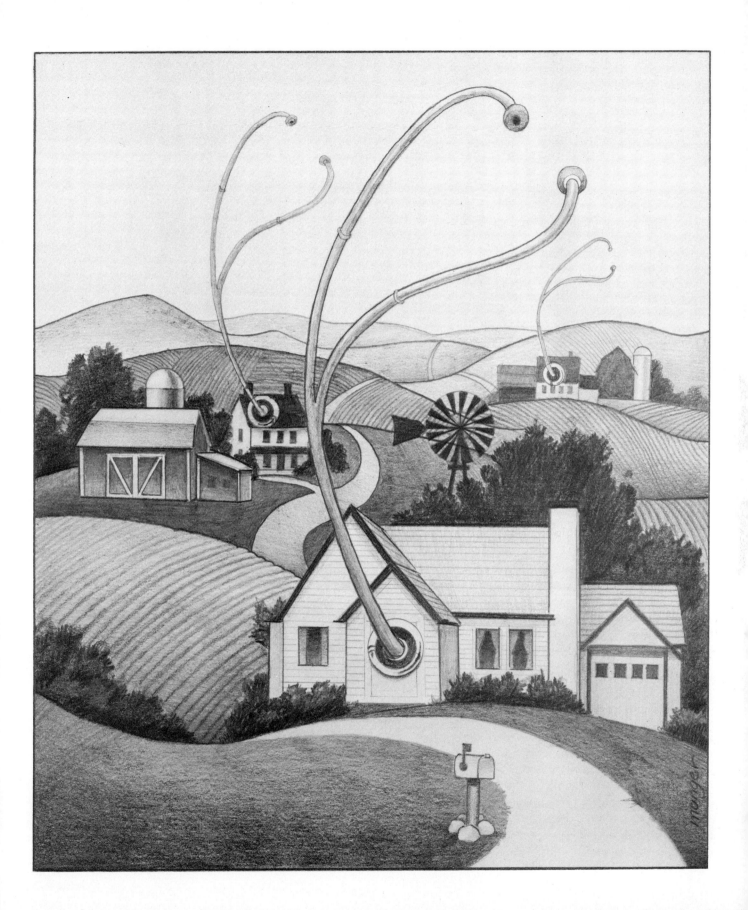

When you need a doctor what do you think about? Do you think about whether or not he is a good doctor, if he makes house calls, or how much he charges? Most people just think of getting well and do not get involved with the credentials, services, or fees of the doctor. However, recently consumer action groups have began to make information about doctors available to the public.

The first such guide was published by the Health Research Group and was limited to doctors practicing in Prince Georges County, Maryland. Other such guides have appeared, many assembled by student and faculty volunteers at local colleges.

The consumer guides list the doctor's training, hospital affiliation and specialty, fees charged for office visits, whether or not he makes house calls and treats emergencies, whether he accepts Medicare and Medicaid patients, and what tests can be provided in the office. Doctors who refuse to provide information are sometimes listed as "un-cooperative."

Why do you think that consumer guides to doctors and services are a good idea? Many doctors feel that the information presented in the guide may be inaccurate or that patients will begin to choose doctors according to the fees they charge and not their competence. Are there any groups in your community that have published this type of guide? If so, which groups are involved?

The consumer guide to doctors is one way of selecting a doctor. But it should only be used as one factor in deciding who will be your physician. In this chapter you will learn about other factors to consider when looking for a doctor, medical specialist, or other health services.

the consumer and the health care team

The public is the consumer when it comes to health care. Most people do not think of themselves as consumers, in this sense,

because of the "mystique" of the health care profession. Many people fear asking their doctor about his credentials or fees. They refrain from asking about the cost of hospital services. People usually become angry about fees after they have received the service. Can you think of any other reasons why people avoid discussing such questions with their doctors?

However, this is beginning to change. People are "shopping around" more for health services and consumers are beginning to make their voices heard through action groups. Such topics as the nursing home scandals, as well as malpractice suits and insurance rates have made people more aware of consumerism involved in health care services.

In order to know what to look for in a doctor or other health professional, one should know something about different medical specialties and the training involved in each area. Many people are unaware of the different types of medical specialists, dentists, and nurses, as well as allied professionals.

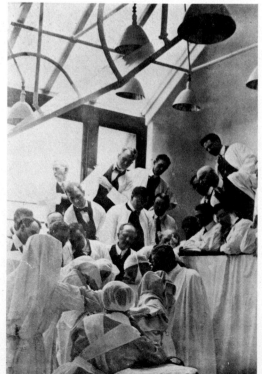

(a)

(b)

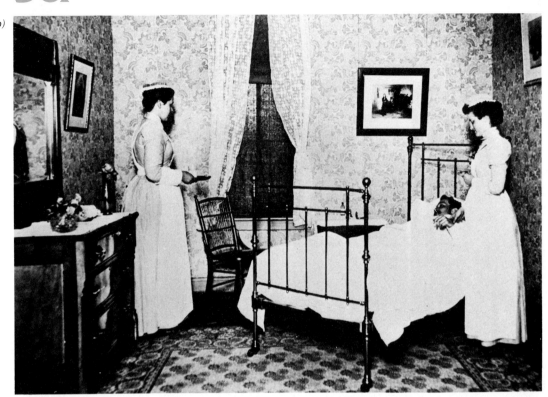

(c)

Early twentieth-century
health care: (a) Dr. Mayo
operating at the Mayo
Clinic, 1913; (b) a private
room at St. Luke's
Hospital, Duluth, 1900;
(c) Dr. Olga Lentz in her
dental office at St. Paul,
1910.

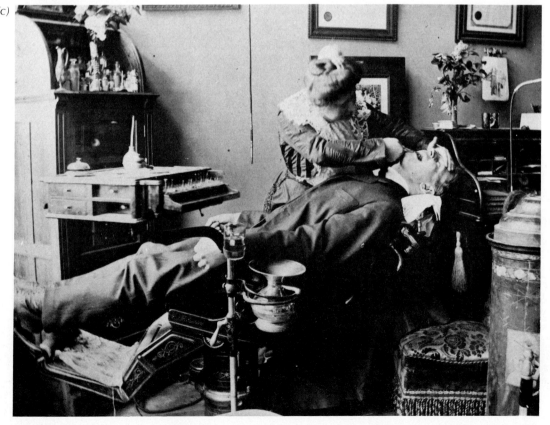

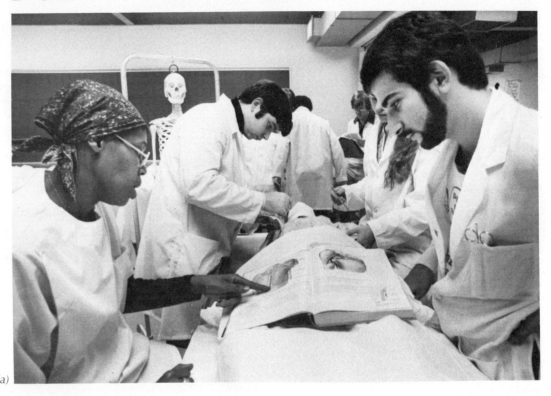

(a)

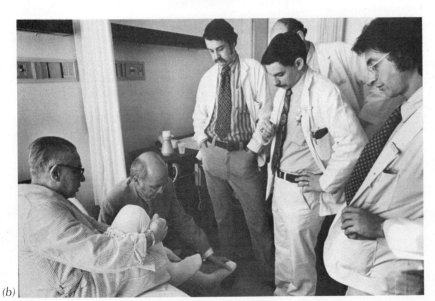

(b)

Portrait of a doctor: (a) medical students, (b) interns, (c) resident, (d) surgeon.

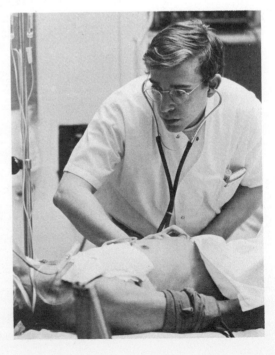

(c)

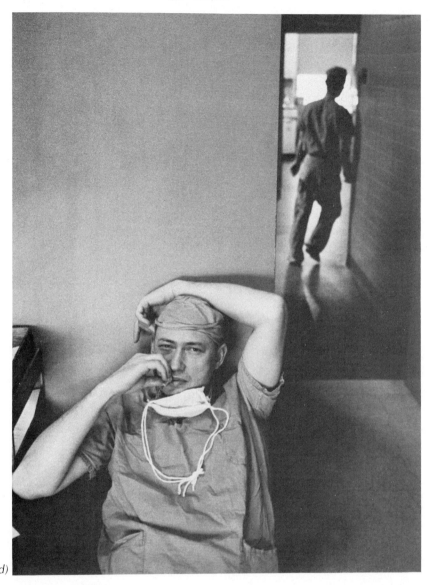

(d)

MEMBERS OF THE HEALTH CARE TEAM

There are a number of people involved in providing health care services. You are probably very familiar with some of these professionals. Others, such as the pathologist, laboratory technician, and physical therapist are probably less familiar to you.

There are two types of physicians, medical doctors and osteopaths. Although professionally "different," their training is similar. A physician spends between eight and ten years in training. The length of time may be longer for certain medical specialties.

Individuals who plan to be physicians must first complete a college curriculum that includes all of the basic sciences. Many of the students are enrolled in a premedical curriculum. Once completed, they apply to medical school. Medical school is usually four years of training and a year of internship. During the internship period, the doctor works in all areas or *services* of the hospital. The doctor is on a rotating schedule where he will get experience in all types of medical practice.

The American Medical Association (AMA), based in Chicago, was organized in 1847 and now has a membership of over 200,000 physicians. Besides working to protect the interests of its members, the AMA serves as an accrediting agent for hospitals, clinics, medical schools, and schools for other health personnel; establishes standards of ethics for physicians; conducts research; grants loans to medical students; and publishes professional journals, such as the *Journal of the American Medical Association,* and consumer materials, such as the magazine *Today's Health.*

The American Osteopathic Association (AOA), based in Chicago, is the osteopaths' professional organization. One of its functions is to accredit colleges of osteopathic medicine. Entrance requirements and training in these colleges are similar to those in other medical schools, but there is more emphasis on manipulative therapy. The AOA estimates that 75 percent of Doctors of Osteopathy (D.O.s) go into general practice.

After the completion of the internship, the doctor may practice medicine or choose to take a residency in a medical specialty. These specialties vary in the length of time needed for training. The doctor also works in the hospital while training in his specialized area. After completing the residency requirement, one can practice that specialty. Some of the common medical specialties are discussed in a later section of this chapter.

An osteopath (D.O.) must complete a similar course of study. However, osteopaths attend schools of osteopathy instead of medical schools. There are presently seven schools in the United States that teach osteopathic medicine. Most osteopaths are in private practice and act as "family doctors" or general practitioners. However, an osteopath may also specialize in a particular medical area. Osteopathic physicians may belong to the staff of general or osteopathic hospitals.

Many people think that osteopaths are limited to manipulative therapy. However, while manipulation may be an important part of the osteopath's treatment, he also uses all accepted diagnostic and therapeutic procedures. Osteopaths and physicians are both recognized as medical practitioners. Their professional organizations have, however, remained apart, though they have united in California. If you wish to find out more about osteopathic medicine, you can write to the American Osteopathic Association, 212 East Ohio Street, Chicago, Ill. 60611.

The physician's assistant (PA) is a fairly recent addition to the medical profession. These individuals are trained to aid the physician in routine and emergency procedures. Most PA programs require a two-year course and are given at medical schools and hospitals.

The Medex is a health care professional who also aids the physician. This program often involves individuals who have some medical training (many have been military medical corpsmen). The *MEDEX* program is designed to respond to: (1) a shortage of people who can deliver primary health care; and (2) an untapped source of medical corpsmen whose

training and motivation are often lost upon leaving the armed services.

The program consists of a 15-month training period that is divided into two phases. The first three months are spent in classrooms and clinical training. The remaining 12 months consists of clinical work under the supervision of a physician and the MEDEX staff. One such program is conducted at Pennsylvania State University, Hershey, Pa.

All of the medical specialists require varying degrees of training beyond the normal internship. Some of the common medical specialists are listed below with a brief description of their functions.

Allergist: Treats people who suffer from allergic conditions that may include asthma and a host of allergies caused by foods, grasses, and other substances.
Anesthesiologist: Gives anesthetic agents to patients prior to and during surgery.
Cardiologist: Diagnoses and treats diseases and disorders of the heart.
Endocrinologist: Diagnoses and treats disorders of the endocrine glands and their secretions.
Family practitioner (general practitioner): Treats the general illnesses and problems of a patient and refers patients to other specialists when necessary.
Gastroenterologist: Specializes in diseases of the stomach and intestines.
Internist: Treats diseases and disorders affecting most of the body.
Neurologist: Diagnoses and treats disorders of the brain and nervous system.
Obstetrician and gynecologist: Diagnoses and treats disorders of the female reproduction system; obstetricians provide care for patients during pregnancy and delivery.
Ophthalmologist: Diagnoses eye diseases and performs eye surgery.
Orthopedic surgeon: Diagnoses and treats bone diseases and disorders.
Otologist, laryngologist, and *rhinologist:* Diagnoses and treats diseases and disorders of the ear, nose, and throat.
Pathologist: Studies cells and tissues of the body and their relation to disease.

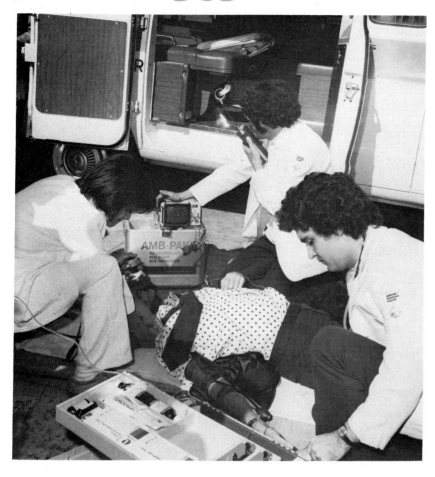

Paramedics with mobile intensive care unit
attending cardiac case.

Pediatrician: Treats the illnesses of children
(usually under the age of 12).
Plastic surgeon: Performs reconstructive and
cosmetic surgery on various parts of the body.
Proctologist: Diagnoses and treats disorders
and diseases of anus, rectum, and intestines.
Psychiatrist: Diagnoses and treats mental
and emotional disorders; may prescribe
drug therapy.
Radiologist: Uses and interprets X rays in
the diagnosis of disease; also uses radioactive
substances in the diagnoses and treatment
of diseases.
Surgeon (general): Performs surgery on
various parts of the body.
Urologist: The diagnosis and treatment of
diseases and disorders of the genitourinary
system.

Now that you are familiar with osteopaths,
physicians, and some of the medical special-

ties, how do you go about choosing the
doctor that is right for you? It is not an easy
process, as one can well imagine. Some
people try many different doctors before
they find one that they are able to relate to
and have confidence in. The following
guidelines will be helpful in choosing a
physician.

1. If you live in a large city, try to find a
   doctor affiliated with a teaching hospital.
2. If the city does not have a teaching hospital, then look for a doctor associated
   with a hospital that has a resident training
   program.
3. A doctor who is board certified (required
   to pass certain examinations in his specialty) is usually considered as particularly
   competent in his field.
4. Consult the county medical society for

366

the names of doctors in your immediate area.

5. Ask friends and co-workers for recommendations about doctors that they have used.

Once you have found a doctor who you think "fits the bill," then make an appointment and do not be afraid to inquire about the way he or she practices medicine. Questions might include those that relate to fees, house calls, response to emergencies, whether or not he or she has a group practice and, if not, who treats the patients if the doctor is not available. If he refuses to answer your questions or does not seem to be open with you, then perhaps you should look for another doctor. Many patients find out too late that they are dissatisfied with their doctor.

It is best to find a good general practitioner or internist. If you need the advice of a specialist, this doctor will most likely refer you to someone of equal caliber. Choosing a doctor is one of the most critical choices you will have to make, so take the time to make the *right* choice.

THE CONSUMER AND SURGERY

All surgery is a serious matter. Many surgical procedures are less complicated than others, but they still include a certain amount of risk. Therefore, surgery should not be performed if it is unnecessary. In recent years, a number of charges have been leveled against the medical profession for performing unnecessary surgery. Some estimates have been made that more than two million operations are performed each year that need not have been performed.

What should you consider before agreeing to surgery? It is always important that an individual get at least one other opinion to confirm the need for surgery. If the opinions disagree, then be sure that your surgeon is qualified. If a surgeon is board certified and a Fellow of the American College of Surgeons (FACS), then you know that he has met strict professional standards.

Try to have the surgery performed at an accredited hospital. Most people think that all hospitals are accredited, but, in fact, only about one-quarter of U.S. hospitals are certified by the Joint Commission on Accreditation of Hospitals (JCAH).

Do not be afraid to ask questions. You have a right to know about your surgery, how it will be done, the type of anesthetic to be used, the risks involved, and what to expect during and following the surgery. Most doctors are more than willing to discuss these matters if patients bring up the questions.

NURSES AS A PART OF THE HEALTH CARE TEAM

Nurses are a vital part of the health care team and they function in many aspects of hospital and community health programs. The registered nurse (R.N.) may function as a hospital nurse, private-duty nurse, public health nurse, armed forces nurse, or in many other capacities. There are three ways to become an R.N. You can attend a two-year school and get an associate arts (A.A.) degree. You can also complete a three-year program in an accredited hospital nursing course. The third way is by taking a four-year program that leads to a bachelor of science (B.S.) degree in nursing. Some schools require a five-year program. Upon completion of any of any of these programs, one may take the examination for state licensing as an R.N.

A licensed practical nurse (L.P.N.) completes a shorter program of training. Most L.P.N. programs take a year, and courses can often be taken at high school adult education programs, hospitals, and community colleges. An L.P.N. can continue his or her education and become an R.N. at a later time. The licensed practical nurse functions at the bedside of the patient. This individual is an adjunct to the physician and registered nurse.

The nurses' aid performs many necessary functions. This individual helps in the feeding, care, and transport of the patients. Nurses'

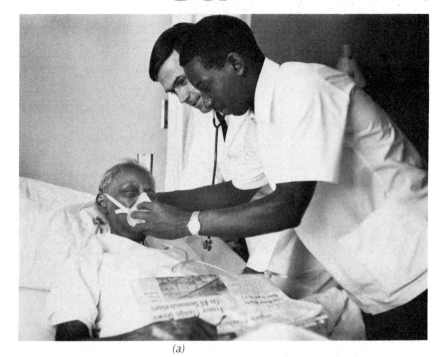

(a)

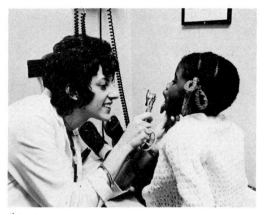

(b)

Nursing: (a) male nurse applying an oxygen mask, (b) nurse practitioner in a pediatric clinic.

aids usually receive on-the-job training while they perform their hospital duties.

A new type of nurse has recently appeared. This is the nurse practitioner. A nurse practitioner is a graduate nurse who takes an additional training course in order to be able to diagnose and treat patients. Some nurse practitioners work without doctors, others are a part of a medical team that includes doctors.

There are presently about 1,500 nurse practitioners in this country. This is a small number compared to the 1.3 million nurses in America. There are about 140 different programs that grant the title of nurse practitioner. The programs of study range from several months to two years.

TECHNICIANS AND THERAPISTS

There are a number of technician and therapist positions in laboratories and hospitals. If you are interested in laboratory work, you want to consider any of these careers: certified laboratory assistant, histology tech-

nician, cytotechnologist, or a medical technologist.

The certified laboratory assistant works in the various laboratories of the hospital and aids in collecting specimens, caring for laboratory equipment, keeping records, and many other duties. The position requires one year of training after high school at a hospital-based school. Most hospitals have on-the-job training programs.

The histology technician works with tissues and the preparation of them for examination by the pathologist. A year of training in a hospital pathology lab is necessary.

The cytotechnologist is involved in the study of cells and their relation to disease. The person must complete a two-year training period and an additional year in a laboratory school.

The medical technologist usually completes four years of college and a hospital training program. This individual is responsible for numerous laboratory tests, analysis, and research.

A health career that is vital to the hospital

is that of the *X-ray technician*. This individual must prepare the patient for X rays, take them, and be constantly aware of safety precautions. Some X-ray technicians are specifically trained in the use of radioactive substances in the diagnosis and treatment of certain diseases. Most X-ray technicians complete a two-year course of study to become a licensed laboratory radiologic technician (L.R.T.).

The inhalation therapist is involved with the administration of oxygen and the equipment used in treating respiratory diseases and problems. The training program usually lasts two years and may be taken at a school or hospital. The course work involves an understanding of the mechanism of breathing as well as clinical practice with respiratory equipment.

PHYSICAL THERAPISTS

Physical therapists are the individuals who aid in the rehabilitation of accident victims, handicapped persons, and those suffering from certain debilitating diseases. Physical therapists teach people how to use artificial limbs and how to walk again after being bedridden for many months.

In order to become a physical therapist, one needs a four-year college program and a clinical intership in a hospital or other facility. One can be licensed to practice physical therapy after passing the state qualifying examination.

DENTISTS AND OTHER DENTAL CAREERS

Dentists are very important members of any

On the frontiers of health: (a) lab technician; (b) physical therapist.

(a)

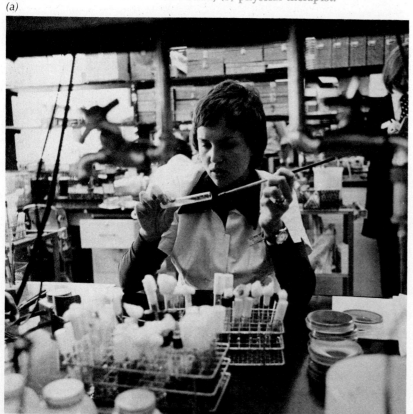

(b)

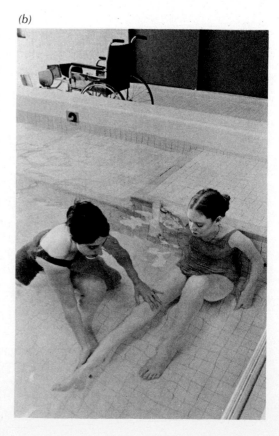

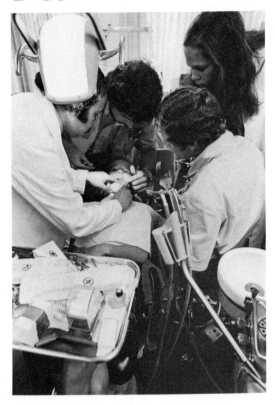

A dental team at work.

health team. Preventive dentistry can save people a lot of problems as they grow older. The dental profession includes a number of specialties that require additional training. A dentist cares for all aspects of the gums and teeth. In order to become a dentist, one first must complete four years of college. In addition, one must attend dental school for four years.

The dental specialties include the following:

1. *Endodontus:* an endodontist is concerned with the prevention, diagnosis, and treatment of diseases and injuries that affect the root of the tooth and related tissue.
2. *Oral surgery:* the oral surgeon uses surgical techniques to remove teeth and correct mouth disorders.
3. *Orthodontus:* the orthodontist is concerned with the development, prevention, and correction of irregularities of the teeth.
4. *Pedodontus:* the pedodontist is concerned

with the treatment of children's dental problems.
5. *Periodontus:* the periodotist is concerned with the treatment and prevention of gum diseases.

Most of you are probably familiar with the *dental hygienist.* This individual usually assists the dentist while he is working. The hygienist also instructs patients in the care of their teeth, professionally cleans the teeth, and takes mouth X rays. The hygienist is a valuable asset to the dentist. In order to become a hygienist, one must complete a two-year college course. Dental hygienists work in hospitals, dental offices, and dental clinics.

Another dental career is that of the *dental assistant.* The dental assistant usually keeps the dentist's records, sterilizes equipment, hands dental instruments to the dentist, develops X-ray film, and orders dental supplies. Dental assistants do not perform work on a patient. Most dental assistants receive one year of training after graduation from high school. However, some programs are two years and the graduate receives an associate arts (A.A.) degree.

Dental technicians are the people behind the scenes. These individuals make dentures, crowns, bridges, dental and orthodontic appliances, and other items needed in dental work. Technicians work in laboratories and this is where they learn their craft. Most on-the-job training lasts between three and four years. Some vocational schools offer this type of career training but the majority of technicians are apprenticed in dental labs.

OPTOMETRISTS AND OPTICIANS

If you are like most people, you may not know the difference between an *optometrist* and *optician.* However, there is a difference in education, function, and training. The optometrist performs visual examinations, fits glasses and contact lenses, and does visual training to correct perception problems. The optometrist may not use medications and will refer patients with eye diseases to an ophthalmologist.

In order to become an optometrist, one must usually take a six-year program of sciences and optometric practice. The graduate optometrist must take the state licensing exam in order to practice in that state.

The optician is the individual who fits glasses and contact lenses according to the prescription of the optometrist or ophthalmologist. Opticians are able to check lenses for the accuracy of the prescription, instruct patients on the use of glasses and contact lenses, fit frames, and make adjustments, if needed. Opticians usually receive on-the-job training.

PSYCHOLOGIST

Psychologists work in all areas of the health field. Some work in research, others in mental hospitals and in school systems. Their work is diverse depending on background, area of specialization, and degree of training. Psychologists are able to administer and interpret psychological tests, collect and analyze data, conduct research experiments, and perform administrative duties.

Most psychologists have a minimum of a master's degree in psychology. However, a doctoral degree is essential for many of the top-level jobs in this field. Some psychologists choose to open a private practice to counsel patients. In most states, one must be certified and licensed in order to enter independent practice.

PODIATRIST

A *podiatrist* is an individual who limits his practice to the study and treatment of diseases and disorders of the feet. There are a number of schools that provide podiatry training. This program usually takes six years. The first two years are completed in a college. The last four years are spent at a school of podiatry.

CHIROPRACTOR

What do you think of when you hear the word *chiropractor?* Many people only think

of bones, but chiropractic practice often extends to the entire body and includes diet, exercise, and various types of therapy. Chiropractors treat their patients mainly by manipulation of body parts, especially the spinal column. Chiropractors are not medically oriented. Their value has been under question by many medical authorities. They are, however, allowed to practice in all but two states. Chiropractors are discussed in greater detail in Chapter 19.

In order to become a chiropractor, one must complete a four-year college curriculum at a school of chiropractic medicine. The degree of Doctor of Chiropractic (D.C.) is awarded at the completion of such a course. State licensure is necessary in most states.

hospitals and other health care facilities

So far in this chapter, we have examined the duties of the people responsible for health care. In this section, the facilities where most of these individuals work are explored.

HOSPITALS

The majority of health care personnel are employed by hospitals. There are two major types of hospitals: the *private hospital* and the *public hospital.* The private hospitals are paid for by contributions and through patient fees. They are *not* supported by taxes. Private hospitals are profit-making enterprises.

The public hospital is tax supported and receives patient fees. It is a nonprofit enterprise. Some public hospitals are run by the federal government (V.A. hospitals), while others are run by state governments (mental hospitals). Most, however, are supported partially by community taxes and contributions.

A teaching hospital is a hospital affiliated with a medical school. These hospitals are called teaching hospitals because the medical students are involved in the hospital. Some authorities feel that teaching hospitals give superior care because of the ongoing research and education at these institutions.

If you have been to a hospital, you are aware of some of the fundamental services of a hospital. In addition to patient services, hospitals provide a service to communities. They offer educational programs, clinics, emergency room services, and numerous other services.

Hospital clinics provide a wide range of health care services to individuals from low and moderate income families. The clinic that provides for prenatal care, pediatric care, venereal disease information and treatment, dental care, and in many cases, mental health services.

NURSING HOMES

Nursing homes have received a great amount of coverage in recent years. The purpose of a nursing home is to provide medical services to those individuals who need long-term care. Most nursing home residents are elderly and require constant care. Some nursing homes are run by churches and other organizations, but the majority are private, profit-making enterprises.

This is where the problem seems to be. Surveys of many nursing homes have found them to be understaffed, unsafe, lacking in cleanliness, and generally below par in services offered. The "nursing home scandal" as it is called has been surveyed by a Ralph Nader group, a subcommittee of the U.S. Senate Special Committee on the Aging, and by numerous state and local groups. All have concluded that many nursing homes are depressing, overcrowded institutions that care little about their patients. Investigations are continuing to try and correct these unfortunate conditions.

CLINICS

Most clinics are a part of a hospital. However, some clinics are independent and established in neighborhoods. Some of these clinics are called Neighborhood Health Centers and were set up by the Office of

Economic Opportunity in order to provide neighborhood health care. This type of health care serves the poor in their own community, so that these people can obtain adequate health services without leaving their neighborhood.

REHABILITATION CENTERS

These centers are often sponsored by organizations devoted to the cure of certain diseases or by private groups. Such centers work with the chronically ill, mentally retarded, physically injured, or otherwise handicapped individuals. Rehabilitation centers teach crippled children to walk, fit artificial arms and legs and train people in how to use them, and generally develop motor coordination.

medical care programs

There are two types of medical insurance programs: private voluntary programs and public programs. The private insurance programs include Blue Cross–Blue Shield and insurance company plans. Blue Cross

Sickle-cell anemia testing at an outdoor program set up by a neighborhood health center.

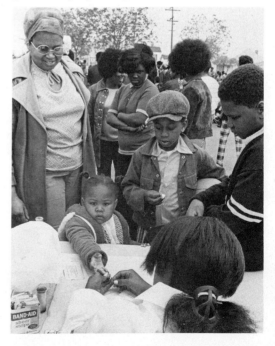

Ralph Nader is the founder of the Center for the Study of Responsive Law, P.O. Box 19367, Washington, D.C. 20036. The group was started in 1969; its stated purpose is to make the federal establishment more responsive to the public interest. The organization includes a Health Research Group which investigates abuses of health and safety. Like the other Nader's Raiders, the group publishes its research findings.

is primarily for medical services and hospitalization while Blue Shield is for surgery. These plans may be paid for by the individual, the company where one is employed, or shared by both.

Medicare and Medicaid are the two public programs available for health service coverage. Medicare is a federally supported program for people over the age of 65. This program pays a large percentage of hospital and doctors' services.

Medicaid is a health insurance program for low-income families. It is supported by the state and federal governments. One must qualify for this plan according to income level.

HEALTH MAINTENANCE ORGANIZATIONS

The HMO is an organization that provides prepaid group health services under one roof. The individual pays a fixed fee, in advance, and for that fee the following services are provided: around-the-clock physician services, emergency care, inpatient and out-patient hospital services, home visits, complete physical examinations, treatment for drug abuse and alcoholism problems, and dental care for children under the age of 12.

There are presently about 175 HMOs in operation and many are well-established in California. A number of health-insurance companies are presently looking into the advantages of starting HMO plans. Federal money is available to some of the HMOs, but in order to qualify they must offer a wide range of services and serve a sufficient number of people.

Many people are opposed to HMOs. The reasons given usually center around the end of the person-to-person relationship that most physicians have with their private patients. Many doctors feel that the HMO will lead to National Health Insurance.

NATIONAL HEALTH INSURANCE

National Health Insurance does not exist in the United States today. However, many plans have been put forth by national leaders. Such a plan would provide all citizens with quality health care at a stipulated premium. It would cover the cost of physician and hospital services as well as *catastrophic* illness. This type of illness is one that is long-term, costly, and often leaves the patient and his family in debt.

You may want to read more about the proposed plans for National Health Insurance. Refer to the "Getting Involved" section at the end of this chapter for an informative article on this subject.

COST OF HEALTH CARE

The cost of health care continues to increase each year. More than 115 billion dollars is spent annually on health care services. However, an attorney for Ralph Nader's Public Citizens Health Research Group recently claimed that many billions spent on health care are wasted on unnecessary surgery, drugs, and X rays.

Because of the excessive cost of medical care, the federal government has passed legislation to monitor the care given under federally supported programs. This legislation established the Professional Standards Review Organizations (PSROs) which may also be involved in monitoring of national health insurance, if it is adopted.

Malpractice insurance is an important component of the rise in medical health costs. Malpractice insurance is an insurance plan purchased by doctors to cover the settlements of malpractice cases, if they occur. However, in recent years there has been a great increase in the number of malpractice claims and the size of the payments to settle the claims. Consequently, insurance companies have substantially increased their premiums for malpractice. Many physicians are unable to keep up with the cost of their malpractice insurance, and some of them have had to stop practicing because of this.

In addition, medical costs to the consumer have risen because of malpractice insurance. Doctors, fearing claims, have had to practice *defensive* medicine. This means that they do tests that may not be necessary or require hospitalization that might have otherwise been avoided. They do this to protect themselves from the possibility of a malpractice claim. Patients may also bear some of the hurt of increased malpractice insurance premiums in the form of more costly visits to the doctor.

THINKING IT OVER

1. Why do many people refuse to consider themselves as consumers when it comes to health care services?
2. Why is *consumerism* important in purchasing health care services?
3. What are some of the major differences between a medical doctor and an osteopath?
4. Discuss the functions of five medical specialists.
5. What are some of the guidelines in choosing a family physician?
6. What should one do before agreeing to surgery?
7. Discuss the various careers of the nursing profession.
8. Discuss the duties of various employees of a hospital laboratory.
9. Discuss the function and training of a physical therapist.
10. What are the functions and training of a dentist?
11. Discuss any three of the dental specialties.
12. Discuss other dental careers that one may choose.
13. What is the difference between an optometrist, ophthalmologist, and optician?
14. What are the functions of a chiropractor? Why are some people opposed to chiropractors?
15. What are the two types of hospitals? How is each supported?
16. What are the functions of a hospital?
17. Why is there a "nursing home scandal?"
18. Discuss the types of private insurance programs that exist today.
19. What is Medicare and Medicaid?
20. How has malpractice insurance increased the cost of medical services?
21. What is an HMO?

KEY WORDS

Health Maintenance Organization (HMO). One-stop health care covered by prepaid fees.

Malpractice insurance. Insurance taken by doctors to protect them against malpractice claims.

Medex. An individual (often a military medical corpsman) who has taken a MEDEX training program to enable him to assist a physician.

National Health Insurance. Proposed plan to insure all citizens for medical services.

Nurse practitioner. A graduate nurse who has taken additional training in order to be able to diagnose and treat patients.

Osteopath. A doctor who attends osteopath school and believes in the manipulation process as one method of treatment.

Professional Standard Review Organization (PSRO). Organization established to monitor health care services that are under federally supported programs.

GETTING INVOLVED
Books and Periodicals

Belsky, Marvin, and Gross, Leonard. *How to Choose and Use Your Doctor.* New York: Arbor House, 1975. How to make your needs known to your doctor.

Health Research Group. *A Consumer's Directory of Prince Georges County (Md.) Doctors.* Washington: Center for Study of Responsive Law, 1975. The Nader group's guide to doctor selection in one county.

"How Good is Your Doctor," *Newsweek,* December 23, 1974. Includes methods of picking a good physician.

Johnson, G. Timothy. *Doctor! What You Should Know about Health Care before You Call a Physician.* New York: McGraw-Hill, 1975. How to go about choosing a doctor.

Wechsler, Henry. *Handbook of Medical Specialties.* New York: Behavioral Publications, 1975. How many doctors specialize in what, and where.

19
HEALTH FRAUD AND QUACKERY

Many of you may not believe that quackery and health fraud are major problems in the United States today. This is certainly not the case as you will see in this chapter. You will learn that many thousands of Americans are victimized each year as they seek relief for various conditions and illnesses.

You will learn how to recognize a health quack and why people seek these quacks. The subject of health fraud through product misrepresentation is also examined. You will learn how self-medication is related to quackery.

Who are the victims of quacks? This chapter explores those who are most likely to be victimized by quacks.

These people include the sick, the poor, the rich, and even the young. Quacks operate in many areas of health care and exploit all ages and socioeconomic groups.

What protection do you have from quacks? Some of the governmental and nongovernmental agencies that are concerned with fraudulent health products and practitioners are discussed. You will also read about how the law deals with such fraud.

In the last section of this chapter, you will examine some of the diseases and conditions that are most affected by quacks. Cancer, arthritis, and obesity are a few of the conditions that quacks exploit. After reading this

chapter, you will have a better understanding of what quackery is, how to recognize it, and how to avoid being taken in by health frauds and quackery.

While reading this chapter, think about the following concepts:

■ The modern-day quack is very different from the "medicine man" of the past.

■ Quacks often flaunt false credentials.

■ People go to quacks because of fear or as a last resort.

■ Self-medication, in some cases, is related to quackery.

■ All types of people may become victims of health fraud and quackery.

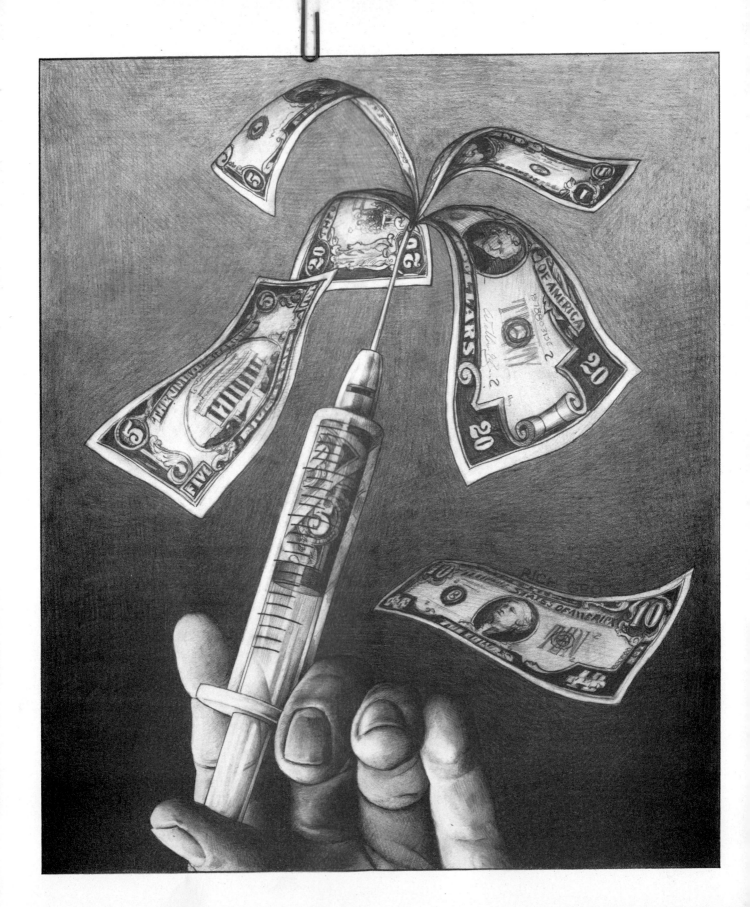

What is quackery? The technical definition of quackery will be given later in this chapter; however, an example may provide the answer to this question. An 82-year-old woman availed herself of a free hearing test sponsored by a hearing-aid promoter. She later reported that the "test" consisted of two salesmen yelling at her in her living room. After this "test," they badgered her into signing a contract. She received an earplug-shaped device that did not work. This is a true experience of someone who has been exploited by a quack.

Hearing aids are very popular among quacks for two reasons. In most states the selling of hearing aids is not carefully restricted by law and a large percentage of older people need these devices. Although some states have started to crack down on fraudulent hearing-aid salesmen, it is still an area in which many quacks operate.

Older people become involved with quacks because they often suffer from such conditions as hearing loss. They tend to look for "fast cures" and cannot get around well enough to shop for the product they need. Many older people cannot afford the "real thing" and think they are getting a bargain from the quack. The so-called bargain often turns out to be worthless and the older person has lost all of his investment.

This is just one of the many areas that are exploited by quacks. Quackery and health fraud are much more common than you may think as you will see in this chapter. You may think that you have never been exploited by a quack; however, reserve judgment until you have finished this chapter.

what is quackery?

Quackery is the use of discredited or unproven methods or devices in diagnosing and/or treating a variety of diseases or other disorders. A quack is an individual or practitioner who uses these methods or devices in deceiving the public. The quack may promote products that are useless for the condi-

tion they are supposed to treat. Other products may be dangerous, even lethal, or they may result in additional physical damage to the victim.

Quacks operate in many areas. Some deal in false cures, often by mail order, for such diseases as cancer or arthritis. Others operate in the area of mechanical quackery. These machines are advertised as the "cure" for many conditions. Some machines are promoted as diagnostic and they are able to analyze one's blood or urine and find out what is wrong with an individual. Some quacks operate in the area of beauty, while others sell useless food supplements and weight control products. Some of the most dangerous quacks operate in the area of psychotherapy and psychic phenomena. As you can see, the health field is a fertile one for the quack.

HOW TO RECOGNIZE A QUACK OR A FRAUDULENT PRACTITIONER

Would you know a quack if you saw one? If you expected a disheveled door-to-door salesperson, you would, in most cases, be unprepared for the present-day quack. Today's quack bears no resemblance to the "medicine man" who used to go from town to town in his wagon.

The quack of today is a businessperson. They often have one or more offices and a number of people working for them. Most quacks try to present a good image and often have many "credentials." Some may have real degrees from accredited institutions, but the majority have mail-order degrees. This is particularly true in the area of psychotherapy. For example, the Universal Life Church of Stockton, California, boasts of having issued a million and a half doctorate degrees at $25 each through its mail-order service. There are many other such "diploma mills" that help to deceive the unwary public. Why do you think one might want a "diploma mill" degree?

When purchasing any health service or product do not be "taken in" by credentials. Read the credentials and find out about the institution that has issued the degree. Many people could have been saved a great deal of money, time, and emotional distress if they had checked this matter out thoroughly before agreeing to services or buying a product.

The American Medical Association has listed the following points on how to recognize a health quack:

1. He often uses a special or secret formula or machine.
2. He may promise or imply quick and easy cures.
3. He may advertise using case histories and testimonials from his patients.
4. He refuses to accept tried or proven methods of medical research.
5. He often claims that medical men are persecuting him and are afraid of his competition.
6. He claims that his methods are better than surgery, X-rays, and medically prescribed drugs.

There are also some general rules that can help you to avoid being exploited by a quack.

1. Do not assume that a published article or advertised claim is legally approved or medically sound. There are numerous health claims and books concerned with health fads that can be dangerous to one's health.
2. Do not automatically accept a physician who is listed in the phone book as a licensed doctor. Check his credentials with the local medical society and be particularly concerned if he complains of persecution by the AMA or FDA.
3. Try to find out as much as possible about any health claim that interests you. You can write to the Food and Drug Administration, Rockville, Md. 20852; the American Medical Association, 535 North Dearborn Street, Chicago, Ill. 60610; or the local chapters of the American Cancer Society, Heart Association, Arthritis

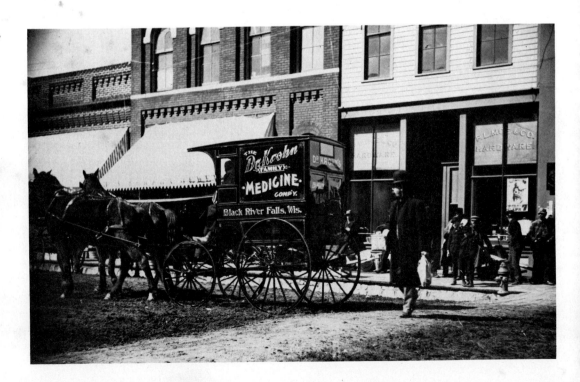

Patent-medicine wagon, Black River Falls, Wisconsin.

Foundation, or Diabetes Association.
Local medical schools and hospitals may
also be of help to you.

why do people go to quacks or use fraudulent products?

In the majority of cases, people go to quacks
or use fraudulent devices or medicines because they lack knowledge and sound judgment. Such people are determined to buy a
product or find a "cure" and they do not
stop to inquire into the practitioner or product. Because many victims of quacks are
gullible or superstitious, they are easy prey
for quacks. In some cases, quacks hire people
who have been "cured" to work for them
and these people offer testimonials to their
services or products. A new victim is often
taken in by such claims. The victim does
not stop to think about how well the "cured"
individual has been paid to sign a testimo-
nial or personally promote a product.

Many people who go to quacks fear the
truth about their illness or condition. It is
not pleasant to know that you may need
an operation or that you may have an incurable disease. Many people go to the quack
as a last resort. They may have tried legitimate medical doctors and had few results.
This is particularly true with diseases, such
as advanced cancer, for which there is no
known cure. The quack offers a final hope
to a person who has tried everything. Sometimes the hope becomes so real that an individual convinces himself that his health is
actually improving. This is more often than
not a very temporary condition.

Some people "fall for" smooth-talking individuals or well-advertised and attractively
packaged items. Many of these products
are health foods, vitamins, food supplements,
and worthless drugs. In many cases, the
product may not be dangerous but false
claims are made about it, and is often sold
at very high prices. Health food advertisements, for example, often claim that they
are better for you because they contain no

Miraculous Cure

Richard D. Creech, of 1062
Second St., Appleton, Wis., says:

"Our son Willard was abso-
lutely helpless. His lower limbs
were paralyzed, and when we
used electricity he could not feel
it below his hips. Finally my
mother, who lives in Canada,
wrote advising the use of Dr.
Williams' Pink Pills for Pale People and I bought some. This was
when our boy had been on the
stretcher for an entire year and
helpless for nine months. In six
weeks after taking the pills we
noted signs of vitality in his legs,
and in four months he was able
to go to school. It was nothing
else in the world that saved the
boy than Dr. Williams' Pink Pills
for Pale People.—*From the Cres-
cent, Appleton, Wis.*

Dr. Williams' Pink Pills for Pale People

are sold by all druggists or direct from
Dr. Williams Medicine Co., Schenectady,
N.Y., postpaid on receipt of price, 50c.
per box; six boxes, $2.50.

preservatives. In most cases, the lack of preservatives encourages spoilage, health foods
are very expensive, and many organic health
foods are ordinary foods that are falsely
labeled.

Time and physical distance are often major
selling points for unscrupulous practitioners.
The elderly and handicapped persons confined to their homes are often victims of
mail-order health cures. The physical distance prevents may persons from finding

out more about the product and from where the product is being sent. Some mail-order houses go out of business "on schedule" many times a year. They often cash checks without completing orders and vacate a location when they suspect that they will be investigated. They may go right back into business under a new name and in a different location. The only thing that remains the same is the product, which may also be renamed.

Quacks offer quick and easy cures. Many people today live a fast-paced life and want their health problems to be "cured" as quickly as possible. They have no time for lengthy medical tests, hospital stays, and prolonged treatments. It is human nature to want to get well quickly. These people are "perfect" victims for the quacks.

Some individuals who go to quacks do so to save money. They feel that the quack is cheaper than legitimate medical treatment. Although health care is expensive, most people can find legitimate health care through clinics and other public programs. Many

people deceive themselves by going to quacks who may continue to raise fees and prolong treatments. In addition, a sick person is losing more than money; he is losing important time that could be used to medically treat his condition.

self-medication and self-diagnosis

Self-medication is the treatment by oneself of medical conditions without consulting a physician. Why are we discussing self-medication in this chapter about quackery? Many people who do treat themselves do so with products offered by quacks. Self-medication and diagnosis is usually done out of ignorance or for many of the same reasons that people choose to go to quacks.

There are different types of self-medication. Of course, one would not expect to visit a doctor every time he had a headache. This is true for other minor conditions that are easily treated by over-the-counter preparations. This is not the type of self-medication

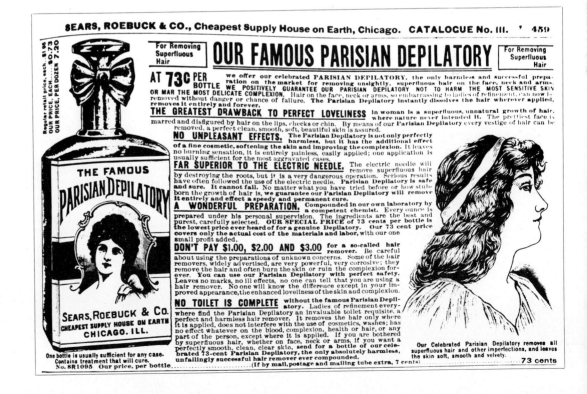

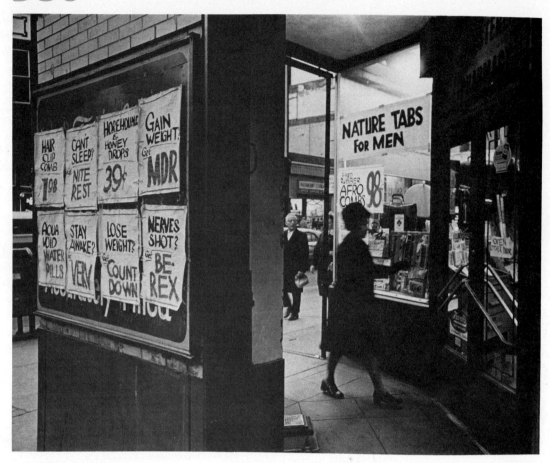

we are discussing here. We are referring to the person who has a persistent condition that should be treated by a physician. This individual often loses valuable time by trying to medicate himself with mail-order products or over-the-counter medications.

There are certain conditions that can be further aggravated by self-medication. Certain medications will mask the true symptoms of a condition. An antacid may make the ulcer sufferer feel better for a short time; but it will not in any way improve the original condition. Many persons incorrectly diagnose their conditions and treat them with the wrong product. By the time they receive medical care, they may have permanently harmed themselves.

Health fraud and quackery are often in the form of products rather than people. Some

of the self-medication products that can be harmful to one's health include over-the-counter drugs, vitamins and food supplements, and aids to weight reduction. Many Americans take large doses of vitamins daily. These "vitamin treatments" have appeared in many best-selling books on the subject of nutrition. Large doses of vitamins have not proven effective in scientific tests and they can be harmful. Vitamin overdose can be particularly severe among children whose growth may be stunted.

One should only self-medicate minor conditions or those with which one is very familiar. We will close this section with the following well-known quotation, "He who has himself for a physician has a fool for a patient." Do you agree?

381

who are the victims of quacks?

As mentioned earlier in this chapter, all types of people are the victims of health fraud and quackery. Elderly individuals often seek quick and convenient cures. It is often easier for a housebound older person to send away for a mail-order product than to seek medical attention. Elderly people are also the ones most often afflicted with such conditions as hearing loss and arthritis. Quacks prey on these conditions because of the large numbers of people who suffer from them and because there is no cure.

However, young people are also victimized by health fraud. Young people are often "taken in" by useless preparations and devices that promote attractiveness. There are cosmetics, dieting aids, and muscle building and breast development products. Many facial creams advertise secret ingredients that "feed" the skin and improve numerous skin conditions. These products may tem-

porarily improve the skin, but they do not produce the long-term effects that are usually claimed by the advertising.

Many women seek products and treatments that will enlarge the breasts. Creams for this purpose, especially those that contain hormones, are useless and can be dangerous. Exercise gadgets fall into the category. Silicone injections for breast enlargement are banned in the United States, but some women go to quacks in other countries for this treatment. Those injections can be extremely harmful to the patient. Why do you think that some women seek such treatment?

Both men and women, but particularly men, spend a great deal of money on hair restoration. There are many methods including implantation (sewing of hair on to the scalp) and hair weaving (attaching and weaving hair to existing strands). Implantation often results in infection and hair weaving may cause further loss of hair and also lead to infection. Both of these methods are expen-

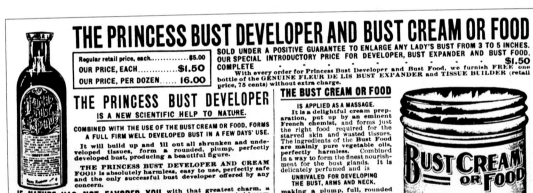

The Food and Drug Administration (FDA) is responsible for evaluating the safety of drugs and medical devices and for preventing the distribution of harmful ones. One of its most notable successes came in the early 1960s, when it deferred approval of thalidomide because it had doubts about the tranquilizer's safety. It was later proved that thalidomide caused serious birth defects; but the FDA's action had prevented it from reaching the U.S. market.

The Federal Trade Commission (FTC) is responsible for stopping unfair and deceptive business practices. That takes in preventing false or misleading advertising of consumer products, including drugs and therapeutic devices. The agency is empowered to take legal action against offenders. If you want to register a complaint, contact the Federal Trade Commission Regional Office nearest you.

sive and are often performed by quacks. The only safe method of hair restoration is transplantation where a trained physician transplants one's own hair to the parts of the scalp that are balding.

Poor people are often victimized by quacks. These people may not be knowledgeable and they try to do the best for their families on their limited incomes. Poor families may add to their diets with high dosages of vitamins or with dietary supplements. They may also look for the quickest and least expensive method of treatment. They may fear the medical establishment and in some cases they may have difficulty in communicating because they speak a different language.

You might think that the rich are protected from such fraud. But this is not so. Wealthy people can afford to seek exotic treatments in far-off places. Such places are often exclusively for the rich and well-known and it is a status symbol to be seen at them. There are many European health spas where individuals are injected with "youth-giving" substances. These places provide all types of health diets and beauty treatments.

There are also many "fat farms" that cater to the rich. These "farms" are often lush resorts where the individual is catered to and pampered. Diet and exercise are the most important features, but beauty treatments are also provided. These places are usually not harmful, though some do promote starvation diets that can be dangerous to certain people. Most people do lose weight but they could have done so for much less money. In addition, this type of weight loss is usually not permanent, as there has been no change in one's eating habits.

protection against fraudulent health products and practitioners

Health quackery is a multimillion dollar business, but there are governmental and nongovernmental agencies that are trying to curtail these practitioners. One such

governmental agency is the Food and Drug Administration (FDA). The FDA is primarily concerned with ingredients and labeling of products, particularly drugs. Along these lines, recent legislation has produced better, more effective labeling. For example, as of January 1, 1974, most packaged foods were required to list nutritional values such as calories, protein, fat content, carbohydrates, vitamins, and minerals. In addition, as of March 31, 1974, all cosmetic labels were required to list ingredients, colors, and possible irritants.

In addition to labeling, the FDA has been involved with the misrepresentation of air-purification systems, alcoholism treatment, anemia preparations, arthritis remedies, baldness cures, cancer treatment, laxative products, cosmetic preparations, diabetes treatments, diagnostic machines, door-bell doctors, eyeglass fraud, health foods, impotency cures, kidney remedies, ulcer cures, and numerous other products and treatments.

The Federal Trade Commission (FTC) is responsible for the control of false and misleading advertising. There have been many recent cases where the FTC has ordered a company to stop advertising a product in a way that claims that one would be cured if he used the product in question. Many of these suits are concerned with such over-the-counter preparations as cold tablets, headache relief pills, and similar products.

The Post Office deals with mail fraud. The American public is bilked in excess of $100 million dollars a year through mail fraud. The mails are used in a wide variety of frauds from quick profit schemes to complex multi-million dollar promotions. Older people are often the main target of mail-fraud schemes. They are also unlikely to report fraud, especially if the amount of money lost is small.

There are many types of mail fraud including false business opportunities, vending machine operations, franchises and distributorships, chain letters, charity rackets, correspondence schools, dance studios, foreign employment, lonely heart clubs, real estate swindles, publishers who promise to publish your book for a fee, unordered merchandise, and work-at-home schemes. Of course, there are legitimate operations in each of these fields, but a large number of fraud cases have been related to these and other mail-fraud areas.

NONGOVERNMENTAL AGENCIES

The American Medical Association and the local medical societies are nongovernmental agencies that fight and legislate against health fraud and quacks. The AMA has a large educational and investigative department that looks into health fraud and publishes pamphlets on the subject. In addition, in their publication *Today's Health* many areas of health fraud are exposed through incisive articles.

State and local medical societies keep updated lists of licensed medical practitioners. One should always check with one of these groups before going to a physician or as an aid in helping one to choose a doctor in a new area. One can also report cases of fraudulent health practice and practitioners to these groups.

Other groups that can be helpful include the National Better Business Bureau, the Consumer's Union, and local consumer action groups. One can check a business by calling the local office of the Better Business Bureau. They will check their files for any complaints against a particular company. Consumer action groups have done an excellent job in public education and involvement. Find out what consumer action groups exist in your community. You might want to become actively involved in one.

The Council of Better Bureaus is the coordinating agency for 150 local bureaus located throughout the United States, Canada, and Mexico. The council hopes to become business's spokesman in the consumer field by establishing a consumer information data bank and setting up mediation panels to handle consumer complaints.

QUACKS AND THE LAW

It is extremely difficult to prosecute a quack because a complaint is usually required. Many people do not wish to get involved in signing a complaint. Some feel that it is embarrassing to have been exploited in this way and others who have invested small amounts of money do not think that it is worthwhile to file a complaint and become legally involved.

It is also difficult to prove the unethical or unlawful practice of medicine. Many quacks cover their steps carefully in order to avoid legal action. Some quacks use trials and lengthy litigations as publicity for their product. Even if they are found guilty, they would have made a great deal of money through the publicity.

Fraudulent health practitioners are hard to track down. They move from place to place, change post-office boxes frequently, or have a false address listed for their business. The address often turns out to be an abandoned warehouse where the fraudulent company was never located.

diseases and conditions commonly treated by quacks

There is probably a quack who will capitalize on any condition to which the human mind or body falls heir. However, there are some conditions, because of their severity or the numbers who suffer from them, that are most readily treated by quacks. Some of these conditions are discussed in the following sections of this chapter.

CANCER

Because there is no "cure" for cancer, people tend to fall for the unscrupulous line rather than face surgery, medical treatment, and hospitalization. There are numerous products sold to "help" cancer patients. One of the best known is Laetrile, a drug made from an extract of apricot pits. The drug costs about two cents per pill to make and is sold for about $1.25 per pill. The drug is illegal in the United States, but can be easily purchased in Mexico. Since 1963, an estimated 5,000 Americans have paid in excess of four million dollars to Dr. Ernesto Contreras, a Mexican physician. Some people claim that Laetrile not only cures cancer, but also prevents it. This is, of course, unfounded

This organization, searching for cancer cures outside the circles of organized medicine, is a proponent of such treatments as Krebiozen and Laetrile.

and these pills can be poisonous to children.

There are numerous other false cancer cures. There are escharotics that are salves used to "draw out" cancer cells from the body. The Hoxsey cancer treatment is a series of common drugs and laxatives. Krebiozen is obtained from the blood of horses who have been injected with a certain substance.

Analysis has shown that Krebiozen consists largely of mineral oil.

There are other so-called cures that consist of grapes, the juice of calves' liver, or other special diets. Some quacks claim that fasting for long periods of time is the answer. There are also many mechanical devices

A machine for the treatment of 29 diseases.

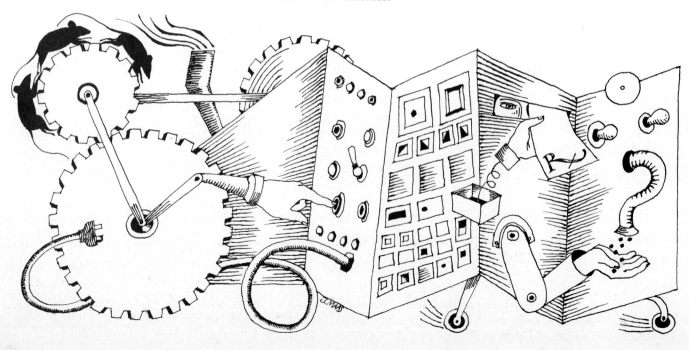

used to induce cancer "cures." One such device was the Detoxacolon, a machine for the treatment of cancer and 28 other diseases. Another device, the Spectro-chrome, treated different diseases through "attuned color waves." Different colors were used to treat different diseases including cancer. Phony cancer cures are harmful for two reasons. They build false hope and, more importantly, they delay treatment. *Time* is the greatest enemy of the cancer patient. Every hour he loses in false treatment could have been used for legitimate medical care.

ARTHRITIS

Arthritis is a painful, disabling disease. Arthritis patients may suffer from deformity of the hands and feet and in extreme cases they may become partially paralyzed. There is no medical cure for arthritis, but advances in treatment have improved the condition of many arthritis sufferers. The arthritic often looks for the fast cure and this is the fact upon which arthritis quacks prey.

The Arthritis Foundation of New York estimates that about 500 million dollars a year is spent on quack arthritis treatment. There are many Mexican doctors who exploit arthritis victims in the same way as they exploit cancer victims. One such doctor "sees" as many as 120 patients during a ten-hour working day and an average examination lasts between seven and ten minutes. Some patients have appointments made many months in advance and still wait in long lines to see the doctor.

These doctors are extremely harmful to their arthritis patients. Patients are examined too quickly to determine the extent of the arthritis or any other condition the patient may have. Drugs are prescribed indiscriminately and the doctor looks only for relief of pain not long-term control or the possibility of further deterioration as a result of the drugs prescribed. There is no follow-up or supervision once the patient returns to his home.

There are many fraudulent devices and medications used by the arthritis quack. In recent years, the copper bracelet was recognized as a "cure" for arthritis. There have also been numerous fad diets that seem to appear every few years. The Arthritis Foundation has stated that no diet can relieve the pain or cure the symptoms of arthritis. There have also been many devices and gadgets including special mittens, electrical vibrators, and copper and zinc discs that are worn in the shoes.

Acupuncture has also been used to treat arthritis as well as numerous other diseases and conditions. Many of the "quack-puncturists" are just that. They are taking advantage of the sudden popularity of acupuncture in this country. Presently, there are few trained, qualified acupuncturists in this country and many arthritis patients have fallen

$500 million is yearly spent by arthritis sufferers on devices such as (a) the Oxydonor ("reverses death into life processes") and (b) the Polorator (electric heat-shocking machine).

(a)

(b)

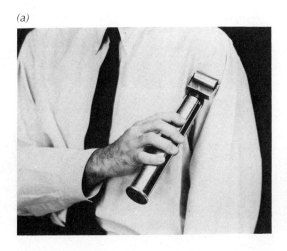

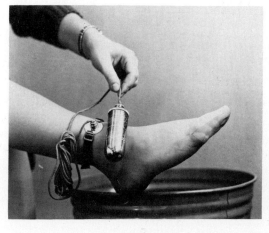

into the hands of unscrupulous, unskilled practitioners. Acupuncture, in the hands of a skilled individual, may help some arthritis sufferers. Unfortunately, few acupuncturists are expert in this area.

PSYCHOLOGICAL QUACKERY

An area of quackery that is often overlooked is the exploitation of the mind. This type of exploitation includes incompetent psychotherapy, phony sex clinics, psychic healers, and psychic surgeons. Let us examine some of the fraud that is rampant in these areas.

Do you know that in most areas of the country anyone can practice psychotherapy, and many of those that do are imcompetent, poorly trained or untrained, or have phony credentials from a mail-order diploma mill? According to the director of the Post Graduate Center for Mental Health, in New York City, more than 100,000 people have suffered psychological damage because of involvement in phony or incompetent encounter groups. It is estimated that in excess of 35 million dollars is spent each year on phony psychotherapy.

Psychotherapy groups of all types have become the fad of the late 1960s and early 1970s. People who never before were involved in therapy joined encounter groups, sensitivity training centers, and sought individual and group therapy. The media is full of "finding yourself" and "how-to-do-it psychology" articles. The time *was* and *is* ripe for the quack therapist.

One of the largest areas of this type of quackery is the phony sex therapy clinic. There is a great demand for knowledge and help in this area and there are a limited number of approved, legitimate clinics. According to Dr. William H. Masters, between 3,500 and 5,000 sex treatment clinics have been established in a recent five-year period. Of these, he estimates that perhaps 100, but most likely only about 50, are legitimate. These 50 offer scientific treatment methods administered by trained personnel.

What about the others? They usually offer superficial sex education and fad approaches to "curing" sexual problems. They use untested, often psychologically dangerous techniques that can add to one's sexual difficulties. They are primarily concerned with money, and a minimum charge of $25 an hour is not unusual. Why do you think that sex therapy clinics have become so popular in recent years?

Another area of psychological quackery is psychic healing. This is the healing of a person through nonmedical methods. There are psychic healers who accomplish this by the "laying-on of hands." Other forms of psychic healing include faith healing and psychic surgery.

In faith healing, the healer usually preaches before a large group. Through faith, a sick person in the audience is said to be healed. You have all heard stories of people dramatically throwing away crutches and walking out of a healing gathering. Few of these cases, however, have been documented. Many times a patient feels strongly that he is healed, but in actuality his condition is unchanged. This may be a simple case of "mind over matter," but it is usually a temporary situation.

Psychic surgery is when the "surgeon" removes an organ or tissue from the body without using surgical techniques. These individuals "operate" in other countries and perpetuate complex hoaxes on their patients. One such "surgeon" known as Dr. Tony is a grammar school dropout who works in Manila. He had jumped bail in Detroit while awaiting indictment on psychic surgery charges.

These healers claim that they "cure" through an energy transfer process. They often seem to extract tissue or blood from the patient; however, under analysis the tissue is from an animal and the blood a fake red-colored preparation. Again, patients who go for such treatment are hurting themselves by putting off or interrupting medical care. In addition, they are psychologically damaged from the experience and the false hope.

OBESITY AND WEIGHT CONTROL

If you recall Chapters 11 and 13, you will remember that millions of people are overweight. This is one of the reasons why quacks are so numerous in the treatment of obesity and in weight control programs. Certainly there are many legitimate products, diets, programs, and practitioners. However, many obesity programs are useless and some may be dangerous to one's health.

There are a variety of exercise and reducing devices. They are always advertised on tele- vision and in magazines and newspapers. These items are fads that disappear almost as fast as they appear. Many devices are promoted because they are "easy." Of course, that is the problem. One cannot expect to lose much weight without expending some energy.

We have discussed diets and diet products in Chapter 13. Most reducing diets are also fads in that they try to make weight loss seem easy and quick. This is also true of dieting aids and food supplements which may deprive one of a healthy diet of good,

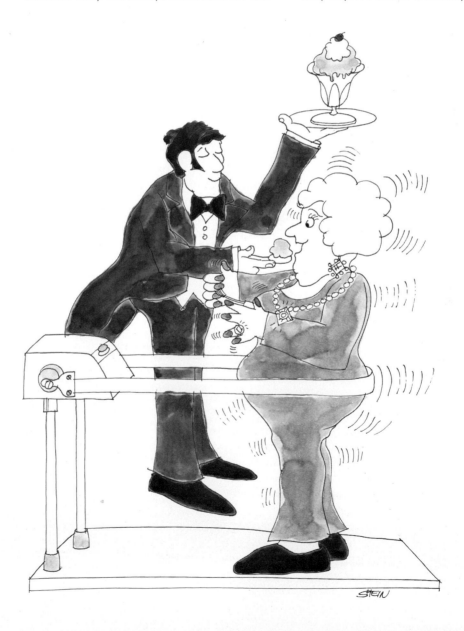

nourishing foods. In order for a dieter to be successful, he must change his eating habits and reduce weight slowly. Weight can only be lost and the loss maintained if a diet is made up of foods that are typically in our diet.

protect yourself

As you can see from reading this chapter, the health quack operates in many different areas. He takes advantage of the terminally ill, the old, the young, the poor, the rich, and the emotionally disturbed. Do you remember the point posed at the beginning of this chapter? "You may think that you have never been exploited by a quack; however, reserve judgment until you have finished this chapter." This was the sentence to which we are referring. How would you respond to this sentence now that you have completed this chapter?

THINKING IT OVER

1. Why are many older people exploited by quacks?
2. Define *quackery.* Can you add anything else to this definition?
3. Discuss the six points listed by the AMA concerning how to recognize a health quack.
4. What are some general rules that can help one to avoid exploitation by a quack?
5. Discuss some of the reasons why people go to quacks.
6. What can be done to discourage people from going to quacks?
7. How is self-medication related to quackery?
8. Discuss some of the ways in which quacks promote attractiveness.
9. How are both the rich and the poor taken in by quackery?
10. Discuss the role of the FDA in protecting the public from health fraud.
11. Discuss the role of the FTC in protecting the public from health fraud.
12. What is mail fraud and how is the public protected from it?
13. What nongovernmental agencies are involved in health-fraud protection?
14. Why is it difficult to prosecute a fraudulent health practitioner?
15. Discuss some of the false "cures" for cancer.
16. How is arthritis treated by the fraudulent practitioner?
17. What is *psychological quackery?* Discuss some examples of this.
18. Why is there so much quackery in the area of obesity and weight control?

KEY WORDS

Detoxacolon. A mechanical device that supposedly could cure cancer and 38 other diseases.

Escharotics. Salves used to "draw out" cancer cells.

Hair weaving. Attaching and weaving hair to existing strands.

Hoxsey cancer treatment. A series of common drugs and laxatives used to falsely treat cancer patients.

Implantation. The sewing of hair onto the scalp.

Krebiozen. A useless serum utilized in treating cancer patients.

Laetrile. A false drug for cancer patients that is made from apricot pits.

Psychic healing. Healing through the mind.

Psychic surgery. "Surgery" without the use of surgical techniques.

Quack. An individual who uses discredited or unproven methods in deceiving the public.

Quackery. The use of discredited or unproven methods or devices in diagnosing and/or treating a variety of diseases or other disorders.

Self-medication. The treatment of oneself for a medical condition without consulting a physician.

Spectro-chrom. A mechanical device that treated disease through "attuned color waves."

Transplantation. The transplanting of one's own hair to the balding areas of the scalp.

389

GETTING INVOLVED
Books and Periodicals

American Medical Association. *A Billion Dollars Worth of Gullibility.* Chicago: American Medical Association, n.d. A pamphlet explaining how much quackery costs in dollar terms.

_____. *Facts on Quacks: What You Should Know about Health Quackery.* Chicago: American Medical Association, 1967. Another attempt to alert people to the dangers of quackery.

Kahn, E.J., Jr. *Fraud: The United States Postal Service and Some of the Fools and Knaves It Has Known.* New York: Harper & Row, 1973. Includes information about mail-order medical frauds.

Kiernan, Thomas. *Shrinks, etc.: A Consumer's Guide to Psychotherapies.* New York: Dial Press, 1974. How to choose the therapy that's good for you, and how to recognize those that are good for nothing.

Masters, William H., "Phony Sex Clinics—Medicine's Newest Nightmare," *Today's Health,* November 1974. An expert writes about legitimate sex therapy clinics.

"Psychological Mayhem," *Today's Health,* February 1974. One of a group of articles from "The Pain Exploiters" series which examines fraudulent psychotherapy. See also the October 1973 (arthritis) and November 1973 (cancer) editions of *Today's Health.*

Plays

Bad Habits, by Terrence McNally, 1974. Comedy involving a zany pair of quacks.

PART VII
ENVIRONMENTAL HEALTH

20 POPULATION DYNAMICS

Population and the problems caused by overpopulation are familiar topics today. In this chapter, you will explore some of the reasons why so much attention is being paid to population and related problems.

You will learn that overpopulation is an underlying cause of other environmental problems. You will explore some of the problems that are related to overpopulation. Over-population is a worldwide situation that is related to pollution, food shortages, and numerous other problems.

You will learn about why there are so many people in the world. You will also explore population growth and the balance of nature. The fact that man is the only animal that can control his environment is also examined. However, there is also a limit to man's ability to continue to control his environment. This will also be discussed in this chapter.

In the last section of this chapter, you will learn about possible solutions to the pollution problem and how man's attitude and behavior toward reproduction has to be modified. You will examine some of the reasons why the U. S. population has leveled off somewhat in recent years and you will read about what the future holds in reference to population and its problems.

While reading this chapter, think about the following concepts:

■ Overpopulation is the underlying cause of other environmental problems.

■ One must experience and "feel" the problems of overpopulation in order to understand them.

■ Overpopulation is a worldwide problem.

■ The United States is one of the largest consumers of food and natural resources although it has a relatively small population.

■ Man has the ability to control his environment although there may be a limit to this control.

■ Overpopulation is both a result of improved health and a threat to good health.

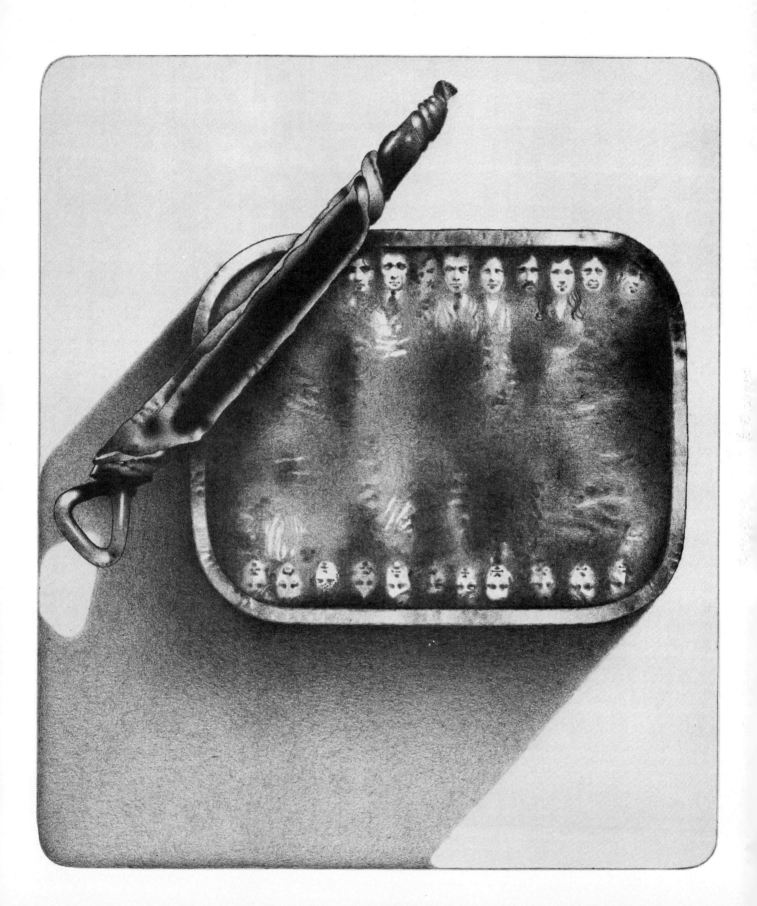

This chapter is concerned with population dynamics. It is about the forces that operate in the area of population. There are many factors involved that most people never consider when discussing population. You may think that a decision of a couple in Minnesota to have a child cannot possibly affect you. However, multiply this decision many millions of times and you are affected and so is the population of the world.

How are you affected? You may not be able to find adequate housing (this is already happening in many parts of the world including certain areas of the United States). You may not be able to buy enough food for your family (this, too, has happened in many countries). You may not be able to find a job (this is happening today in the United States and many other countries— unemployment is extremely high for both blue-collar and white-collar employees).

If you have enough to eat, have a place to live and a steady job, you may still be suffering from problems related to overpopulation. You may not have connected these situations to overpopulation, but many are related. For example, in parts of California students do not have outside recess because of the pollution problem. The air pollution is "unsafe" for people. Why is this related to overpopulation? Too many people and cars and too much industry to meet the needs of the people have resulted in a serious air pollution or "smog" problem.

Air pollution is only one of myriad problems that stem from overpopulation. Have you been caught in rush-hour traffic recently or have you experienced blackouts or brownouts? Do you wait in long lines in stores, board "packed" subways and buses, or live in the overcrowded cities? In what other ways is your life directly affected by overpopulation? After reading this chapter, you will have a better understanding of the dynamics of population and how each of us are affected by overpopulation.

overpopulation and the environment

Overpopulation, sometimes referred to as "people pollution," is the underlying cause of our other environmental problems. There are more cars, planes, and factories causing the air to be polluted. Solid wastes and other wastes contribute to water pollution. In addition, overpopulation has resulted in an increase of noise and stress. These are only a few of the pollution problems related to an abundance of people. The subject of pollution is explored in detail in Chapter 21.

When we take a drive in the country or relax in a spacious backyard, it is difficult to realize that we have population and pollution problems. Many of you have probably taken camping trips and wondered what the "fuss" was all about in relation to overpopulation. Many people in this country do not experience the problems of overpopulation firsthand. In order to understand these problems one must "feel" the problem. For example, try to swim or fish in a polluted body of water; or you might try to breathe in polluted air. Have you ever seen smog from a plane or taken a walk through a crowded neighborhood? These are "feeling" experiences that enable one to understand what the problem really entails.

Many Americans who do not experience an overpopulation problem feel that there is none. They are not aware of the suffering of their fellow Americans and millions of people in other countries. The United States, or parts of it, can no longer be viewed in an isolated manner. We belong to a world of nations, many of which are so overpopulated that their people cannot survive. As you will see in the next section of this chapter, overpopulation is a worldwide problem and each country has a responsibility to this problem.

overpopulation—a worldwide problem

There is a theory of "doubling time" for population. This simply means that the

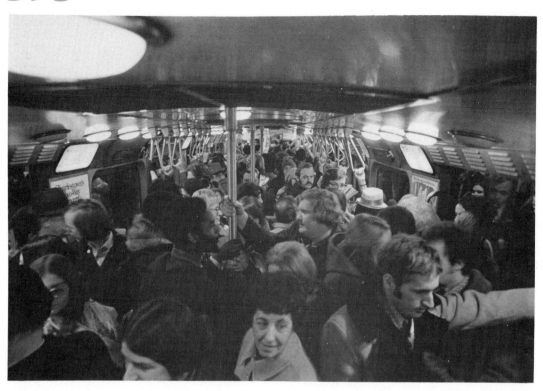

Rush hour in Boston.

world's population doubles every so many years. As you will see from the statistics that follow, the doubling time has continued to decrease so that while at one point it may have taken 1,000 years to double the world population, today it may take as little as 35 years. This is a frightening theory to consider.

In 1650, there were about 500 million people in the world. It took about 1,000 years to attain this doubling from 250 million to 500 million. In 1850, 200 years later, the population had doubled to one billion. In 1930, only 80 years later, the population had doubled once again to two billion. In April 1976, the population of the world reached the four billion mark; the doubling times seem to be about 35 years. This means that by the year 2000, there will be more than seven billion individuals in the world.

At the current rate of increase, the world population adds 200,000 people each day! That is the size of many major cities. For example, one could populate an entire city the size of Des Moines, Iowa, in one day. If the population continues to follow the doubling time theory then there may be 10 billion persons inhabiting the earth in the year 2025. Would you want to live in that type of society?

The United States has not been lagging behind in the population explosion. In 1900, the U.S. population was 76 million; it had doubled by 1950 to 152 million. By 1970, the total was increased to about 205 million. Today it is about 210 million. You may have read how the U. S. population growth is now about 1.1 percent annually. One should not relax because of this statistic as the birth rate has not yet equalled the death rate. In addition, the American population is very young. One out of every three North Americans is under the age of 15. This suggests the possibility of another baby boom when these young people begin to have families.

Doubling time in the underdeveloped coun-

Paul R. Ehrlich is a
professor of biology at
Stanford University.
He is especially con-
cerned with the biology
of population. The
earth's population has
far outstripped its
resources; and Dr.
Ehrlich believes that
the only way to prevent
millions of people from
starving to death is to
lower the birth rate—
if not voluntarily, then
by compulsion.

tries is from 20 to 50 years as compared to doubling time in the developed countries which is from 50 to 200 years. The population growth appears to be slowest in the industrialized countries. Europe for example has a growth rate of 0.8 percent a year as compared to the growth rate of Latin America which has the fastest growth, about 2.9 percent per year. Africa is adding to the population at the rate of about 2.6 percent annually, followed by Asia (excluding Russia) with an annual growth rate of 2.3 percent.

Latin America, Africa, and Asia have a combined population in excess of 2.7 billion people; this is nearly three-fourths of the world's population. It is predicted that by the year 2000, more than 81 percent of the world's population will be living in these three areas.

All of these statistics may be somewhat confusing; but they are concrete examples of population growth and where it is occurring. What is important to remember is that population trends on the whole are not showing signs of markedly slowing down. This is an alarming prospect because the parts of the world are interdependent and what happens in one part of the world will be felt in all the other parts.

THE PROBLEM OF CONSUMPTION

The United States, although having a relatively small proportion of the world's population, is one of the largest consumers of resources. For example, Americans throw away more food, per person, than many people have to eat in other parts of the world. We throw away other things besides food. In one recent year, Americans discarded 40 million tons of paper, 200 million tires, 76 billion containers, 38 billion bottles, 78 billion cans, and junked 7 million cars.

Americans are also huge energy users. The American population of 210 million uses more energy than the combined 500 million people in the other industrialized nations. Some experts have estimated that about 25 percent of this energy is wasted. Americans consume more than 50 percent of the world's natural resources.

As one can see from these statistics concerning consumption, the average American is very involved with the world population problem. Americans are consuming food and resources in a much greater amount than the population warrants. This so-called "conspicuous consumption" deprives populations of other countries from getting their "fair share" of the world resources.

In relation to food and the consumption of food resources by Americans, consider the following example. American livestock is well fed in order to improve the quality of meat and to cut down on grain and other food reserves. Livestock are fed grain, soybeans, milk products, fish meal, and wheat germ. In a recent year, it was estimated that American livestock consumed the protein equivalent of six times our human consumption. It is also estimated that we annually feed our livestock as much grain as all the people in China and India eat in one year.

This protein waste goes one step further when you consider that the average American eats about twice the protein his body can use. In fact, Americans consume so much protein that our livestock population could be reduced by one-quarter and still provide every American with a half pound of meat a day. This would be sufficient to meet the protein requirement without considering protein obtained from nonmeat sources such as beans, nuts, grains and other products.

Food is only one area of American consumption. However, it is a most important area as many millions of people in the world are either starving or at the brink of starvation. This subject is explored in greater detail later in this chapter.

WHY ARE THERE SO MANY PEOPLE IN THE WORLD?

The population grows like interest paid in a bank—it is compounded. More people

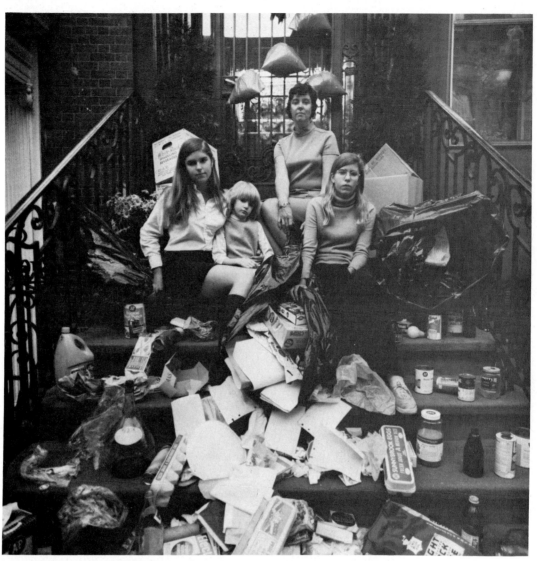

An American family
with one week's worth
of garbage.

continue to reproduce more people just as more money in the bank produces more money. Without controls the population continues to increase.

Thomas Malthus wrote a population essay in 1838 from which many of our present-day population theories have been derived. Malthus wrote that although food production increases arithmetically, human population increases geometrically. This simply means that under normal conditions, population size increases faster than the food

supply. A struggle for existence then becomes obvious. It was Charles Darwin who concluded that, based on the Malthusian theory, there is a tendency toward overpopulation in nature and resultant competition for food and shelter. The Malthus essay resulted in Darwin's well-known theories of survival of the fittest and natural selection. *Survival of the fittest* means that those organisms that best adapt to their environments tend to survive. *Natural selection* means that those organisms that are best adapted to survive and reproduce will do so and produce or-

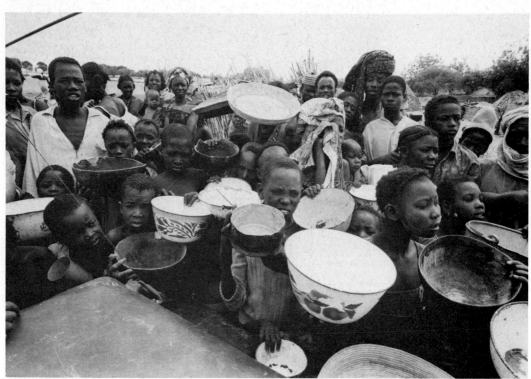

In some parts of the world people are starving for want of grain, and in other parts cattle are fattened on grain to feed the affluent.

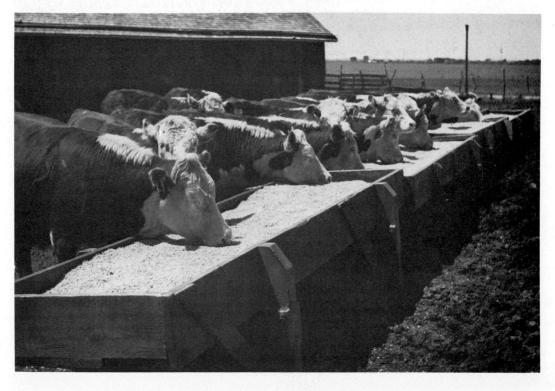

ganisms that are better able to survive. How do you think these theories apply to present-day human situations? Do you think they are valid when applied to the human population?

There are so many people in the world because as long as the birth rate exceeds the death rate, there will continue to be overpopulation. What are some of the reasons for this? One reason is that medical science has given us the ability to keep people alive longer. People are living longer today than ever before, and more people are either cured of serious illness or their illnesses are controlled so that they can live longer. Large epidemics that once killed thousands of people have been practically eliminated. In addition, infant mortality is down in most countries. Many areas that do suffer from health problems are also helped by the larger community of nations.

Because of these reasons, overpopulation continues to exist. This brings us to a discussion of zero population growth (ZPG). This topic was introduced in Chapter 10. Zero population growth is defined as the point at which the number of births equal the number of deaths and the population remains stationary. This "break-even" point is thought to occur at 2.1 children per family in the United States. The birth rate is presently below 2.1 and is only about 1.9. This is the lowest birth rate ever experienced in this country.

The lowered birth rate does not mean that we automatically reach ZPG. In order to reach this the population must "level off" after a long period of time. Fluctuations in the birth or death rate can markedly affect the resulting population. However, it is anticipated that if the United States continues its present birth rate and immigration rate, a population plateau will be reached sometime in the first half of the twenty-first century.

Let us examine some of the reasons for the decrease in birth rate in the United States. Many people are deciding to have fewer children because of the publicity given to

ZPG and other population theories. Economic restraints have also affected the reduction in birth rate. People are finding it more and more difficult to "make ends meet" and a large family places a strain on the budget.

Birth control methods have been improved and the wide use of birth control pills has also contributed to the reduction in population growth. In addition, there are a number of organizations that disseminate birth control and family planning information and services. Liberalized abortion laws have also contributed to lower birth rates. It is interesting to note that recent United Nations' statistics reveal that the most liberal abortion laws exist in the highly industrialized nations. If you recall, from an earlier section of this chapter, population growth in general is slowest in these nations.

Another aspect of ZPG is that women in this and other countries are choosing to have fewer children or in many cases no children. Women, now liberated by advances in contraceptive technology and by the women's movement are considering careers other than motherhood. For example, the proportion of working women has increased from 30 to 43 percent in the past 20 years or many women feel that they no longer have to choose between a career and a family. Smaller families make this a realistic possibility.

How will the attainment of ZPG affect us? Schools will be affected; in fact in many areas of the country they are already affected. Fewer students mean that there is a need for fewer teachers and classrooms. It will enable teachers to have smaller classes and to teach a variety of special classes in specific areas of interest. There will be more individual teaching possible with a lower student-to-teacher ratio. There, of course, will have to be a change in the number of teachers being prepared for this career. Many colleges have already noted a decrease in the number of students preparing to be teachers.

Zero population growth will also affect the environment. It has been estimated that one American child places as much strain on the world environment as 50 children born in India. Reducing our population may not lessen the environmental strain, however, unless there is a concentrated effort to do so. It is likely that we will have to decrease the amount of resources consumed and give technology a chance to "catch up" with the problems of the environment. A recent government study estimated that by the year 2000 the consumption of minerals would be 9 percent less with two-child families than it would be with three-child families. The demand for recreational facilities, according to the same report, would be decreased by 30 percent.

Other benefits are also listed by ZPG proponents. They predict that incomes will increase and there will be more spendable income. They also feel that taxes will level off as less taxes are needed to provide schools and services and there are a greater number of adults (from the postwar baby boom) to pay these taxes. They also feel that the median age in this country will be 37 instead of 28. This will result in a combination of age and experience that will lead to better education, higher family income, increased productivity, and greater job security. Crime rates are also expected to decrease; most crimes are committed by younger people and crime often results from poor living conditions that can be related to population density.

All of this may sound like ZPG is the answer for the future, but there is also a negative side. When discussing such a complex question, one must consider all the countries in the world and realize that they may not choose to have ZPG. Some countries see their power in numbers, especially those countries that are underdeveloped economically. There is also the problem of economic growth. Many people feel the ZPG may also result in ZEG (zero economic growth). This combination of factors has implications for the United States as well as the rest of the world.

It is impossible to predict the future concerning these matters. The best that can be done is to consider all the alternatives and estimate the results. The population problem cannot be examined in an isolated way. The entire world is involved. The future population policy of the world should perhaps best be discussed in a worldwide forum. Can you think of any ways in which all nations could participate in formulating world population policy?

population growth and the balance of nature

Population growth is intertwined with the balance of nature. What man does on earth can upset plant and animal growth. Man, unlike other animals, controls his environment. Only a limited number of animals can survive in a limited environment. In many areas, man has encroached upon the natural habitats of animals and as a result their populations have been greatly reduced.

As a result of the overpopulation of the human species, many species of wildlife have become endangered and extinct. The threat of man comes from legal and illegal slaughter and man's need to continue to cultivate new land for food. This cultivation, in turn, reduces the land available for the animal population. Other threats to wildlife include

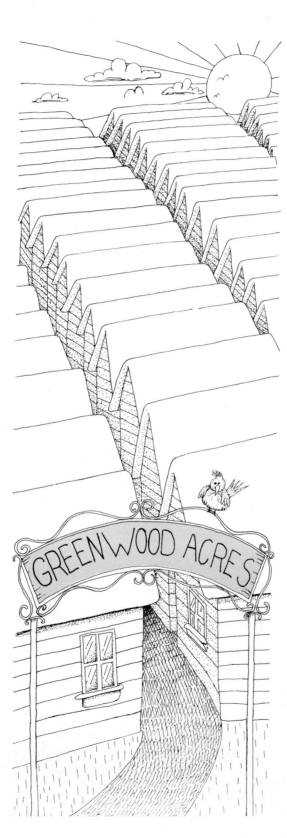

pesticides and other chemicals, pollutants, zoos, the pet trade, and the demand for animals to be used in scientific research.

The International Union for Conservation of Nature and Natural Resources lists more than 1,000 types of animals threatened with extinction. Among these creatures are 100 that are native to the United States. For example, in the 1860s the Lewis and Clark expedition reported that they saw great numbers of California condors. Today, there are only about 40 or 50 of these birds in existence.

The human population is not completely ignoring the problem. There are many conservation groups that have become increasingly vocal about the problem. In 1973, delegates from 80 countries met to agree upon an international pact to eliminate commerce in a number of endangered species. However, only seven countries have ratified the pact which requires ten ratifications in order to go into effect.

The United States has become actively involved in the preservation of animals with the passage by Congress of the 1973 Endangered Species Act. Under this act, the Department of Interior gives absolute protection to any species that is considered endangered and guarantees protection to animals that are considered by experts to be threatened.

The acts of the United States and other nations are only a small beginning, as much damage has already been done to the wildlife and the land that they once inhabited. You may be interested in joining a local group that is involved in wildlife preservation. Find out about the groups in your area and perhaps one will share your common interest.

MAN AND FOOD

Man controls his environment to grow food, use other resources, and build shelter. We have discussed the use of resources and food to some extent in this chapter. However, the use of food is a topic that must be discussed further because it is basic to survival. Food is so important and in such short supply that many millions of people face starvation in the near future. United Nations food experts have noted that 32 countries in the world are desperately short of food. These countries have difficulty in purchasing the grain, fertilizer, and petroleum products that would help them to avoid mass starvation. There is a possibility that 700 million of the total 900 million population of these countries may starve.

In order to discuss these serious food-related problems, the World Food Conference was held in Rome during November 1974. Dr. Henry Kissinger delivered the keynote address in which he said, "The food problem has two levels—first, coping with food emergency, and second, assuring long-term supplies and an adequate standard of nutrition for the growing population." He also stated that "at the present growth of 2 percent [population], the gap between what the developing countries produce themselves and what they will need will rise from 25 million to 85 million tons by 1985."

In past years, the United States and other food-producing countries were depended upon for their large reserves of grain. However, grain reserves have been steadily dwindling until there is only enough grain left to provide for 26 days of consumptions at present rates. The conference did agree that there is a definite need for an international reserve of food supplies.

The conference also agreed to a two-pronged attack on the world's deteriorating food situation. One part of the plan is concerned with relieving the United States and other countries of the major responsibility of having the only grain reserves. This would mean organizing an international food reserve. The second part of the plan calls for the United States and other nations to become actively involved in helping the developing areas of Asia, Africa, and South America to increase their food production. Farming experts feel that the potential is there; what is needed is capital and expertise.

A number of scientists object to the plans and conclusions of the World Food Conference. One ecologist at the University of Wisconsin thinks that the delegates to the conference failed to face the possibility that the world's "carrying capacity" may have already been exceeded. The "carrying capacity" refers to the total number of people that can be fed using available resources. This ecologist feels that any increase in food production will only aggravate the decline of the quality of life unless population is brought under control.

It may be considered that while international cooperation is essential to build up a grain reserve and to help underdeveloped countries produce their own food, population must also be simultaneously controlled. There is a need to control population growth so that the increases in population do not counteract any advances in food supplies.

possible solutions to the population problems

In this chapter, we have discussed many of the problems that are created by and related to overpopulation. Some of the solutions to these problems are discussed in this section. As you read these solutions, think about how effective you think they might be. Also, think about any other solutions you might recommend.

One solution would be to modify man's behavior and attitude toward reproducing. Education must reach more people and concentrate on the problems of overpopulation. Once people are aware of the problems, they may be more willing to practice birth control and by so doing limit their own families. Although birth control programs have been very successful in some countries, they have failed miserably in many other countries. It is not enough to provide the means of contraception; the population must appreciate the goals of such a program and understand the need for it.

In addition, information and birth control services must be made available to all who desire it. All children should be "wanted." If children were planned and wanted, the

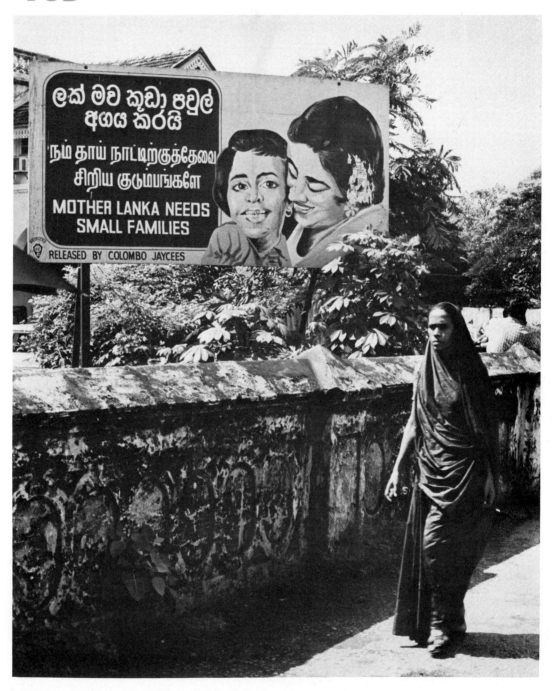

Sri Lanka's propaganda
war on overpopulation.

problem would be greatly reduced. In addition, a program of birth control would make the abortion issue much less complex. Fewer people would need to seek an abortion if they were educated concerning family planning and contraception.

Another solution is an economic one. Under present American tax law, a large family receives favored status. The more children one has, the greater the tax deductions. In addition, large families are also favored in college loans and other financial aid programs. Many people qualify for financial assistance only if they have a large number of children. Tax laws should be restructured so that one is not "punished" for being single or childless. Presently, the single person and the childless couple pay more taxes than the married person or the couple with children who earn the same income.

Life styles in this country have been changing as we discussed in Chapter 10. More and more people are choosing not to marry, or if they do marry to do so at a later age. In addition, many people who do marry choose to have no children or perhaps only one child. It is important that the general population be more accepting of these life styles. Acceptance in the long run will help to further stabilize the population growth. Less people will succumb to the social pressures that, in many cases, cause them to marry and have children.

Because of a change in life style, better birth control methods, and more liberalized abortion laws, the United States' population has leveled off somewhat. However, as pointed out in this chapter, there is still much more to do before a no-growth population is reached.

Overpopulation is a result of improved health but is also a threat to good health. Overpopulation has increased because of advances in medical science, improved technology, and a greater interest in the health of people. However, these improved conditions have contributed to the expansion of populations. It can be best described as a "vicious cycle."

There has been great criticism of the United States and other developed countries because of their affluence in a time of crisis in other parts of the world. This is not an easy problem. The issues are complex and involve a multitude of political and economical factors. The answers need to be found, but only through worldwide cooperation can this be accomplished.

THINKING IT OVER

1. Give some examples of how overpopulation is an underlying cause of other environmental problems.
2. What is meant by "feeling" the problems of overpopulation? Give an example of your own.
3. In what ways is overpopulation a world-wide problem?
4. What is meant by *doubling time?*
5. What is the present doubling time of the world population? Is it expected to increase or diminish?
6. In which countries does the population increase the fastest? Explain why this is so.
7. Is the United States considered a large consumer of natural resources? Explain your answer.
8. Discuss some of the reasons why there are so many people in the world.
9. Discuss Malthus' theory concerning population.
10. Define and discuss Darwin's theories of *natural selection* and *survival of the fittest.*
11. Discuss some of the reasons why populations continue to grow so rapidly.
12. What is ZPG? How does it relate to current population problems?
13. How does population affect the balance of nature?
14. Discuss some of the conclusions of the World Food Conference.
15. Discuss some possible solutions to the population problems.

KEY WORDS

Carrying capacity. The total number of people that can be fed using available resources.

Conspicuous consumption. The overconsumption of food and other natural resources in quantities not justified by the size of the population.

Doubling time. The number of years it takes for the world population to double.

Natural selection. Those organisms that are best adapted to survive will reproduce and their offspring will be better able to survive.

Struggle for existence. A competition for food, shelter, and survival.

Survival of the fittest. The organisms that are best adapted will survive and reproduce; the least adapted will die.

World Food Conference. A group of nations
that met in November 1974 to discuss
world food problems.
Zero Economic Growth (ZEG). A cessation
of economic growth that may result from
ZPG.
Zero Population Growth (ZPG). ZPG results
when the birth rate equals the death rate.

GETTING INVOLVED

Books and Periodicals

Borgstrom, George. *The Food and People
Dilemma*. North Scituate, Mass.: Duxbury,
1973. Food and population in the poor
and the rich countries.
Ehrlich, Paul R. *Population Bomb*. New
York: Ballantine, 1971. The dangers of
uncontrolled population growth.
Klein, Rudolf, "The Trouble With a Zero-
Growth World," *The New York Times
Magazine,* June 2, 1974. The problems of
a no-growth world.
Norton, Eleanor Holmes. *Population Growth
and the Future of Black Folk*. New York:
Planned Parenthood Foundation, pamphlet 1380, n.d. Ms. Holmes rebuts the
notion that zero population growth is
antiblack.

Movies

Soylent Green, with Charlton Heston, 1973.
What will happen if the population continues to grow, and food becomes very
scarce? We hope this isn't the answer.
Distributed by Metro-Goldwyn-Mayer,
Films Incorporated.
Z.P.G., with Oliver Reed, Geraldine Chaplin,
1972. Births have been outlawed because
of overpopulation; but one couple decides
to have a baby anyway. Distributed by
Paramount, Films Incorporated.

21
POLLUTION

We have all heard the word pollution, but what does it really mean on an individual basis? How does pollution affect you and how do you contribute to it? These and other related questions will be explored in this chapter.

You will examine the relationship between the management and mismanagement of the environment and pollution. The contribution of technology to pollution is also examined. Major forms of pollution are discussed and their impact on our way of life is studied. These major forms of pollution include air, water, pesticide, radiation, food, noise, land, and social pollution.

In the final section of this chapter, the future and pollution are discussed. What the individual can do is examined. Groups that are interested in fighting pollution are discussed. The group process of solving pollution problems is also examined. After reading this chapter, you will have a better understanding of pollution and the problems posed by it.

While reading this chapter, think about the following concepts:

■ The management and mismanagement of the environment are related to pollution.

■ Technology has, in many cases, added to the pollution problem while contributing to a better way of life.

■ Man has manipulated the environment for convenience, as well as necessity.

■ Social pollution is reflected in environmental pollution.

■ In order to improve present-day environmental conditions, individuals must learn to sacrifice to some degree.

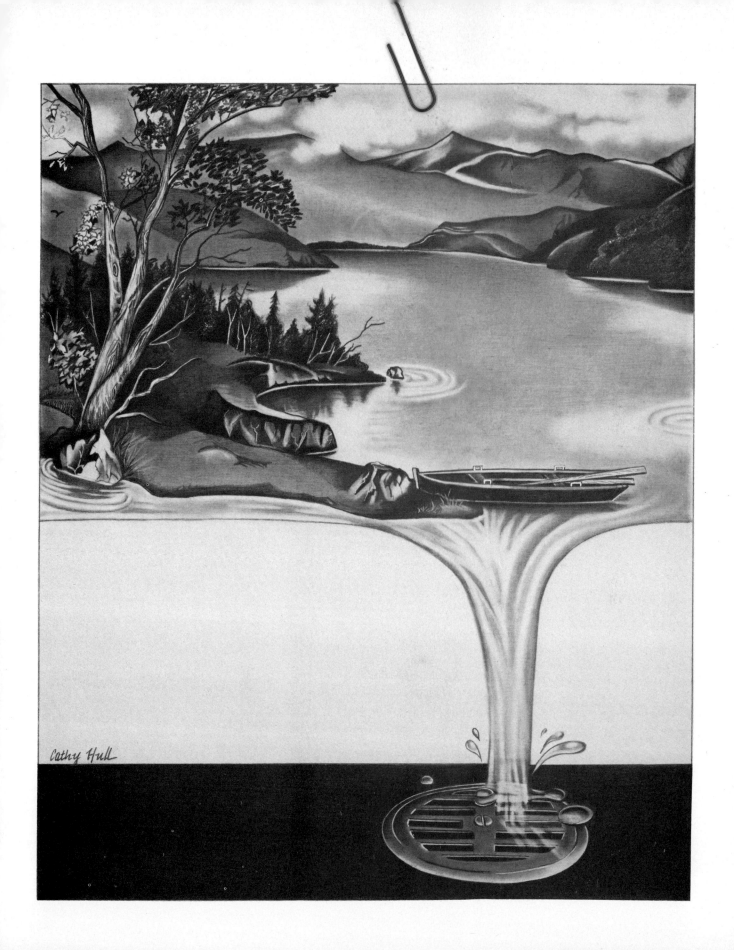

Cathy Hull

In April 1972, the U. S. Environmental Protection Agency published a survey of pollution in the drinking water of communities located in the lower Mississippi River area. These communities derived their drinking water from the Mississippi River. New Orleans was one of the cities in the survey.

The drinking water that came out of the taps in New Orleans was found to contain small quantities of 66 organic chemicals. Eight of these chemicals are considered highly toxic or potential carcinogens. It was also pointed out that chlorine used to purify the drinking water was a component of some of the substances identified as dangerous.

This situation is not considered to be an isolated one. Carcinogens have appeared in the drinking water of Evansville, Indiana; Washington, D. C.; San Francisco; and in other communities that border on the Ohio and Mississippi Rivers. The problem cannot be taken lightly. The Environmental Defense Fund, a private organization, issued a report on the Louisiana situation and concluded that the cancer mortality rate in New Orleans could be cut by 15 or 20 percent if the dangerous chemicals were removed from the drinking water.

At present, there is no federal law that requires a water system to comply with Federal standards adopted in 1962 by the U. S. Public Health Service. These standards only apply to interstate water carriers such as planes, trains, and buses. In many states that have adopted the 1962 standards, they either are not enforced or used as guidelines. A 1973 survey of 446 water systems in six states was conducted by the General Accounting Office. The six states included in this survey were Maryland, Massachusetts, Oregon, Vermont, Washington, and West Virginia. The survey revealed that three-quarters of the systems had never been tested for chemical content and about the same number of systems failed to adequately test for bacterial contamination.

In many communities, it is difficult to find people with adequate training in chemistry and microbiology to assure water quality.

In many states, the budget alloted for water treatment facilities and employees is minimal. Most state health departments are extremely understaffed and a Maryland official described their water inspection program as "horrible" to a Ralph Nader task force.

There is hope that the approval of a new Federal Safe Drinking Water Act will allow for the establishment of mandatory national standards for drinking water by the Environmental Protection Agency. You may be interested in finding out about your community drinking water and the safeguards utilized to protect it. You may also want to investigate your state's inspection program to find out if it is satisfactory.

the management and mismanagement of the environment

No part of nature exists alone. Each part of nature is interdependent on all of the other parts. No matter what we do as individuals, a larger group affects our surroundings in some way. The ecology of the earth is affected every day by the acts of human beings. Ecology may be defined as the study of the relationship between organisms and their environments. Ecology is a relatively new science and much is still unknown in this area. Therefore, in many situations it is difficult to predict how our surroundings or environment will be affected by a particular event.

There are some basic principles of ecology that will help you to understand the normal life cycles of nature. In many cases, people think they are only affecting one aspect of the environment, while in reality they may be affecting an entire natural cycle. It is important to keep in mind the following question, "What effect will a certain action have on all living things it comes into contact with and what will be the short- and long-term effects on the quality of life?"

Consider the following ecological principles as a foundation for the remainder of this chapter.

1. Most living things are organized into communities of mutual support; these communities are called ecosystems. The survival of the entire ecosystem is dependent on each member of that system. When one species is destroyed or greatly reduced, the ecosystem as a whole suffers. In turn, the survival of each member of the system is directly related to the survival of the entire ecosystem.

2. The greater the ability of a species to adapt, the better are the chances of survival. This was discussed in Chapter 20 in relation to *survival of the fittest.*

3. An ecosystem containing a large variety of species is more stable than one having a few species. This allows the ecosystem to continue to function even if one species is endangered or annihilated.

4. The natural cycles that involve all species include food chains, breathing cycles, nitrogen cycles, and many more that are too numerous to mention.
   a. In a *food chain,* different species serve as food for other species. All parts of the chain are interdependent. When one part is destroyed, the other parts are affected and the environment is altered.
   b. The *breathing chain* involves the gases essential to life. Animals breathe in oxygen and breathe out carbon dioxide. Plants take in carbon dioxide and give off oxygen. Both types of organisms are dependent on one another. Without animals, plants would not survive and vice-versa.
   c. The *nitrogen cycle* involves the wastes of animals that are broken down and decomposed by bacteria into nitrogen compounds. These compounds are essential for plant growth. Animals are dependent on the plants that have grown from the nitrogen compounds. This is a natural cycle; that is, if altered, results in disruption of the ecosystem.

5. A most essential, though often overlooked, principle of ecology is that nothing can ever be truly discarded. When we throw something away, we are just putting it into a different place in the environment. For example, if you burn rubbish, the smoke that is produced will affect the air. The residue will affect the soil balance. Often the immediate effects are not seen, but they slowly build up until serious damage is caused.

6. Another principle of ecology is that nothing is "for ever." Natural resources, once used, are gone and cannot be replaced. We learned that this was true in the use of land for fuel production. We are also learning it is true in the case of oil as reflected by the *energy crisis* presently being experienced.

These natural laws existed long before man. If one respects the principles of ecology and the related natural cycles, there is some insurance that pollution problems would be minimized. However, man has, in most cases, chosen to ignore these principles and today we are living with the result.

Technology has had to manage and control the environment in order to support more life. In doing this, man has cleared acres of land, built many thousands of factories, and produced consumer items that have added to the environmental problem. One of these consumer items is the automobile. Man has also had to look for new sources of energy in order to prevent the depletion of known sources.

Technology has acted to benefit man in many instances. However, this technology has also manipulated the environment for convenience, as well as necessity. Examples of this include throw-away containers of all types, too many automobiles, and pleasure vehicles. It is not uncommon to find two or more cars in the driveways of suburban homes. Many people own power boats, motorcycles, snowmobiles, and numerous other pleasure vehicles. These vehicles use much needed gasoline and, at the same time, they pollute the air with the exhausts from their engines.

One can conclude that "nature's way" has been managed for necessity and mismanaged for pleasure and convenience. Most people do not stop to think about the environment when they are out on their boat. They may be *aware* of the problem, but being aware is not enough. Each person must be emotionally involved in the real problems of environmental imbalance and what can happen as a result of it.

If you recall Chapter 20, you will remember the statement that one must "feel" overpopulation in order to appreciate the problem. The same is true for pollution. As with overpopulation, pollution is a problem that can be approached on an individual level. Each person can do a great deal within his own environment to begin to change things for the better.

major forms of pollution

Most of you are probably all too familiar with the major forms of pollution. Each of these major forms will be briefly discussed in the following sections. If you desire to know more about any of these forms of pollution, consult the "Getting Involved" section at the end of this chapter or your college or community library.

AIR POLLUTION

What do we mean when we use the term *air pollution?* It can be defined as man-made contamination of the outdoor atmosphere. It differs from occupational pollution which is defined as pollution of the air within a mine, factory, or other industrial setting. There are many different types of pollutants. Some are natural and others are man-made. Natural pollutants include pollen, dust, carbon dioxide, viruses, bacteria, and fog droplets. Man-made pollutants include exhaust from engines, factory by-products, aerosols, smoke, fumes, gases, and numerous other products of advanced technology.

In order to understand the nature of air pollution, we will examine the three categories of air contamination. These categories include attrition, vaporization, and combustion.

Attrition is the wearing or grinding down by friction. It occurs in every aspect of one's life. Every time you run on your shoes you are wearing them down. Think of other situations that apply to attrition. However, in terms of air pollution, attrition may be thought of as the dispersal of particulates (particles of solid or liquid matter) into the atmosphere. Attrition processes that result in air pollution include sanding, grinding, demolishing, drilling, and spraying. A number of industries contribute to pollution through the process of attrition.

Vaporization is the change of a substance from a liquid to a gas. Vaporization may occur under heat or pressure or by the natural evaporation of volatile substances. A volatile substance is one that will evaporate at normal temperatures. Vaporization of matter is a major cause of odors in the atmosphere.

Combustion is the third contributor to air pollution. Combustion is simply the process of burning. Chemically speaking, it is the combination of certain substances with oxygen resulting in the production of energy. Many fuels are burned to produce energy and the products of combustion contaminate or pollute the air that we breathe.

One of the most dangerous contributors to the air pollution problem is the aerosol. This is the product that dispenses your hair spray, deodorant, shaving cream, perfume, food products, and numerous other "spray" products. The problem is in the product used to propel the aerosol substance. This chemical is called *fluorocarbon* and scientific evidence suggests that it is destroying the ozone layer of the atmosphere. The ozone layer protects us by preventing most of the ultraviolet rays of sun from reaching earth.

Ultraviolet rays are extremely dangerous to man and other forms of life. Such conditions as excessive wrinkling, skin cancer, and cataracts could be caused by increased ultraviolet rays. In extreme cases, the rays could cause death by breaking down matter and causing genetic mutation or change.

There has been much controversy about

this issue. The proponents of aerosols state that research is still in its early stages and the possibility of danger is still many years in the future. The opponents want an immediate ban on the use of these substances. They feel that enough information is already known to warrant the banning of these products. They also feel that the longer we wait to act, the greater the danger to human life. At present little is being done to halt the use of these products. In fact, in the year since the scientific results were published, there has been a 10 percent increase in the production of these products. This figures out to be about six million more aerosol cans produced this year as compared to last year.

The chemical pollution of the atmosphere is a subject that is not well understood. Presently, there are about 50,000 industrial chemicals in common use. The federal government regulates only 450 which were found to be potentially harmful or dangerous. It has been estimated that 3,000 new chemicals are introduced each year. One can see that the numbers alone prevent sufficient study to determine whether or not these chemicals are dangerous. In addition, the danger, as in the case of the aerosols, often does not become evident until after many years of use.

THERMAL INVERSIONS

You may have experienced an <u>inversion</u> without realizing it. A thermal inversion occurs when the surface air is cooler than a layer of air above it and it cannot rise and mix. This phenomenon of cooler surface air trapped by a layer of warm air is called an inversion. An inversion results in the surface air containing pollutants remaining close to earth and causing intense air pollution. Refer to Figure 21-1 for a diagram of a temperature inversion.

Inversions are usually affected by the season of the year and tend to occur in the fall and winter. The major inversions of our time have occurred during these months. One such disaster occurred in the New York Metropolitan area during Thanksgiving weekend of 1966. During this period, a choking air settled over the city and the carbon monoxide level reached the danger point. Citizens were asked to voluntarily stop using their cars, and apartment owners were asked not to operate incinerators and to keep furnaces burning low. Fortunately, a mass of cool air blew the smog out by Sunday of that weekend.

Another serious air pollution episode occurred in Donora, Pennsylvania, in October 1948.

Figure 21-1
A thermal inversion. (a) At midday the sun's rays warming the earth create an unstable condition—the warmest air at the bottom moves freely upward. At night the cool earth cannot heat the surface air enough to penetrate the warm air layer above. (b) As a result, the surface air, and the pollutants it contains, remains close to the earth.

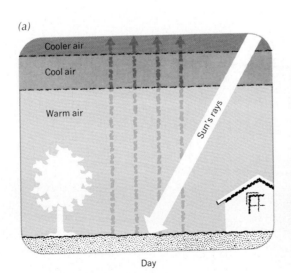
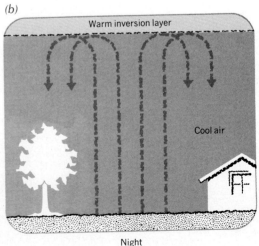

Donora is an industrial community on the banks of the Monongahela River. In this area, a high pressure ozone had left the air fairly stationary for a period of five days. A temperature inversion had trapped the ground air and all the particles and gases in it. The polluted air could not rise and became so contaminated that several thousand people became ill and many had to be hospitalized. Twenty people died as a result of this inversion.

There have been many other disastrous inversions and many communities are constantly surrounded by a smog layer. One of the best known smog areas is Los Angeles, California. Industry and a great number of automobiles have contributed to the situation. The weather pattern and topography of this area also adds to the smog situation.

HEALTH EFFECTS
OF AIR POLLUTION

Many people are affected by air pollution. As you can see from the discussion of inver-sions, many people have died as a result of air pollution. The major effect on health appears to be the action of irritant materials on the respiratory tract. Those materials that are involved include sulfur oxides, nitrogen dioxide, and ozone.

Many studies have been conducted over the years on animals and animal tissue exposed to various irritants common in polluted air. The results of these studies suggest these conclusions.

1. Certain irritants can either slow down or stop the action of the *cilia* (hairlike cells that line the airways and propel the mucus out of the respiratory tract).
2. The slowing down or stopping of the cilia creates a health hazard in that the body cannot remove the dirt and bacteria-laden mucus from the respiratory tract.
3. Irritants in the air have been found to increase and/or thicken the mucus in the respiratory tract.
4. Irritants can cause constriction of the air passages.

Smog over L.A.

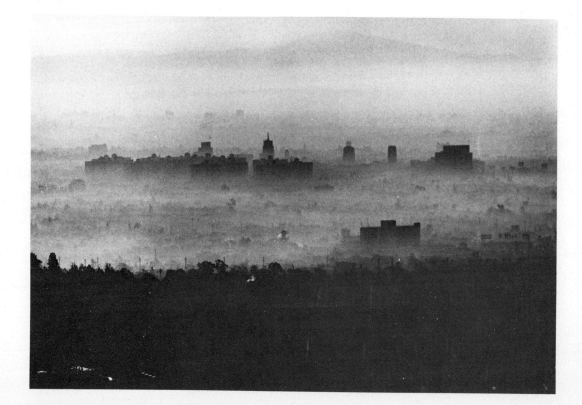

5. They may also cause swelling or excessive growth of the cells that line the air passages.
6. Respiratory infection may result from one or more of these reactions because breathing may become more difficult and bacteria and other microorganisms are not removed from the respiratory system in an efficient manner.

Air pollution also contributes to acute and chronic respiratory diseases. Coughing, an acute condition, is often reported to increase during and following high-pollution periods. Acute nonspecific upper respiratory diseases, which include colds and other conditions, also appear to increase in symptoms during peak air pollution periods. Many people show symptoms of the common cold following exposure to air pollution. The weakening of the body's defenses to acute respiratory disease has also been linked to air pollution.

Chronic respiratory conditions include bronchial asthma, chronic bronchitis, and pulmonary emphysema. All of these conditions are affected by air pollution. Bronchial asthma results from an abnormal constriction of the bronchioles accompanied by an increased production and thickening of mucous secretions. Polluted air is thought to be one of the stimuli capable of causing an asthma attack. In New Orleans, for example, epidemic outbreaks of asthma have been linked to air pollution.

In cases of chronic bronchitis, a lasting or recurrent cough is symptomatic. British researchers have extensively studied the relationship between air pollution and chronic bronchitis. In one three-year study, they found a significant relationship between death rates from chronic bronchitis and sulfur concentration in the air. In another six-year study, the researchers found that mail carriers were absent from work more often because of chronic bronchitis when they worked in polluted areas. In the areas of heaviest pollution, there were three times as many absences as in lower pollution areas. A third five-year study indicated that there was a high relationship between chronic bronchitis and the amount of acid in the rain and snow (thought to be produced from the mixing of sulfur oxide with moisture to form sulfuric acid).

Air pollution also affects the eyes. You may have experienced a burning, tearing sensation when exposed to air pollution. Often these symptoms result from smog and sulfur dioxide. Permanent eye injury has not been shown, but the symptoms are often painful and annoying. Air pollution has also been linked to dizziness, headaches, blurred vision, and a slowing-down of responses. These reactions may result from increases in carbon monoxide in the air.

Some pollutants have been found to be *carcinogenic* or cancer-causing. This is so in the case of lung cancer. A number of conditions contribute to the disease and air pollution is thought to be one of these conditions. In some cases, researchers believe that the slowing down of the cilia caused by pollutants allows certain cancer-causing substances to remain in contact with the respiratory tract cells over a longer period of time. This contact could result in cancer. Cases of lung cancer have been shown to occur more often in highly polluted areas than in less polluted areas. Some research also exists that links pollutants in the atmosphere to skin cancer.

OTHER EFFECTS
OF AIR POLLUTION

There are numerous other effects of air pollution that are not directly related to health of humans. Air pollution also affects the health of animals, particularly animals that are usually kept outside of the home such as livestock. In many of the air pollution disasters, animals became ill or died as a result of exposure to the atmosphere.

Pollution also affects vegetation. In many areas, crops have been destroyed by air contamination. Sulfur dioxide and fluorides are some of the chief offenders. In fact, vegetation can be examined to determine what

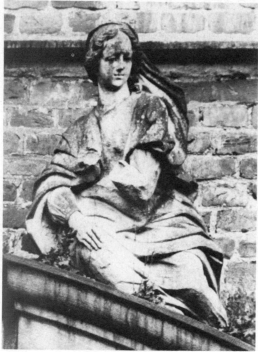

(a)

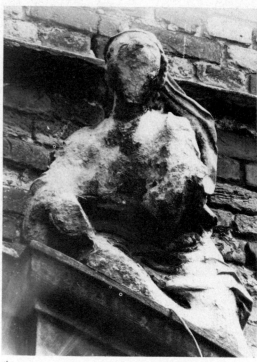

(b)

This 275 year old sculpture shows (a) 206 years of normal damage and weathering: 1702-1908; (b) 60 years of damage done by heavy pollution: 1908-1968.

substances caused the vegetation to die. Some industrial plants keep a variety of vegetation in the grounds as an aid in controlling their own emissions into the atmosphere. The vegetation indicates the level of pollution in a short period of time.

Pollution also causes erosion and corrosion of buildings, homes, and monuments. Steel, iron, zinc, brass, copper, nickel, and lead have been found to corrode faster in highly industrialized areas. The degree of deterioration has been found to be proportional to the amount of a certain pollutant present. Books are often damaged by the sulfuric acid in the air. In addition, fabrics, leather, textiles, rubber, and paints are all affected in some way by air pollution.

Air pollution has an important effect on visibility. Did you ever notice a gray or brownish sky in midday? It can seriously affect how well one can see distance. The danger of this is self-explanatory. Automobile collisions increase and many involve large numbers of cars. In addition, air travel becomes hazardous and airports may have to cease operations. A burning dump often

causes such severe smoke that numerous cars are involved in pile-up collisions.

What about the economic effects of air pollution? The total estimated cost of air pollution is about 16 billion dollars a year in damage to people and property. The cost to fight air pollution has been estimated at about $113 billion over the next ten years. Air pollution can be related to cost in terms of higher medical costs, increased loss of livestock, increased maintenance costs, higher cleaning costs, greater job absenteeism, higher food bills, lowered real estate values, reduced crops, and more expensive industrial equipment.

The cost of air pollution is high in terms of people, animals and plants, structures, and of course, in dollars. Air pollution is a double threat: to our health and our way of life. Air pollution, like other forms of pollution, must be met head-on now; it is something that we cannot *afford* to overlook or wait for.

WATER POLLUTION

As you will recall from the beginning of the chapter, water pollution is a serious problem. It affects the water we drink, the water of the lakes and rivers, and the oceans around us. Water pollution affects food supplies, recreational activities, land areas adjacent to waterways, and industries that utilize large quantities of water.

One of the greatest problems of present-day water pollution is sewerage treatment. Many communities have sewerage treatment plants; but many of these are not equipped to handle the newer chemical pollutants or the increase in demand for sewage treatments. As a result, most sewage is dumped into rivers after undergoing minimal treatment.

"Treated" sewage is only one aspect of the problem. Raw sewage is that material that enters the streams, rivers, and oceans without having undergone any treatment. Industrial sewage that enters directly into a waterway further complicates the problem of water pollution.

What are some of these pollutants? One of the major offenders is the phosphates. If

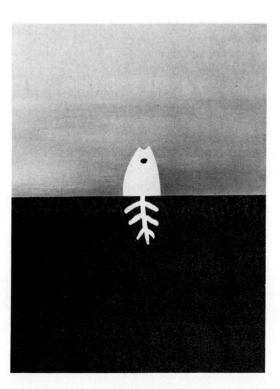

you read the label on your detergent, you may find that phosphates are listed as active ingredients. Many newer products advertise "no" or "low" phosphates, a recent reaction to the growing water pollution controversy. Phosphates contribute to the death of life in bodies of water. This process is called eutrophication.

Eutrophication causes lakes and rivers to "die." Of course, a body of water cannot die in the literal sense, but the plants and animals within that lake or river can die, resulting in a stagnant body of water. In the eutrophication process, the phosphates that reach the body of water act as a nutrient for certain kinds of algae and waterweeds. This affects the natural cycle of life in the body of water. The algae and weeds grow excessively and the water becomes green, murky, and often has a foul odor. The decaying algae remove oxygen from the water which causes many fish to die. Plant life begins to overtake the body of water hastening the "aging process" of the lake or river. Eventually the lakes develop swamp-like areas that will, in time, turn into land.

Farming wastes are also major contributors to water pollution. These wastes include sediment from soil erosion, animal wastes, pesticides (to be discussed later in this chapter), and chemical fertilizers. The effluent of these wastes enters the rivers and further contributes to water pollution. Areas that are many hundreds of miles from industrial plants and large cities are often polluted by farming wastes.

Nuclear power plants are another source of water pollution. They create thermal pollution which is the heating of the water that they return to the rivers. Often, the water being returned is 20 degrees warmer than the natural river temperature. This action disrupts life patterns in the river by altering spawning habits of fish, producing excessive plant growth, diminishing oxygen supplies, and killing fish. Radioactive pollutants are also a danger from nuclear power plants. They will be discussed later in the chapter.

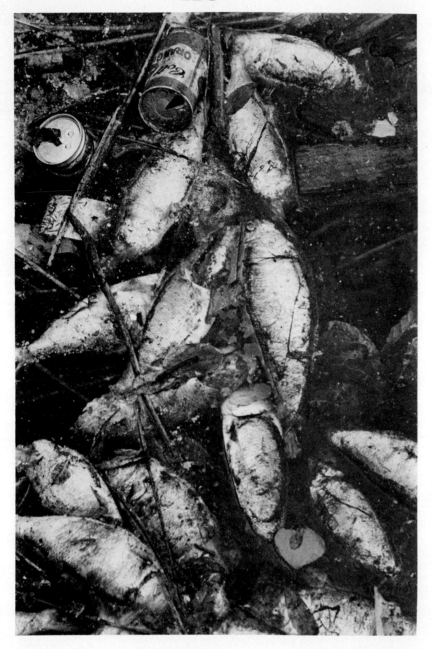

PESTICIDES

The pesticide problem was first brought to national attention by the book, *Silent Spring* by Rachel Carson published in 1962. Though this book is not recent, the information it contains about pesticides still holds true today. In *Silent Spring,* Rachel Carson wrote about the widespread effect of chemical pesticides on every aspect of our life and how they are both a health and pollution hazard.

At one time, DDT and similar products (chlorinated hydrocarbons) were widely used. They were designed primarily to destroy insect pests, but the residues of these products continue to exist threatening humans, plants, and animals. DDT has been associated with the death of fish and birds and has produced certain symptoms in humans. The Federal Aviation Agency has reported that pilots who spray DDT on fields have suffered from uneasiness, insomnia, drowsiness, dizziness, paralysis, mental confusion, depression, and numerous other symptoms.

Another type of dangerous pesticide was recently banned by the Environmental Protection Agency. In the spring of 1974, sales of vinyl chloride pesticides were banned for use in the home, food handling establishments, hospitals, and other enclosed areas. Products containing vinyl chloride were recalled from store shelves. About 28 products were affected by this decision. Vinyl chloride is a chemical strongly suspected of causing a rare form of liver cancer. This condition has been diagnosed in 12 workers involved in the conversion of vinyl chloride to the plastic, polyvinyl chloride.

There are a number of pesticides that should be avoided. These pesticides include DDT, BHC, dieldrin, chlordane, lindane, heptachlor, endrin, aldrin, Silvex, toxaphene, endosulfan, DDVP, and any compounds containing arsenic, lead, or mercury. The compounds have a lasting effect on the environment.

You may think that there are no safe pesticides, but there are a number of safe, effective products available. A few of these products include Sevin (effective for household and garden pests); Melathion (effective for a variety of pests), Pyrethin (effective for caterpillars and aphids), Diazinon (effective for most garden pests), and Methaldehyde (effective for slugs and snails).

RADIATION

Radiation was briefly mentioned in our discussion of water pollution. There are three

The Environmental Protection Agency (EPA) was created in 1970 to coordinate government efforts to improve the environment. Air pollution, water pollution, and noise pollution all come under the agency's control. Recently the EPA has been busy establishing automobile emission standards.

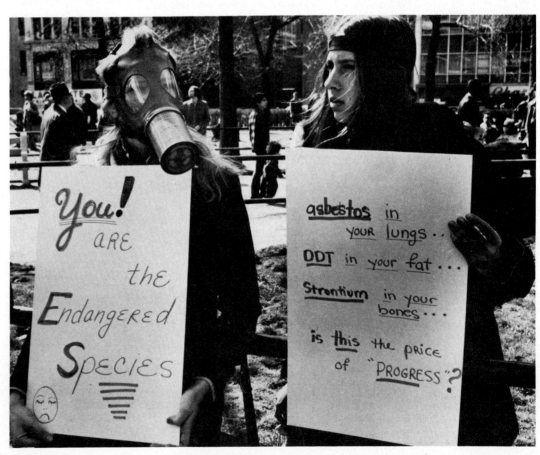

major uses of radiation: *therapeutic* (in the treatment of cancer and other diseases), *industrial,* and in *nuclear power plants.* There has been an ongoing controversy concerning the dangers of radiation. The "escape" of radioactive materials into the environment could have disastrous, even fatal, results. The life of most radioactive materials is quite long; one such material, plutonium-239, has a lethal period of tens of thousands of years.

The results of a large nuclear accident at a nuclear power plant would be unimaginably disastrous. Ten years ago the Atomic Energy Commission (AEC) estimated that such an accident could cause 45,000 deaths, a greater number of serious injuries, billions of dollars in property damage, and radiation contamination of an area the size of Pennsylvania. Though such accidents are termed "highly unlikely" by the AEC, the potential danger does exist and radiation pollution could cause death, cancer, other diseases, and serious genetic defects.

FOOD ADDITIVES

As you may recall from Chapter 12, *food additives* are substances that are intentionally or unintentionally added to food products. Review Chapter 12 for a discussion of food additives and organic foods. You may also want to review the section on the FDA in Chapter 19. The FDA acts to protect us from food additives in food.

NOISE POLLUTION

Noise pollution surrounds us in many cities. The noise of car engines, honking of horns, building and demolition equipment, subway noises, and other noises too numerous to mention are a part of the environment of most large cities. Noise pollution, however, can occur around your own home. A high volume on a stereo or radio, motorcycles, and lawn mowers all contribute to noise pollution. Physical damage may occur to the ear, causing partial or temporary deaf-

ness. In addition, one can also suffer from psychic damage. This stress can be related to the *Selye general adaptation syndrome* that was discussed in Chapter 4. Noise pollution and other types of pollution add a certain amount of stress to our lives that can result in physical illness.

POLLUTION OF THE LAND

There are many aspects of land pollution that should be considered. Man has planted and replanted the land until, in many areas, the soil has been depleted of important nutrient materials. In addition, many forest lands have been cut down to make way for roads, homes, and industry. Many natural areas have been converted into asphalt and concrete. Strip mining (the mining of coal or other materials by "stripping" off the soil to expose a section of material to be mined) has continued although it is considered ecologically unsound.

Another vital aspect of land pollution is *littering.* Littering is a serious problem that has changed the cities and countrysides of many areas. Most people overlook the fact that littering is a form of pollution. It has been estimated that the cost of picking up litter is in excess of one billion dollars per year. Things that are thrown away remain where they are placed. Glass and aluminum are replacing tin cans and these materials do not disintegrate or rust away. Plastics, too, will not just disappear once they have become litter. Litter pollution builds upon itself.

What can we do to eliminate part of the litter problem? Advertising campaigns and public education programs are helpful, but they are not enough to rid us of this problem. Some states began antilitter programs that are working. In Oregon, the state legislature banned pop-top cans and no-deposit, no-return bottles. Oregon citizens must pay deposits on their containers. The deposits act as an incentive to return bottles and clean up the litter. The result has been worth it; the volume of cans and bottles in state-wide

The Sierra Club was founded in 1892. Even in those days our wildlands were in danger; and so the club helped to create the National Park Service and the Forest Service. Now its areas of concern include pollution in cities as well as in wilderness areas, the protection of endangered species, and the dangers of overpopulation. The club has branches all over the country. It sponsors trips and outings to wilderness areas, and produces films and books about the environment.

Keep America Beautiful, a national nonprofit organization, aims to control litter. It researches new methods of litter control, grants awards for successful programs, and does a lot of public service advertising. One famous ad shows a Cherokee Indian (Iron Eyes Cody) crying at the sight of the littered land.

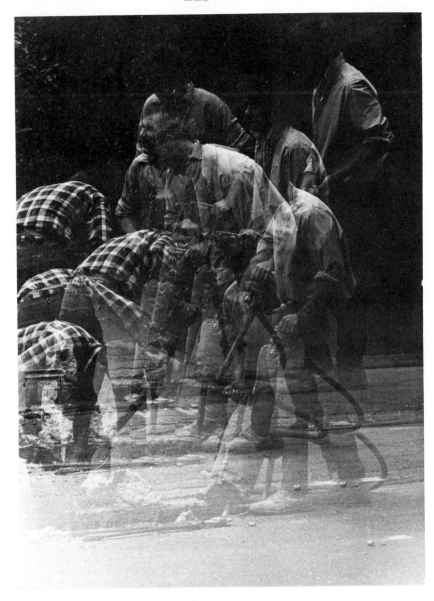

Noise pollution unlimited; here, a jackhammer symphony shatters the already cacophonic urban scene.

litter has been reduced by 92 percent in the past three years.

In the state of Washington, a "Model Litter Control Act" was passed in 1972. The Act was designed to stop all littering through education and citizen participation groups. The Act imposes fines of up to $250 for littering. Cars and boats without litterbags are fined $10. In addition, a tax has been levied against the gross sales of industries that contribute to litter. These industries include bottlers, newspaper publishers, paper manufacturers, and supermarket chains. These tax levies help to pay for the antilitter program. Does your state have an active antilitter program or legislation concerning littering? You may be interested in finding out what is being done to eliminate litter in the local, state, and national levels.

SOCIAL POLLUTION

Social pollution is not a *new* form of pollution. It is one with which you are probably

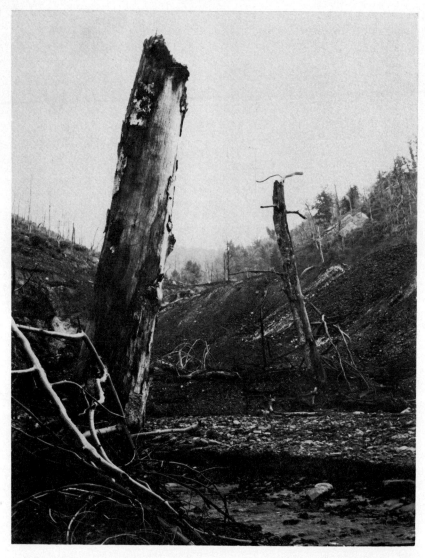

Land pollution, one species: strip mining in Appalachia.

familiar. Social pollution is simply a lack of concern for others. This lack of concern leads to all forms of pollution. People who "do not care" will litter, add to water pollution, buy products that add to the pollution problem, and, in general, disregard legislation enacted to protect the environment. Social pollution combined with overpopulation is the underlying cause of many of our pollution problems.

where do we go from here?

What has been done to improve environmental pollution? The air quality of many areas has been improved in the past few years. Many large industrial plants have installed smoke-reduction devices. Improved emission controls on automobiles have also helped to reduce air pollution. However, problems still exist, particularly in congested areas. Washington, D.C., Los Angeles, and the New York metropolitan area continue to exhibit a worsening in air quality.

There has been some improvement in water pollution conditions; but most lakes and rivers remain unchanged. Under recent legislation, 30,000 industrial plants are being required to reduce dumping of pollutants into the water. The Environmental Protection

Agency predicts that most U.S. rivers and lakes will be relatively clean by 1976; the more polluted waterways will take until the mid-1980s.

Solid wastes are still very much of a pollution problem. However, some solutions are offering improvement. These solutions include recycling, burning of wastes to produce energy, and collecting and disposing of garbage in more efficient ways. For example, the city of Chicago plans to build a 13.5 million dollar facility that will handle about 2,000 tons of trash a day. This plant is expected to produce enough shredded refuse to replace 5,300 tons of coal per week and will generate enough electricity to serve 50,000 homes. The solution to the solid waste problem may be found through recycling plants that produce both reusable matter and energy.

As far as pesticides are concerned, the current picture appears somewhat brighter. The use of several chemicals has been restricted or banned and DDT is prohibited except in a few cases. Research is being conducted to find new, more effective, and environmentally safe pesticides.

The individual can also participate in cleaning up pollution. One can use returnable bottles, pick up after himself and others, be willing to buy produce that is slightly less than perfect, and avoid wastefully packaged products. People can also sacrifice some comfort as in the case of a reduction of energy. Thermostats can be turned down, air conditioners can be used less frequently, and cars can be driven only when necessary.

The accomplishment of these goals is a long-term project. In order to solve pollution problems, individuals must learn to respect themselves and others. Solving these problems is a group process. An individual can help, but without the backing of others, accomplishment will be limited. One must keep in mind the principle discussed at the beginning of this book: "I'm O.K. — You're O.K." We have a responsibility to ourselves and to others and society will in turn reap the benefits from this mutual responsibility.

THINKING IT OVER

1. How would you define the terms *ecology* and *ecosystem?*
2. Discuss some of the principles of ecology.
3. Discuss the natural cycles or chains found in the environment.
4. How has technology controlled the environment to support more human life?

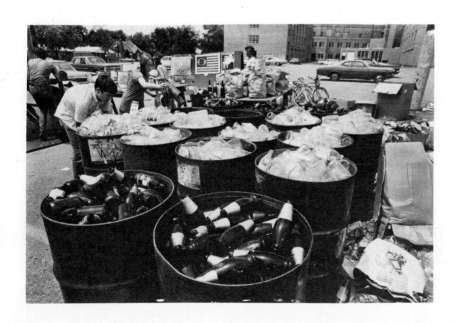

Bottle roundup at recycling center.

5. How has man manipulated the environment for convenience as well as necessity?
6. Discuss some of the components of air pollution.
7. What is a thermal inversion? Explain and draw a diagram.
8. Discuss an air pollution disaster related to a thermal inversion.
9. What are the three categories of activities that contribute to air pollution?
10. Discuss some of the health effects of air pollution.
11. What are some of the problems of water pollution?
12. What is the difference between raw and treated sewage?
13. What is meant by the process of *eutrophication?*
14. What is *thermal pollution?*
15. Discuss a dangerous pesticide and how it affects the environment and our health.
16. Discuss the three major uses of radiation. Why is the use of radioactive materials potentially dangerous?
17. What is noise pollution? How does it affect our stress level?
18. Discuss littering and what can be done to control it.
19. What is *social pollution?*
20. Discuss some of the areas of progress in the fight against pollution.

KEY WORDS

Attrition. Wearing or grinding down by friction; a contributing factor to air pollution.

Breathing chain. The interdependence of plants and animals through the process of breathing.

Combustion. The production of energy through burning; a contributing factor to air pollution.

Ecology. The interdependence of organisms and their environment.

Ecosystem. Natural communities of mutual dependence and support.

Eutrophication. The destruction or "death" of a body of water usually caused by phosphate pollution.

Food chain. The natural dependence of different species of life on each other for food.

Nitrogen cycle. The decomposition of matter and release of nitrogen compounds.

Ozone layer. A layer of the atmosphere that prevents most of the sun's ultraviolet rays from penetrating through to earth.

Particulates. A particle of solid or liquid matter.

Raw sewage. Sewage that has not been treated.

Social pollution. A lack of concern for others.

Strip mining. The stripping of land for mining purposes.

Thermal inversion. The phenomenon of a layer of cool air trapped by a layer of warmer air so that the bottom layer containing pollutants cannot rise.

Thermal pollution. The heating of water before it is returned to a river; often occurs at nuclear power plants.

Vaporization. The change of a substance from a liquid to a gas; a contributing factor to air pollution.

GETTING INVOLVED

Books and Periodicals

Environmental Quality Staff, California Institute of Technology. *Smog, A Report to the People.* Los Angeles: Ward Ritchie, 1972. The harmful effects of air pollution.

Graham, Frank, Jr. *Since Silent Spring.* Boston: Houghton Mifflin Company, 1970. Discusses the contributions of Rachel Carson's *Silent Spring* and what has happened in the area of pesticides since then.

Schaeffer, Francis. *Pollution and the Death of Man.* Wheaton, Ill.: Tyndale House, n.d. Pollution can be disastrous . . .

Sierra Club. *Space for Survival: How to Stop the Bulldozer in Your Own Back Yard.* New York: Simon and Schuster, n.d. What you can do to preserve space.

Movies

Alone in the Midst of the Land, 1970. A short that dramatizes the ultimate effects of pollution. Distributed by the National Broadcasting Company, Films Incorporated, Twyman.

The American Wilderness, 1971. A plea for preservation of our remaining wilderness areas. Distributed by National Broadcasting Company, Films Incorporated.

The Everglades, 1971. A short about industry threatening this Florida wilderness area. Distributed by National Broadcasting Company, Films Incorporated.

No Blade of Grass, with Nigel Davenport, 1970. A polluted environment leads to disaster, and a peaceful family finds that it will kill for self-preservation. Distributed by Metro-Goldwyn-Mayer, Films Incorporated.

Say Goodbye, 1972. A sad documentary about animals threatened with extinction. Distributed by Films Incorporated.

The Slow Guillotine, 1969. Pollution in Los Angeles. Distributed by National Broadcasting Company, Films Incorporated.

Wolves and the Wolf Men, 1972. The documentary credited with initiating wildlife preservation legislation. Distributed by Films Incorporated.

EPILOGUE

The Minnesota Indoor Clean Air Act makes it illegal to light a cigarette, cigar, or pipe in public anywhere in that state, unless the area has been designated as a smoking area. More than 30 other states have passed similar laws to protect the nonsmoking public from the smoking public.

The Environmental Protection Agency estimates that millions of Americans have suffered a hearing loss as a result of noise pollution. Noise has been listed as a factor in fatigue and weight loss as well as hearing loss.

What do these two recent news stories have in common? Both of them present an environmental problem that is affecting the individual. However, if you look closely at these stories, you will also note that the individual, in both cases, initiated the problem.

In the case of the antismoking law, it is the individual smoker and groups of smokers who have caused the nonsmoker to protest smoke pollution. It is a vicious cycle of the individual affecting the environment and, in turn, that environment affecting the individual.

The same is true for the second story concerning noise pollution. The individual contributes to the noise that pollutes the environment and, in turn, adversely affects other individuals.

This book began with a study of the individual and his mental–emotional state. It then proceeded to discuss many aspects of health science that affect the individual. The book concluded with an examination of how the individual affects his environment. It has been clearly demonstrated that man does affect his environment and that environment affects man.

Let us take this cycle one step farther. We have seen that although environmental problems and concerns are worldwide and affect large segments of society, solutions often boil down to each individual and how he feels about himself.

Do you recall the discussion of "I'm OK—You're OK?" A person who has attained this life position feels good about himself and, in turn, is able to feel good about others. This person is less likely to be affected by his environment than a person who does not feel good about himself.

An example of this is the effect that stress can have upon an individual. A person who feels good about himself will be less affected by the destructive aspects of stress. This individual is less likely to be classified as a "Type A" (one who runs a greater risk of suffering a heart attack). He would also be less prone to other stress symptoms such as high blood pressure, ulcers, and severe headaches.

The individual who feels good about himself will relate better to the people around him. His emotional health is directly related to his physical and social health. He will have a more positive effect on his environment if he feels "O.K." about himself.

One may conclude that the theme of this book has been that the individual affects the environment, and the environment, in turn, affects the individual; however, an individual who feels good about himself can affect his environment in a positive manner. If more individuals reacted in this way, the world would certainly be a healthier place in which to live.

FILM DISTRIBUTORS

Abkco Industries, Inc.
1700 Broadway, New York, N.Y. 10019

American Cancer Society
Local unit, or 219 East 42 Street, New York, N.Y. 10017

American Heart Association
Local unit, or 44 East 23 Street, New York, N.Y. 10010

American Lung Association
State or local Christmas Seal Association, or 1740 Broadway, New York, N.Y. 10019

American Osteopathic Association
Order Department, 212 East Ohio Street, Chicago, Ill. 60611

Argosy Film Service
1939 Central Street, Evanston, Ill. 60201

Association-Sterling Films
Executive Offices, 866 Third Avenue, New York, N.Y. 10022

Avco Embassy Pictures
1301 Avenue of the Americas, New York, N.Y. 10019

Budget Films
4590 Santa Monica Boulevard, Los Angeles, Calif. 90029

Cassavetes, John
c/o Director of Public Relations, United Artists, 729 Seventh Avenue, New York, N.Y. 10036

Charand Motion Pictures
2110 East 24 Street, Brooklyn, N.Y. 11229

Cine-Craft Co.
1720 West Marshall Street, Portland, Ore. 97299

Cinema International Corporation
Rijswijkstr. 175, P.O. Box 9255, Amsterdam W3, The Netherlands

Cinema V Distributing, Inc.
595 Madison Avenue, New York, N.Y. 10022

Clem Williams Films
2240 Noblestown Road, Pittsburgh, Penn. 15205

Columbia Cinemateque
711 Fifth Avenue, New York, N.Y. 10022

Contemporary/McGraw-Hill Films
1221 Avenue of the Americas, New York, N.Y. 10020

Films Incorporated
4420 Oakton Street, Skokie, Ill. 60076

Hurlock Cine-World
13 Arcadia Road, Old Greenwich, Conn. 06870

Institutional Cinema Service
915 Broadway, New York, N.Y. 10010

Ivy Films/16
165 West 46 Street, New York, N.Y. 10036

Kit Parker Films
12 Carmel Valley Center Building, Carmel Valley, Calif. 93924

Lederle Laboratories
Division of American Cyanamid Co., Film Library, Danbury, Conn. 06810

Lewis Film Service
1425 East Central Street, Wichita, Kan. 67214

Macmillan Films
34 MacQuesten Parkway South, Mount Vernon, N.Y. 10550

Metro-Goldwyn-Mayer, Inc.
1350 Avenue of the Americas, New York, N.Y. 10019

Modern Sound Pictures
1402 Howard Street, Omaha, Neb. 68102

Mogull's Camera & Film Exchange, Inc., 235 West 46 Street, New York, N.Y. 10036

Mottas Films
1318 Ohio Avenue NE, Canton, Ohio 44705

National Audiovisual Center (General Services Administration)
Order Section, Washington, D.C. 20409

National Broadcasting Co., Inc.
30 Rockefeller Plaza, New York, N.Y. 10020

New Yorker Films
43 West 61 Street, New York, N.Y. 10023

Paramount Pictures, Inc.
240 West 60 Street, New York, N.Y. 10023

Planned Parenthood Federation of America, Inc.
810 Seventh Avenue, New York, N.Y. 10019

rbc Films
933 North LaBrea Avenue, Los Angeles, Calif. 90038

Roa's Films
1696 North Astor Street, Milwaukee, Wis. 53202

Select Film Library
115 West 31 Street, New York, N.Y. 10001

Swank Motion Pictures
201 South Jefferson Avenue, St. Louis, Mo. 63166

"The" Film Center
915 Twelfth Street NW, Washington, D.C. 20005

The Movie Center
57 Baldwin Street, Charlestown, Mass. 02129

Trans-World Films
322 South Michigan Avenue, Chicago, Ill. 60604

Twyman Films
329 Salem Avenue, Dayton, Ohio 45401

United Artists 16
729 Seventh Avenue, New York, N.Y. 10036

United Films
1425 South Main Street, Tulsa, Okla. 74119

Universal 16
445 Park Avenue, New York, N.Y. 10022

Walter Reade 16
241 East 34 Street, New York, N.Y. 10016

Warner Brothers
Non-Theatrical Division, 4000 Warner Boulevard, Burbank, Calif. 91503

Welling Motion Pictures
80 Meacham Avenue, Elmont, N.Y. 11003

Westcoast Films
25 Lusk Street, San Francisco, Calif. 94107

Wholesome Film Center
20 Melrose Street, Boston, Mass. 02116

Willoughby-Peerless, Inc.
110 West 32 Street, New York, N.Y. 10001, or 415 Lexington, New York, N.Y. 10017

PHOTO CREDITS

ILLUSTRATION CREDITS

CHAPTER ONE
3: Edward A. Butler. 5: Vivian Cohen. 17: Abner Grayboff.

CHAPTER TWO
27: Rich Grote. 32: Guy Smalley. 34: Bob Shein.

CHAPTER THREE
39: Steve Marchesi. 47: Bob Shein.

CHAPTER FOUR
57: Cathy Hull.

CHAPTER FIVE
73: Rich Grote. 78: Abner Grayboff.

CHAPTER SIX
103: Cathy Hull. 116: Bob Shein.

CHAPTER SEVEN
121: Cathy Hull. 137: Guy Smalley.

CHAPTER EIGHT
155: Steve Marchesi. 161: Guy Smalley. 167: Abner Grayboff.

CHAPTER NINE
175: John Sovjani.

CHAPTER TEN
209: Steve Marchesi.

CHAPTER ELEVEN
233: Andrew Moszynski. 237: Guy Smalley. 240: Vivian Cohen.

CHAPTER TWELVE
251: Rich Grote. 258: Guy Smalley. 260: Julie Maas. 262: Bob Shein.

CHAPTER THIRTEEN
271: Andrew Moszynski. 276: Abner Grayboff.

CHAPTER FOURTEEN
291: Cathy Hull. 300: Guy Smalley. 302, 303: Vivian Cohen.

CHAPTER FIFTEEN
309: Nancy Munger. 310: Bob Shein.

CHAPTER SIXTEEN
325: Cathy Hull. 333: Guy Smalley.

CHAPTER SEVENTEEN
341: Edward A. Butler. 343: Guy Smalley.

CHAPTER EIGHTEEN
359: Nancy Munger.

CHAPTER NINETEEN
375: Rich Grote. 384: Julie Maas. 387: Bob Shein.

CHAPTER TWENTY
393: Steve Marchesi. 401: Guy Smalley.

CHAPTER TWENTY-ONE
407: Cathy Hull.

INDEX

Papanicolau, George N., 351
Pap test, 343, 351–352, 355
Parasitic worms, 328, 338
Parents Without Partners, 225–226
Pauling, Linus, 258, 312
Pavlov, Ivan, 6–7
Peer group, 13–15, 24; and obesity, 277; pressure, 77–78; and smoking, 108
Penis, 178–80, 195, 206
Permanent Central Narcotics Board, the, 123
Permissiveness, 162–163
Personality, 2; and body build, 5–6; and community, 13–15; development, 28–29; disorders, 48; and environment, 4, 6; and family, 11–13; and Freudian theory, 16–18; and heredity, 4; and self-actualization, 20; and self-concept, 18–19; and sex-roles, 15-16
Personality types, 299–301, 306, 307, 425
Personal values, 35, 37
Pesticides, 416, 417, 420, 421, 422; and cancer, 417
Peyote, 144, 150
Phobias, 47–48, 55
Phosphorus, 257
Physical dependence, 118; on cocaine, 139; on drugs, 132, 136, 140–141, 149; on nicotine, 106–107
Physical fitness, 232, 234, 236–248, 249; and automation, 236, 248; and flexibility, 240–241, 248; and total fitness, 234, 236, 248, 249
Piaget, Jean, 10
Pipes: and death rate, 112; use of, 107
Placenta, 187, 192, 206
Planned Parenthood Federation of America, 194–195
Planned Parenthood—World Population, 404
Pneumonia, 308, 313
Poison Control Centers, 259
Polio, 321
Pollution, 392, 401, 406, 408, 418; air, 394, 406, 410, 412, 420, 422; and cancer, 408, 413, 417, 418; and disease, 413; effects of, 413–414; and environment, 406, 408, 418; food, 406, 418; improvement of, 420–421, 422; land, 406, 418; and littering, 418–419; and man, 406, 408–410, 418, 422; noise, 406, 418,

419, 422, 425; radiation, 406, 415, 417–418, 422; social, 406, 419–420, 422; and stress, 422; and technology, 409, 421; water, 406, 408, 414, 415, 420–421, 422
Polygamy, 210, 228
Population, 392, 394–397, 399–400, 401, 402; and balance of nature, 400–401; and consumption, 396; and doubling time, 395–396; and food, 401–402; and medical science, 404
Pornography, 156–157, 171, 172
Postpartum depression, 192, 205, 206
Potassium, 257
Potentiation, 124, 149, 150
Pregnancy, 174, 176, 186, 187, 192, 205–207; and marijuana, 139; and "morning sickness," 186; subsequent to infertility, 202; and weight, 186–187
Premarital sex, 159–160, 172
Prescription drugs, 127–128, 133, 149, 150
President's Council on Physical Fitness and Sports, 236–237, 245
Professional Standards Review Organizations (PSROs), 372–373
Prohibition, 79–80
Projection, 64, 68
Promiscuity, 156, 171, 172
Prostitution, 169, 172
Proteins, 252–253, 254–255; and amino acids, 252–253, 268
Protozoans, 327, 338
Psilocybin, 144
Psychoanalysis, 18, 25, 51
Psychosis, 42, 46, 55
Psychosomatic disease, 46, 55
Psychotherapy, 51
Psychedelics, see Hallucinogens
Psychoactive drugs, 127–128, 150
Psychological dependence, 118; on cocaine, 139, 142; on drugs, 133, 136, 140–141; on marijuana, 138; on nicotine, 106–107
Psychological needs, 29–30
Pulmonary diseases, 308, 310–315, 316
Pylorospasm, 85

Quackery, 340, 354–355, 374, 376, 388; and the FDA, 382, 388; how to recognize, 376–377; and the law,

383; and obesity, 374; psychological, 386, 388; victims of, 376, 378–379, 381

Rabies, 321, 327
Rationalization, 64, 68
Regression, 65, 66, 68
Rehabilitation Centers, 371
Repression, 64, 68
Resuscitation, 290, 302–303
Rheumatic heart disease, 290, 291, 305, 307
RH factor, 174, 193, 207
Rickettsiae, 327–328, 338
Right to Life Committee, the, 203, 205
Rogers, Carl, 19
Rosenman, Ray, 300, 307
Rubella, 328, 338
Rubeola, 328

Sabin vaccine, 321
Sadism, 169, 172
Salk, Jonas E., 321
Salvation Army, 96, 98
Sanger, Margaret, 194
Save-a-Life League, 49
Schizophrenia, 41, 42–44
Secularism, 159, 172
Self-medication, 379–380, 388
Selye, Hans, 58, 68; and noise pollution, 418
Sex determination, 184–186, 205; and amniocentesis, 186, 205
Sex education, 163–164; 171, 176
Sexism, 217–218
Sex roles, 15–16, 25
Sex stereotyping, 217–218
Sexual behavior, 154, 156, 160, 162, 171, 196, 198; and counseling, 227; and the double standard, 161–162, 172; after sterilization, 201; teaching about, 164
Sexuality, 9, 40
Sexual revolution, 154, 157, 171, 172; in marriage, 217–218
Sheldon, William H., 4, 6
Shettles, Landrum B., 185
SIECUS (Sex Information and Educational Council of United States, Inc.), 176
Sierra Club, the, 418
Single persons, 208, 213, 225–226, 227